COMPREHENSIVE PSYCHIATRY REVIEW

The accreditation process for psychiatry in the United States is considered one of the most difficult among all medical specialties. Although many board review books in psychiatry exist, this is the first fact-based resource with comprehensive coverage and an easy-to-read design that can be used for both written and oral review. Dr. William Weiqi Wang has developed a concise, outline-oriented format supplemented with case studies to prepare residents for the oral and written psychiatry boards. Each chapter can stand alone and is presented in "bite-size" clusters to facilitate easy absorption of the material. A section at the end of the book includes 150 board-style questions and answers. This book is a necessity for anyone who plans to score aggressively on the American Board of Psychiatry and Neurology (ABPN), Psychiatry Resident-In-Training Examination (PRITE), and even the United States Medical License Examination (USMLE), and for medical students who want to pursue a career in psychiatry.

William Weiqi Wang, M.D., Ph.D., is an attending psychiatrist at SSM St. Joseph Health Center, an affiliate faculty member at St. Louis University, and Director of Medical Education at the Olivette Institute, St. Louis, Missouri.

Comprehensive Psychiatry Review

William Weiqi Wang

Olivette Institute, St. Louis, Missouri

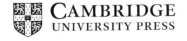

CAMBRIDGE
UNIVERSITY PRESS

CAMBRIDGE UNIVERSITY PRESS
Cambridge, New York, Melbourne, Madrid, Cape Town, Singapore,
São Paulo, Delhi, Dubai, Tokyo

Cambridge University Press
32 Avenue of the Americas, New York, NY 10013-2473, USA

www.cambridge.org
Information on this title: www.cambridge.org/9780521106450

First published 2010

Printed in the United States of America

A catalog record for this publication is available from the British Library.

Library of Congress Cataloging in Publication data
Wang, William Weiqi, 1962–
    Comprehensive psychiatry review / William Weiqi Wang.
        p. ; cm.
    Includes bibliographical references and index.
    ISBN 978-0-521-10645-0 (pbk.)   1. Psychiatry–Outlines, syllabi, etc.
    2. Psychiatry–Examinations–Study guides.   I. Title.
    [DNLM: 1. Psychiatry–Outlines. WM 18.2 W246c 2009]
    RC457.2.W36   2009
    616.890076–dc22   2009011756

ISBN 978-0-521-10645-0 Paperback

To Lini and Will

Contents

Introduction

Open to any page and read just a small passage and you will learn or be refreshed with a tangible amount of psychiatric knowledge without having to linger on the rest of the book. *Comprehensive Psychiatry Review* is a book you can benefit from whether you have a few hours to read several chapters or a few minutes to read just a few lines.

This book is designed for the busy mental health professionals who have the need and desire to be updated in medical knowledge, but often not the time for vigorous and uninterrupted study. This book provides those enthusiastic learners an easy, quick, and efficient way of learning. This book should be particularly helpful for test preparation for the ABPN examinations and PRITE. It should also offer a distinct advantage for medical students who desire to score aggressively in the USMLE, and those who target a successful career in the field of psychiatry. This book may further provide a learning opportunity to benefit mental health clinicians who consistently strive for better patient care.

In 50 chapters this book fosters a collection of clinically relevant and important information drawn from major textbooks and other authoritative sources. Each chapter starts with an introductory text that provides a brief review of the current understanding of the topic, followed by the main bullet-style text. The information is clustered in "bite-size" portions to facilitate immediate absorption. Each item is designed to be read independent of the rest of the book. The items are alphabetically listed and can be found and refound easily. The text is further enriched with many figures, diagrams, mnemonics, and historical trivia. The design of this book is intended to facilitate easy learning and memorization. However, readers should be cautioned that some of the mnemonics are created not for scientific accuracy, but as an optional instrument to assist memorization. Multiple choice questions are provided at the end of the book for self-assessment.

The selection of content proved to be an arduous task. To find a field consensus of required knowledge for both the clinical need and the test requirement, I scanned through a huge volume of material including major textbooks, published review books, old PRITE test questions of the past 10 years, papers of Continuous Medical Education (CME), and unpublished syllabi of the Board review courses. I also consulted the content outline from ABPN as a generally accepted guide of coverage. The contents are further filtered on the basis of clinical relevance, testability, proneness to confusion, and difficulty for memorization. Through such scrutiny I established a continuously updated database of study material, from which the final product was composed. The "book knowledge" provided here is of moderate depth and is believed to be adequate as a foundation upon which clinical competency can be built.

Psychiatry is now in its most exciting era. The influx of new information has never been of the same volume and speed in history. While providing a new horizon of patient care, the proceedings of science also place a greater burden on clinicians for continuous learning. I hope this book will serve as an efficient learning guide and an alternative resource in the world of traditional textbooks. It is my belief that when equipped with adequate instruments, absorbing a vast volume of knowledge in a relatively short period of time is a mission possible.

William W. Wang, M.D., Ph.D.

1 Functional Neuroanatomy

Once upon a time, psychiatric conditions were divided into "organic" and "functional," based on whether there was an observable structural or chemical deviation. This categorization is no longer meaningful. Scientific researches continue to find more and more anatomical structures that have a tangible connection to the neuronal functions with which most psychiatrists are concerned: mood, thought, cognition, behavior, and also movement and sensation. Changes in these structures, often at microscopic scale, may have significant impact on mental function. Knowledge of these anatomical structures is essential in understanding the biological aspect of psychiatry.

The general organization of the central nervous system is presented in Figure 1–1. Anatomy of the spinal cord is not reviewed here because of its relatively limited application in common psychiatric disorders. Selected topics on spinal cord anatomy are reviewed in Chapter 43, in combination with spinal cord diseases.

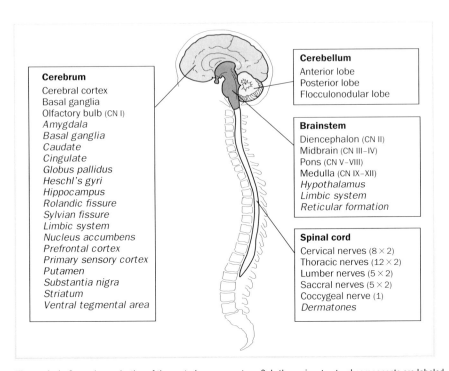

Figure 1–1 General organization of the central nervous system. Only the major structural components are labeled. Structures described in this chapter are listed in italic font.

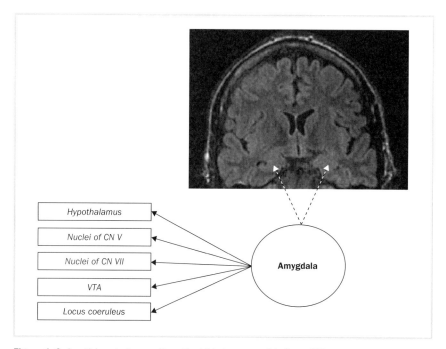

Figure 1–2 Amygdala output connections. The inlet shows amygdala in an MRI coronal section. Abbreviations: MRI stands for magnetic resonance imaging; VTA stands for ventral tegmental area.

Amygdala: anatomy (Figure 1–2)

From Greek, "almond."

▶ Groups of neurons deep within the medial temporal lobes
▶ An essential part of the limbic system
▶ Involved in memory, emotional reactions, and appetite conditioning
▶ Output to:
  ▷ Hypothalamus: activation of the sympathetic nervous system
  ▷ Nuclei of the trigeminal nerve (CN V) and facial nerve (CN VII): facial expressions
  ▷ Ventral tegmental area (VTA): activation of dopamine
  ▷ Locus coeruleus: activation of norepinephrine

Amygdala: roles in anxiety and fear

▶ Mediates learned fear responses
▶ Directs the expression of certain emotions
▶ Exerts influence on the cortex
▶ Damage to the amygdala may ablate the ability to distinguish fear and anger
▶ Positron emission tomography (PET) shows that harm avoidance is associated with increased activity in the right amygdala and other structures

Auditory system

▶ Peripheral system:
  ▷ Changes of air pressure form sounds
  ▷ Vibration of tympanic membrane

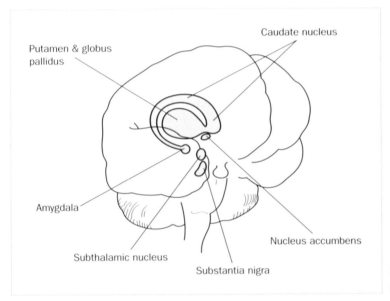

Figure 1–3 Components of basal ganglia.

    ▷ Vibration is transmitted through ossicles to the endolymph of the cochlear spiral
    ▷ Vibrations of the endolymph move cilia on hair cells
    ▷ Hair cells generate neural impulses
▶ Central system:
    ▷ Neural impulses travel through cochlear nerves to cochlear nuclei (brainstem)
    ▷ Then the impulses travel to the medial geniculate nucleus (MGN, at thalamus)
    ▷ MGN projects to the primary auditory cortex (Heschl's gyri)

Basal ganglia (Figure 1–3)

▶ Anatomical components:
    ▷ Putamen
    ▷ Caudate nucleus
    ▷ Nucleus accumbens
    ▷ Globus pallidus
    ▷ Subthalamic nucleus
    ▷ Substantia nigra
▶ Function (consists of a series of circuits that are associated with a variety of functions):
    ▷ Motor control
    ▷ Cognition
    ▷ Emotions
    ▷ Learning

Caudate nucleus

▶ Anatomy:
    ▷ Part of basal ganglia
    ▷ Together with putamen, forms the dorsal striatum
    ▷ Separated from the lenticular nucleus by the internal capsule

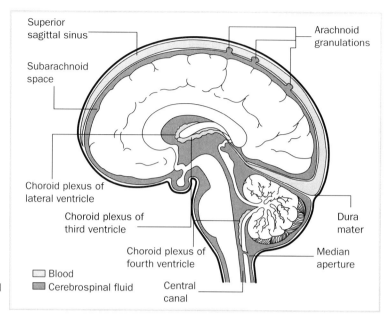

Figure 1-4 Flow of cerebrospinal fluid.

▶ Function:
  ▷ Important part of the learning and memory system
▶ Neurochemistry:
  ▷ Highly innervated by dopamine neurons
  ▷ These neurons originate mainly from the VTA and the substantia nigra

Cerebellum function

▶ Activated before a planned – or even imagined – movement
▶ Modulates the tone of agonistic and antagonistic muscles
▶ Predicts the relative contraction needed for smooth motion

Cerebrospinal fluid: formation and absorption (Figure 1-4)

▶ Formation:
  ▷ Choroid plexuses of lateral, third, and fourth ventricles
▶ Flow:
  ▷ Choroid plexuses
  ▷ Ventricles
  ▷ Median aperture (foramen of Magendie) or lateral apertures (foramina of Luschka)
  ▷ Subarachnoid space
▶ Absorption:
  ▷ Through arachnoid granulations, also known as arachnoid villi
  ▷ To the superior sagittal sinus or venous lacunae

Cingulate

▶ Anatomy:
  ▷ A gyrus between the corpus callosum and the cingulate sulcus
  ▷ An integral part of the limbic system

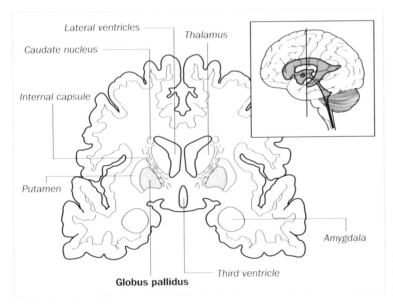

Figure 1–5 Coronal cut shows globus pallidus and its surrounding structures.

▶ Function:
  ▷ Emotion formation and processing
  ▷ Learning
  ▷ Memory
  ▷ Unconscious priming

Glial cells

▶ Astrocytes:
  ▷ Most common type of glial cells
  ▷ Nutritional support to neurons
  ▷ Deactivation of neurotransmitters
  ▷ Integration with the blood-brain barrier
▶ Oligodendrocytes:
  ▷ Appear only in the central nervous system
  ▷ Form myeline sheaths
▶ Schwann cells:
  ▷ Appear only in the peripheral nervous system
  ▷ Form myeline sheaths
  ▷ Remove cellular debris

Globus pallidus (Figure 1–5)

▶ Anatomy:
  ▷ A subcortical structure
  ▷ A major element of the basal ganglia
  ▷ Forms the dorsal striatum
▶ Function:
  ▷ Involved in the regulation of voluntary movements at a subconscious level
  ▷ Probably involved in physiological pace-making

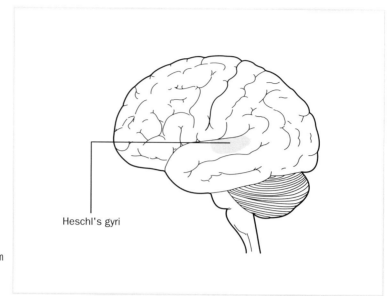

Figure 1–6 Heschl's gyri, the primary auditory cortex. It is the first cortical structure to process incoming auditory information from the medial geniculate nucleus (MGN).

Heschl's gyri (Figure 1–6)

Richard Heschl (1824–1881) was an Austrian anatomist.

▶ Also known as the transverse temporal gyri or Heschl's convolutions
▶ Located bilaterally in the primary auditory cortex in the superior temporal gyrus
▶ Receives auditory stimuli from the contralateral ear
▶ Supplied by the middle cerebral artery

Hippocampus

From Latin, "sea horse."

▶ Located in the medial temporal lobe
▶ Part of the limbic system
▶ Plays an important role in memory and spatial navigation

Hypothalamus

▶ Anatomy:
  ▷ Located below the thalamus, just above the brain stem
  ▷ Occupies the major portion of the ventral region of the diencephalon
▶ Function:
  ▷ Links the nervous system to the endocrine system via the pituitary gland (hypophysis)
  ▷ Synthesizes and secretes hypothalamic-releasing hormones, and these in turn stimulate or inhibit the secretion of pituitary hormones
  ▷ Regulates certain metabolic processes and other autonomic activities – body temperature, hunger, thirst, and circadian cycles

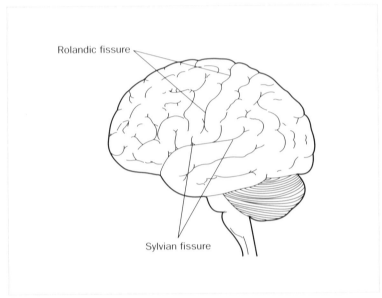

Figure 1-7 Rolandic fissure and Sylvian fissure.

Important brain fissures (Figure 1–7)

Luigi Rolando (1773–1831) was an Italian anatomist.
Franciscus Sylvius (1614–1672) was a German-Dutch physician and anatomist.

▶ Rolandic fissure:
  ▷ Also known as the central sulcus or fissure of Rolando
  ▷ Separates the parietal lobe from the frontal lobe, and the primary motor cortex from the primary somatosensory cortex
▶ Sylvian fissure:
  ▷ Also known as the lateral sulcus or lateral fissure
  ▷ Divides the frontal and parietal lobes from the temporal lobe

Limbic system

▶ Anatomy (major components as listed):
  ▷ Amygdala
  ▷ Cingulate gyrus
  ▷ Hippocampus
  ▷ Hypothalamus
  ▷ Mammillary body
  ▷ Nucleus accumbens
  ▷ Orbitofrontal cortex
  ▷ Thalamus
▶ Function:
  ▷ Pleasure
  ▷ Sexual arousal
  ▷ Health consciousness
  ▷ Not completely understood

Nucleus accumbens (Figure 1–3)

▶ Location: the head of the caudate and the anterior portion of the putamen
▶ Neurobiological role:
  ▷ Reward
  ▷ Pleasure
  ▷ Addiction
▶ Neurotransmitter:
  ▷ Mainly gamma-aminobutyric acid (GABA)
  ▷ Some cholinergic interneurons
▶ Associated with the action of addictive drugs such as cocaine and amphetamine; almost every drug abused by humans has been shown to increase dopamine levels in the nucleus accumbens

Prefrontal cortex

▶ Anterior part of the frontal lobes, generally involved in executive function (regulating thoughts and actions in accordance with internal goals)
▶ Orbitofrontal cortex:
  ▷ Decision making
  ▷ Emotion and reward
  ▷ Part of the limbic system
▶ Medial prefrontal areas
  ▷ Planning complex cognitive behaviors
  ▷ Personality expression
  ▷ Moderating appropriate social behavior

Primary sensory cortex

▶ Lateral postcentral gyrus in the parietal lobe
▶ Roughly overlaps with Brodmann areas 3, 1, and 2
▶ Receives the thalamocortical projection from the sensory input fields

Putamen (Figure 1–3)

From Latin, "shell."

▶ Anatomy:
  ▷ Part of basal ganglia
  ▷ Dorsal striatum
  ▷ Outermost part of the lenticular nucleus (the inner part is globus pallidus)
▶ Function:
  ▷ Not well defined
  ▷ Likely to play a role in reinforcement learning

Reticular formation

▶ Also known as the reticular activating system
▶ Anatomy:
  ▷ Centered in the pons, connected to the thalamus, hypothalamus, cortex, and cerebellum

▶ Function:
  ▷ Arousal and motivation
  ▷ Maintaining the state of consciousness
  ▷ Circadian rhythm

Reward system

▶ Primarily involves the mesolimbic and mesocortical dopamine pathway
▶ Anatomical structures include VTA, nucleus accumbens, substantia nigra, and prefrontal lobe

Substantia nigra (Figure 1–3)

From Latin, "black substance."

▶ A heterogeneous portion of the midbrain
▶ A component of basil ganglia
▶ Center of dopamine production
▶ Plays a central role in the reward system and addiction

Striatum

▶ A subcortical structure of telencephalon, it consists of:
  ▷ Putamen
  ▷ Caudate nucleus
▶ Striatum is the major input station of basal ganglia

Ventral tegmental area

▶ Also known as ventral tegmentum
▶ Is part of the midbrain
▶ Consists of dopamine, GABA, and glutamate neurons
▶ Is part of two major dopamine pathways
  ▷ The mesolimbic pathway, which projects to the nucleus accumbens
  ▷ The mesocortical pathway, which projects to cortical areas in the frontal lobes
▶ Functions:
  ▷ Part of the reward system
  ▷ Emotion and security motivation
  ▷ Avoidance and fear-conditioning

2 Neurochemistry

The synthesis, metabolism, transportation, interaction, and other behaviors of neuro-chemicals play important roles in mental activities. Two major categories of neurochemi-cals are studied in psychiatry: neurotransmitters and neuroactive drugs. This chapter reviews the important neurotransmitters, which include

▶ Acetylcholine
▶ Dopamine
▶ Gamma-amino butyric acid (GABA)
▶ Glutamate
▶ Glycine
▶ Histamine
▶ Melatonin
▶ Norepinephrine
▶ Serotonin

Acetylcholine synthesis and metabolism (Figure 2–1)

Theodor Meynert (1833–1892) was a German-Austrian neuropathologist and anatomist.

▶ Location
  ▷ Basal nucleus of Meynert at basal forebrain
▶ Precursors
  ▷ Acetyl-CoA and choline
▶ Metabolism
  ▷ Breaks down to acetyl-CoA and choline
  ▷ Catalyzed by acetylcholinesterase in the synaptic cleft

Adrenergic α-1 antagonism: clinical effects

▶ Sedation
▶ Orthostatic hypotension
▶ Priapism

Adrenergic α-2 receptor

▶ Presynaptic receptors provide negative feedback on the release of serotonin and norepinephrine
▶ Agonists – decreases serotonin and norepinephrine release
  ▷ Clonidine – sympatholytic action; helpful in opiate withdrawal
▶ Antagonists – increases serotonin and norepinephrine release

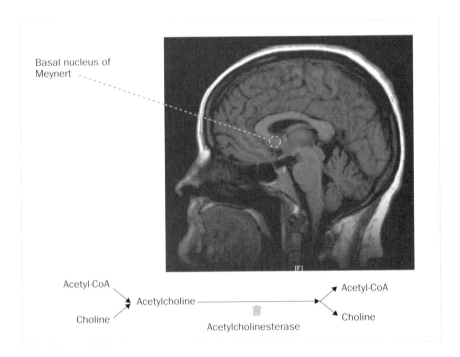

Figure 2–1 The location of basal nucleus of Meynert on MRI medium sagittal cut, and metabolic pathways of acetylcholine. MRI, magnetic resonance imaging.

▷ Yohimbine – reversal of selective serotonin reuptake inhibitor (SSRI)-induced sexual side effects, probably by raising norepinephrine tone
▷ Mirtazapine –antidepressant, known to have minimum sexual side effects

Biogenic amine neurotransmitters

▶ Catecholamines
  ▷ Dopamine
  ▷ Norepinephrine
  ▷ Epinephrine
▶ Serotonin
▶ Acetylcholine
▶ Histamine

Cellular location of neurotransmitter synthesis

▶ Neurotransmitters are synthesized in the neuron
▶ Peptide neurotransmitters are synthesized in the body of neuron cell, also known as soma
▶ All other neurotransmitters are synthesized in the presynaptic axon terminal, also known as bouton

Direct-coupled ion channels (See Figure 2–2 on page 12)

▶ Ion channels are part of the receptors
▶ Binding of a ligand directly changes the ion channel

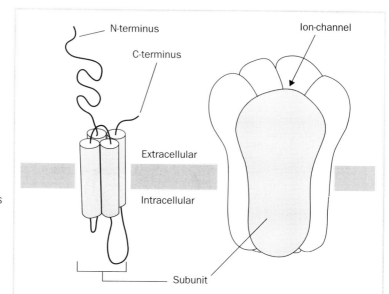

Figure 2-2 Direct-coupled ion channels. Each subunit is a single peptide that crosses the cell membrane four times, which forms four transmembrane domains. Both C-terminus and N-terminus are located in extracellular space. A direct-coupled ion channel receptor usually composes of 4–5 subunits.

▶ No second messengers are involved
▶ Typically constructed with multiple subunits, each has 4–5 transmembrane domains
▶ Fast in response to neurotransmitter activities
▶ Examples of direct-coupled ion channel receptors
  ▷ Nicotinic cholinergic
  ▷ 5-HT3
  ▷ GABA-A
  ▷ Glutamate receptors

Dopamine synthesis

▶ Synthesized from tyrosine
▶ Rate-limiting enzyme is tyrosine hydroxylase

Dopaminergic nuclei: localization

▶ Substantia nigra – supplies to nigrostriatal pathway, associated with extrapyramidal syndrome (EPS)
▶ Ventral tegmental area (VTA) – supplies to mesolimbic-mesocortical pathway, associated with antipsychotic effects and reward system
▶ Hypothalamus, including the arcuate and periventricular nuclei – supplies to tuberoinfundibular pathway, associated with prolactin regulation

Dopaminergic receptors

▶ All are membrane-anchored, G-protein linked receptors
▶ Subtypes – D1, D2, D3, D4, D5
▶ Activation of D1 and D5 results in an increase in cyclic adenosine monophosphate (cAMP)
▶ Activation of D2, D3, and D4 receptors results in a decrease of cAMP

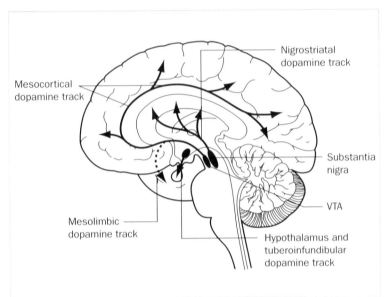

Figure 2–3 Dopaminergic nuclei and pathways.
VTA, ventral tegmental area.

Dopamine tracts and physiological function (Figure 2–3)

▶ Nigrostriatal – blockade is associated with EPS and Parkinsonism
▶ Mesolimbic – blockade is considered the key mechanism for the remission of psychotic symptoms
▶ Mesocortical – blockade is associated with cognitive deficits
▶ Tuberoinfundibular – physiologically, dopamine inhibits prolactin secretion through this tract; antagonism causes prolactin elevation

GABA receptors (See Figure 2–4 on page 14)

▶ GABA-A – direct-coupled receptor with chloride channel; has binding sites for GABA, benzodiazepines, and barbiturates
▶ GABA-B – G-protein coupled receptor
▶ GABA-C – direct-coupled receptor with ligand-gated chloride ion channel

GABA synthesis

▶ Location – found only in central nervous system (CNS)
▶ Precursor – glutamate
▶ Rate-limiting enzyme
  ▷ Glutamic acid decarboxylase (GAD) is the enzyme
  ▷ Pyridoxine (vitamin B6) is the cofactor

Glycine

▶ An inhibitory neurotransmitter
▶ A mandatory adjunctive neurotransmitter for glutamate activity

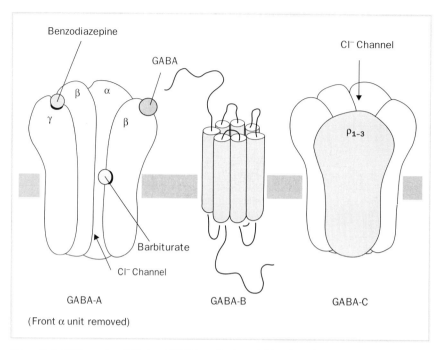

Figure 2–4 GABA receptors. GABA-A and GABA-C are direct-coupled ion channel receptors with chloride ion channel, composed of five subunits. Binding sites of GABA, benzodiazepines, and barbiturates are shown in GABA-A receptor. GABA-C receptors are composed of a variety of combination with ρ1, ρ2, and ρ3. GABA-B receptors are G-protein coupled receptors. GABA, gamma-amino butyric acid.

G-protein coupled receptors (Figure 2–5)

▶ Characteristic seven transmembrane domains
▶ Uses second messengers
▶ Functions as a regulator to slow ion channels or modulatory receptors
▶ Examples of G-protein coupled receptors
  ▷ Cholinergic – muscarinic
  ▷ Dopamine – D2
  ▷ Norepinephrine – α-1, α-2, β
  ▷ Serotonin – 5-HT1a, 5-HT1C, 5-HT2
  ▷ Opioid – all types
  ▷ Substance P-NK

Histamine blockade: clinical effects

▶ Allergy relief
▶ Hypotension
▶ Sedation
▶ Weight gain
▶ Decreased gastric acid production

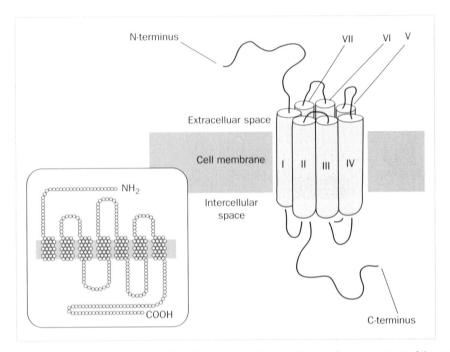

Figure 2–5 The Schematic structure of G-protein linked receptor shows the approximate arrangement of the seven trans-membrane domains. The inlet shows the wiring of the polypeptide where each little ball represents one amino acid. The polypeptide is genetically sequenced so that most lipophilic amino acids are clustered in seven sections, which facilitates the anchoring of the receptor on the highly lipophilic cell membrane.

Inhibitory and excitatory neurotransmitters

▶ The major inhibitory neurotransmitter are GABA and glycine
▶ The major excitatory neurotransmitter is glutamate

Melatonin

▶ Secreted by the pineal gland
▶ Has synapses and receptors at suprachiasmatic nucleus (SCN) of the hypothalamus
▶ Plays an important role in circadian regulation
▶ Receives positive feedback from increased sleep drive in the evening
▶ Receives negative feedback from the retinohypothalamic tract

Monoamine oxidase

▶ Two subtypes of monoamine oxidase (MAO) – MAO-A and MAO-B.
▶ Both MAO-A and MAO-B appear in CNS
▶ MAO-A also appears in liver and intestine, where it breaks down tyramine from food
▶ When MAO-A is inhibited, tyramine-rich food can cause surge of tyramine in blood and hypertensive crisis may occur

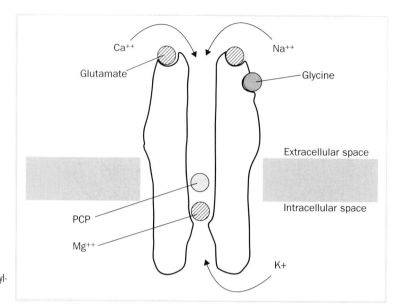

Figure 2–6 NMDA receptor and its ligands.
PCP, phencyclidine; NMDA, *N*-methyl-D-aspartate receptor.

Muscarinic vs. nicotinic acetylcholine receptors

▶ Mechanism of action
  ▷ Muscarinic receptors are G-protein coupled receptors
  ▷ Nicotinic receptors are direct-coupled ion channels
▶ Subunits
  ▷ Muscarinic receptors are single unit proteins contain seven transmembrane domains
  ▷ Nicotinic receptors are constructed with five subunits – two α subunits, one β, one γ, and one δ.

N-methyl-*D*-aspartate (NMDA) receptor (Figure 2–6)

▶ One of the five major types of glutamate receptors
▶ When activated by two molecules of glutamate and one of glycine, opens the integrated Ca^{++} channel to allow influx of calcium
▶ Blockade by Mg^{++} and PCP
▶ Plays a key role in learning and memory
▶ Down-regulation of receptor may cause psychosis
▶ Drugs bind to NMDA receptor – memantine, acamprosate

Norepinephrine synthesis (Figure 2–7)

▶ Norepinephrine (NE) – located at locus ceruleus in upper pons
▶ Conversion from dopamine catalyzed by dopamine-hydroxylase
▶ Rate-limiting enzyme is tyrosine hydroxylase, same as dopamine

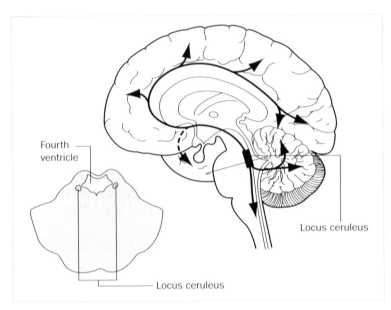

Figure 2-7 Norepinephrine nucleus and major pathways.

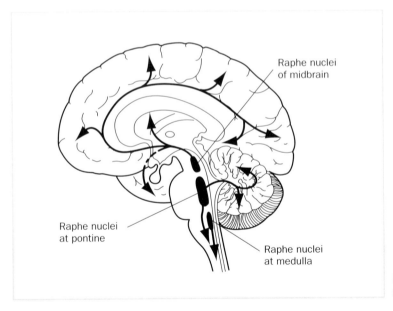

Figure 2-8 Serotonergic nuclei and projections.

Opioid regulation of dopaminergic reward system

▶ Dopamine in the mesolimbic system originates in the VTA of the midbrain, and projects the nucleus accumbens, and releases in the nucleus accumbens
▶ Tonic control by activation of opioid receptors
  ▷ Activation of μ and Σ receptors increases dopamine activity, and produces euphoria
  ▷ Activation of κ-receptor decreases the dopamine activity, and produces dysphoria

Selected serotonin receptors with clinical relevance

▶ 5-HT1a – antidepressant and anxiolytic action
▶ 5-HT1d – target of antimigraine drug sumatriptan
▶ 5-HT2a – target of atypical antipsychotics, as well as hallucinogens
▶ 5-HT2b – gastrointestinal tract (GI) regulation
▶ 5-HT2c – GI as well as anxiety and seizures

Serotonergic nuclei: localization (Figure 2–8)

▶ Serotonin is produced by neurons located in two areas
  ▷ Raphe nuclei, located at upper pons and midbrain
  ▷ Caudal locus ceruleus

Serotonin receptor distribution and proposed clinical relevance

▶ Basal ganglia – agitation, akathisia
▶ Brainstem and GI – nausea, vomiting
▶ Limbic system – insomnia, sedation
▶ Spinal cord – sexual side effects
▶ Cranial vasculature – migraine

Serotonin synthesis

▶ Location – median and dorsal raphe nuclei in pons
▶ Precursor – tryptophan
▶ Rate-limiting factor – availability of tryptophan

3 Neurophysiology

According to classical antiquity, physiology concerns about the "nature" of living organism, which refers principally to the interplay between structure and function. Parallel with the technological advancement, neurophysiology has achieved great progress in the past century. At the microscopic level, the boundary between biochemistry and neurophysiology often becomes blurred, a phenomenon pleasantly accepted in the world of biological science.

While a systemic coverage of neurophysiology is beyond the scope of this book, this chapter reviews a few important topics of neurophysiology relevant to clinical psychiatry. Two topics covered with more details are memory and studies on arousal and wakefulness.

Apoptosis vs. necrosis (See Figure 3–1 on page 20)

▶ Apoptosis is programmed cell death. It
  ▷ Involves expression of specific genes
  ▷ Has no inflammatory response
  ▷ May be prevented by neurotrophins
  ▷ Is associated with development, and neurodegenerative disease
▶ Necrosis is a cell death process due to external damage. It
  ▷ Has no expression of specific genes
  ▷ Has inflammatory response
  ▷ May be enhanced by neurotrophins under certain conditions
  ▷ Follows acute insult or injury

Arousal and wakefulness: *anatomy*

▶ Related anatomic regions
  ▷ The ascending reticular activating system
  ▷ The intralaminar nuclei of the thalamus
  ▷ The cortex
▶ Pathological effect of lesion
  ▷ Small lesions of the ascending reticular activating system may have significant effects on conscious status
  ▷ Only large, bilateral cortical lesions may cause significant change in alertness
  ▷ Persistent vegetative state – disconnection of the thalamus and the ascending reticular activating system

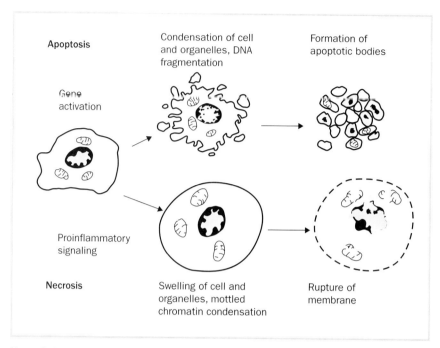

Figure 3–1 Apoptosis vs. necrosis.

Arousal and wakefulness: *electrophysiology*

▶ Thalamus and cortex fire rhythmical electric bursts at 20–40 Hz
▶ Ascending reticular activating system stimulates the thalamus and coordinates the oscillations of cortical regions
▶ Degree of the synchronization of electro-neuronal activity is positively related to the level of wakefulness
▶ Altered electro-neuronal activity
  ▷ Sleep and drowsiness – asynchronous electro-neuronal activity
  ▷ Stupor and coma – absence of electro-neuronal activity

Evoked potential (EP)

▶ Surface (scalp) recordable electrical potentials from the brain following stimuli
▶ Stimulation may be visual, auditory, somatosensory, or cognitive
▶ Gating phenomenon – when two identical stimuli were given to a normal individual in short time (less than 1 second), the EP to the second stimuli is reduced
▶ P300
  ▷ A positive wave that occurs about 300 milliseconds after a sensory stimulus
  ▷ Source – the limbic system
  ▷ Decreased amplitude is found in individuals with schizophrenia, and children with schizophrenic parents
▶ N100
  ▷ A negative wave that occurs about 100 milliseconds after a stimulus
  ▷ Smaller and delayed in schizophrenia
  ▷ No deficiency in gating was found in schizophrenia

- P50
  - ▷ A positive wave recorded 50 milliseconds after an auditory stimulus
  - ▷ Smaller and delayed, with no gating in schizophrenia

Excitotoxicity

John Olney is a contemporary U.S. psychiatrist and neuroscientist at Washington University in St. Louis.

- A pathological process of neuronal damage by excessive glutaminergic activity
- The process
  - ▷ Excessive stimulation of glutamate receptors
  - ▷ Opens the calcium channels in glutamate receptors
  - ▷ Prolonged high intraneuronal concentration of calcium and nitric oxide
  - ▷ Intracellular cascades subsequently activate many proteases and finally destroy the neuron
- John Onley discovered the toxic effect of glutamate, a phenomenon thought to be restricted to retina, occurred throughout the central nervous system (CNS); he also coined the term
- Excitotoxicity is believed to be involved in any neuronal damage, including stroke, injury, and neurodegererative diseases, as well as debilitating mental illness such as schizophrenia.

Hypothalamic-pituitary-adrenal axis (HPA) and mental disorders

- Hormones
  - ▷ Hypothalamic – corticotropin-releasing hormone (CRH)
  - ▷ Pituitary – adrenocorticotropic hormone (ACTH)
  - ▷ Adrenal – cortisol
- The hormonal response pattern depends on
  - ▷ Nature of the stressor
  - ▷ Individual's coping ability
  - ▷ Physical condition – pain, sleep status, etc.
  - ▷ Social status
- Pathological alterations in hypothalamic-pituitary adrenal (HPA) functioning are seen in
  - ▷ Mood disorders
  - ▷ Posttraumatic stress disorder
  - ▷ Dementia of the Alzheimer's type
  - ▷ Substance-related disorders
- HPA changes in depression
  - ▷ Elevated cortisol
  - ▷ Failure of dexamethasone suppression
  - ▷ Enlarged adrenal size
  - ▷ Elevated sensitivity to ACTH
  - ▷ Blunted ACTH response to CRH
  - ▷ Elevated CRH

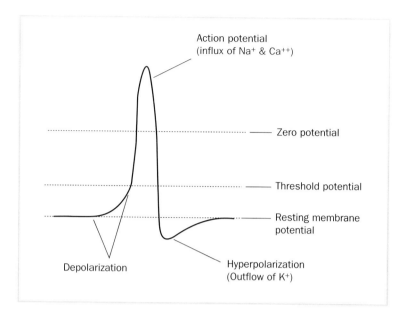

Figure 3-2 Action potential.

Mechanism of action potential (Figure 3-2)

▶ Resting potential neurons: –55 to –70 mV
▶ Na-K-ATPase pump moves Na⁺ out and K⁺ in against their concentration gradient, and maintains the resting potential
▶ Depolarization – reducing the cytosol negative charge, makes the cell membrane ready to have action potential
▶ The action potential starts with depolarization by rapid influx of Na⁺
▶ Ca⁺⁺ also has a higher concentration outside of cell, and enters cell during action potential with Na⁺; Ca⁺⁺ involves in many cytosol activities, also activates repolarization by outward K⁺ current
▶ The outward K⁺ current causes hyper polarization, and transiently decreases cell membrane excitability after an action potential

Memory: *declarative memory* (Figure 3-3)

▶ Also known as explicit memory
▶ Facts, events, and associative learning
▶ Requires conscious awareness and concentration
▶ Impaired after brain injury
▶ Structures involved
  ▷ Hippocampus
  ▷ Orbitofrontal cortex
  ▷ Parahippocampal gyrus

Memory: *formation and storage*

▶ Anatomical regions
  ▷ Hippocampus and surrounding medial temporal lobe

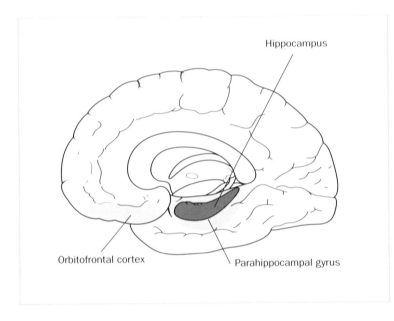

Hippocampus

Orbitofrontal cortex   Parahippocampal gyrus

Figure 3–3 Structures associated with declarative memory are shown in the median cut of the brain with brainstem removed – orbitofrontal cortex, hippocampus, and parahippocampal gyrus.

- ▷ Cortex
- ▷ Cerebellum
- ▶ Mechanism of storage
  - ▷ Formation of connections between synapses
  - ▷ Quantity of connections is related to the retaining of information
  - ▷ Increased time-allowed memorizing and repeated recall of a memory may help establish more connections and hence better memory
- ▶ Smell and emotion
  - ▷ Both are connected to the hippocampus
  - ▷ Tend to be long term
- ▶ Effects of stress
  - ▷ Moderate stress – causes increase in adrenaline, which enhances learning and memory
  - ▷ Severe stress inhibits learning and memory
- ▶ Effects of mood
  - ▷ Happy mood enhances memory
- ▶ Prelinguistic memory
  - ▷ Before the age of 3–5 years, when the language learning is initiated
  - ▷ Only memories associated with strong emotion (traumatic) or with smell are likely to be remembered

Memory: *nondeclarative memory* (See Figure 3–4 on page 24)

- ▶ Also known as implicit memory
- ▶ Skills, habits, and nonassociative learning
- ▶ Does not require conscious awareness and concentration
- ▶ Usually remains intact after brain injury
- ▶ Structures involved
  - ▷ Basal ganglia
  - ▷ Limbic system
  - ▷ Perceptual cortex

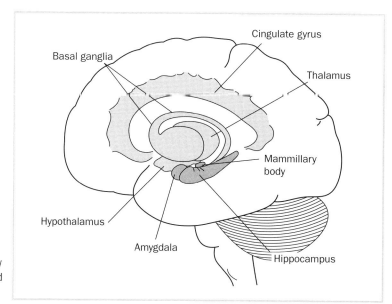

Figure 3-4 Major structures involved in nondeclarative memory – basal ganglia, limbic system, and perceptual cortex (not labeled).

Memory: *short term vs. long term*

▶ Short term (primary memory)
  ▷ Includes immediate memory, working memory, and buffer memory
  ▷ Adversely affected by emotion, stress, and quantity of input
  ▷ Capacity of short-term memory is limited
▶ Long term (secondary memory)
  ▷ Includes recent memory, recent past memory, and remote memory
  ▷ Has much higher capacity in the quantity of information to be stored

Memory: *working memory*

▶ Ability to store information for several seconds while awaiting the related cognitive operations
▶ Anatomy
  ▷ Neurons in the dorsolateral prefrontal cortex
  ▷ Left frontal cortex
▶ Function
  ▷ Associated with goal-directed behavior

Myelination and demyelination
Theodor Schwann (1810–1882) was a German physiologist.

▶ Myelin
  ▷ A phospholipid layer surrounds the myelinated axons of neurons
  ▷ Supplied by Schwann cells for peripheral neurons, and oligodendrocytes in CNS
▶ Function of myelin layer
  ▷ Provides electrical insulation for the axons
  ▷ Increases the speed of neuronal conduction
  ▷ Provides guide for regrowth of injured neuronal fibers

▶ Demyelination may occur in
  ▷ Neurodegenerative diseases
  ▷ Autoimmune diseases

Neuromuscular synapses

▶ Also known as neuromuscular junctions
▶ Connection between the axon from motor neuron and the muscle fibers
▶ Each muscle fiber is innervated by a single neuron
▶ Each motor neuron innervates multiple muscular fibers, in the estimated range of 2000

Neuronal migration

▶ Mission of migration
  ▷ Postmitotic neurons need to move to their adult locations in the cortex to function properly
▶ Direction guidance
  ▷ Guided by astrocytic glial fibers
▶ Time
  ▷ Prominently in the first and second trimesters
▶ Heterotopia – neurons reside in ectopic positions because of failure in migration; neuronal heterotopias may be associated with pathology of
  ▷ Epilepsy
  ▷ Mental retardation
  ▷ Learning disability
  ▷ Schizophrenia

Neuronal pruning and reinforcement

▶ Synaptogenesis forms five-fold excess of synaptic connections needed for normal brain function
▶ Synapses serve no relevant function are eliminated in the process of pruning
▶ Synaptic pruning reinforces repeatedly activated neural circuits
▶ N-methyl-D-aspartate (NMDA) type of glutamate receptors may mediate the process of synaptic reinforcement

Primitive reflex circuit

▶ Neuronal circuit with direct linkage between sensory pathways and motor pathways
▶ No conscious awareness is required
▶ Local, all-or-none
▶ Does not generate any purposeful behavior

Resting potential (Figure 3–2)

▶ Electric potential across cell membrane when there is no active changes
▶ Usual resting potential is –70mV, with negative charges inside the cell
▶ Maintained by a variety of ion channels and ion transporters
▶ Na^+/K^+-ATPase plays a major role in maintaining a higher Na^+ level outside of the cell and K^+ level inside of the cell

Synaptogenesis: *critical times*

▶ Synaptogenesis occurs in high rate from second trimester to 10 years of age
▶ The peak of synaptogenesis
  ▷ Within the first 2 postnatal years

Triphasic waves

▶ An electroencephalogram (EEG) pattern found in hepatic encephalopathy (about 50%) and other metabolic encephalopathies
▶ Characteristics
  ▷ High-amplitude, positive waves preceded and followed by low-amplitude negative waves
  ▷ Repeated in short runs at a rate of 1–2 Hz
  ▷ Bilaterally synchronous
▶ Proposed pathophysiology
  ▷ Dysfunction of the thalamocortical relay neurons
  ▷ Abnormalities in glutamate metabolism

4 Child and Adolescent Development

The basic assumption in the theories of developmental psychology states that human life follows a series of defined stages, and that every stage has its own principle and specific task, and that successful completion of the stage-specific task is fundamental for the development to proceed smoothly. Though adjustment at times is needed with new data available, these theories are still in large held authoritative in mainstay psychiatry. Jean Piaget's, Sigmund Freud's, and Eric Erikson's are among the most established schools, as compared in Figure 4–1. These theories, along with other theories regarding child and adolescent development, contributed to our current understanding of human development and the problems occurring during the process from birth to death.

Adolescence stage: *classical theories* (See Figure 4–1 on page 28)

Jean Piaget (1896–1980) was a Swiss psychologist.
Erik Erikson (1902–1994) was a German psychologist.
Sigmund Freud (1856–1939) was an Austrian neurologist and psychiatrist, founding father of psychoanalysis.

- ▶ Jean Piaget
  - ▷ Formal operational stage (11–adulthood)
  - ▷ Deals with concepts and ideas
  - ▷ Abstract, deductive, and conceptual thinking
  - ▷ Synthesis, integration of traits, attitudes, and impulses to create a total personality
- ▶ Erik Erikson
  - ▷ Identity vs. role confusion (11–20 years)
  - ▷ Struggle to develop ego identity
  - ▷ Group identity
  - ▷ Hero worship
  - ▷ Ideology
- ▶ Sigmund Freud
  - ▷ Adolescence (12–18 years)
  - ▷ Sexual development approaches mature stage

Attachment

John Bowlby (1907–1990) was a British psychoanalyst.

- ▶ Emotional and behavioral dependence to caregiver or provider
- ▶ Develops in infant stage (ages 6 weeks–3 years) and lasts through adult life
- ▶ Derived from John Bowlby's cognitive theory

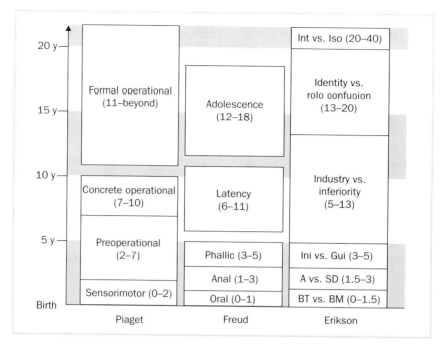

Figure 4–1 Developmental stages from birth to early adulthood – a comparative chart of theories by Jean Piaget, Sigmund Freud, and Eric Erikson.

A vs. SD, autonomy vs. shame and doubt; BT vs. BM, basic trust vs. basic mistrust; Ini vs. Gui, initiative vs. guilt; Int vs. Iso; intimacy vs. isolation; Y, years.

▶ Four types of attachment style are identified; Type B–D are also called "insecure attach-ments," and are associated with development of personality disorders
  ▷ Type A – secure attachment: child protests the mother's departure and quiets on the mother's return
  ▷ Type B – avoidant attachment: little to no signs of distress at the mother's departure and no visible response to the mother's return
  ▷ Type C – ambivalent attachment: sad on the mother's departure but warmed up to a stranger, and ambivalent signs of anger on mother's return
  ▷ Type D – disorganized attachment: lack of coherent response, often stereotypes upon the mother's return after separation

Behavioral milestones for a 2-year-old

▶ Building an eight-cube tower
▶ Climbing stairs
▶ Domestic mimicry
▶ Playing interactive games
▶ Pulling on clothes
▶ Referring to self by name
▶ Separation anxiety is diminishing
▶ Using fifty words and word combinations

Behavioral milestones for a 3-year-old

▶ Building a ten-cube tower
▶ Drawing a circle
▶ Feeding self
▶ Going up stairs using alternative feet
▶ Putting on shoes
▶ Riding tricycle
▶ Unbuttoning
▶ Understanding on taking turns

Behavioral milestones for a 4-year-old

▶ Brushing teeth
▶ Copying a cross
▶ Counting three objects
▶ Playing cooperative game
▶ Walking down stairs
▶ Washing and drying face

Behavioral milestones for a 5-year-old

▶ Controlling sphincters
▶ Drawing a square
▶ Drawing a recognizable person
▶ Counting ten objects
▶ Dressing and undressing self
▶ Playing competitive games

Classical theories associated with developmental stage of preschool years (Figure 4–1)

▶ Erik Erikson
 ▷ Initiative vs. guilt (3–5 years).
▶ Jean Piaget
 ▷ Preoperational stage (2–7 years) – object permanence, egocentricity, magical thinking, associative logic
▶ Sigmund Freud
 ▷ Latency (6–puberty) – repression of sexual interest, formation of superego

Concrete operational stage

▶ From Jean Piaget's developmental theory
▶ 7–11-years-old
▶ Rational and logical thought
▶ Concept of conservation (water in a tall cup has the same volume as in a bowl)
▶ Ability to understand someone else's point of view

Correlation between behavior and neurological maturation

▶ Basal ganglia and cortical motor circuits – maturation is in parallel with
  ▷ Social smiling (1–4 months)
▶ Limbic system – maturation of the major fiber tracts (6–12 months) is in parallel with
  ▷ Attachments (ages 6 weeks–3 years)
  ▷ Separation anxiety (9–18 months)
  ▷ Stranger anxiety (6–8 months)
▶ Thalamic projection to the auditory cortex – maturation is in parallel with
  ▷ Language (~2 years).
▶ Prenatal androgenization of the hypothalamus is correlated to
  ▷ Gender difference in physical aggressiveness starting in early childhood
▶ Hypothalamic-pituitary-gonadal axis – maturation is in parallel with
  ▷ Sexual desire and functioning in adolescence

Egocentrism

▶ From Jean Piaget's developmental theory
▶ Children see themselves as the center of the universe; they are unable to take the role of another person
▶ Characteristic for children in the preoperational stage

Erikson's social developmental model (Figure 4–1)

▶ Erikson focused on the boundary between the child and the environment and assumed psychological development and crisis occurring in sequential stages (epigenetic) expanding the entire life cycle
▶ Successful resolution of phasic crisis will result in a favorable outcome, called "virtues."
▶ There are eight stages, or phases in the entire life
  ▷ Basic trust vs. basic mistrust (birth–18 months); virtue – hope
  ▷ Autonomy vs. shame and doubt (18 months–3 years); virtue – will
  ▷ Initiative vs. guilt (3–5 years); virtue – purpose
  ▷ Industry vs. inferiority (5–13 years); virtue – competence
  ▷ Identity vs. role confusion (13–20 years); virtue – fidelity
  ▷ Intimacy vs. isolation (20–40 years); virtue – love
  ▷ Generativity vs. stagnation (40–60 years); virtue – care
  ▷ Ego integrity vs. despair (60 years and older); virtue – wisdom

Gender Identity

▶ Psychological and behavioral identity related to masculinity and femininity
▶ Starts to establish by 2–3 years of age
▶ Factors help shaping the gender identity
  ▷ Cues and experiences from people surrounding
  ▷ Physical characteristics
  ▷ Parental and cultural attitudes
▶ People usually develop a secure gender identification along with their biological sex; however, gender identity and sex are not always congruent to each other

Gender role

▶ Conscious behavior to disclose the person's gender identity
▶ Built up cumulatively through
  ▷ Casual learning
  ▷ Explicit instruction and inculcation
  ▷ Biological attributes – male hormones may have sensitized the nervous system to absorb lessons of masculine behavior more easily.

Good-enough mothering

Donald Winnicott (1896–1971) was a British psychoanalyst.

▶ From Donald Winnicott's object-relation theory
▶ Key ability of a good-enough mother
  ▷ Ability of conscious and unconscious adaption to the baby at different developmental stages
  ▷ Ability of mature object relations
  ▷ Ability of holding, handling, and object-presenting
▶ Transitional object is another important concept of Winnicott's

Imprinting

Konrad Lorenz (1903–1989) was an Austrian ethologist and zoologist.

▶ A form of phase-sensitive learning
▶ In certain developmental phase, organisms may learn certain behavior pattern rapidly and maintain the behavior for long time (imprinted)
▶ Popularized by Konrad Lorenz with his geese study
  ▷ During the critical period of the first 36 hours after hatching, geese may imprint on the first moving stimulus they saw
  ▷ Famously demonstrated by showing geese imprinted on Lorenz himself; they followed him around as if he was the mother goose
▶ The theory was applied by some to the influence of parental role model

Infantile amnesia

▶ Most people cannot recall events that happened before 5 years of age
▶ This phenomenon is probably caused by the lack of language-based retrieval of prelinguistic memory

Jean Piaget's developmental stages (Figure 4–1)

▶ Sensorimotor (0–2 years)
▶ Preoperational (2–7 years)
▶ Concrete operational (7–11 years)
▶ Formal operational (11 years onward)

Language milestones

▶ Before 8 months
  ▷ Vegetative sounds (0–2 months)

▷ Vowel sounds (2–6 months)
▷ Babbling (6–8 months)
▶ Around 1 year is the transition from listening to talking; word comprehension starts 8–10 months; word production starts 11–13 months
▶ Around 2 years is the transition from simple word production to word combinations (20–24 months) and grammar (2½ years)

Object constancy

▶ A concept from object relations theory
▶ The capacity to maintain a lasting relationship with a specific object, and rejecting any substitute for such an object
▶ Usually refers to children's inner memory of a secure relationship with mothers
▶ This is the stage when children can relate to another person in his or her own right
▶ Not to be confused with "object permanence"; the latter is a concept in Jean Piaget's cognitive development theory

Object permanence

▶ The awareness that objects continue to exist even when not visible
▶ Jean Piaget found infants achieve this awareness at the age of 8–9 months, during sensorimotor stage (0–2 years)

Object relations theory

Otto Kernberg (1928–) is an Austrian-born U.S. psychiatrist.
Melanie Klein (1882–1960) was an Austrian-born British psychologist.
Margaret Mahler (1897–1985) was a Hungarian-born U.S. psychiatrist. She is also known for her separation-individualization theory of child development.

▶ Derived from psychoanalytic theory; pioneers include
▷ Otto Kernberg
▷ Melanie Klein
▷ Margaret Mahler
▷ Donald Winnicott
▶ It emphasizes interpersonal relations, primarily in the family, especially between mother and child
▶ The idea is that the ego or self exists only in relation to objects
▶ "Object" refers to the person that is the target of feelings or intentions, usually a loved one
▶ Kernberg's triad – an object relation consists of three parts
▷ Self-representation
▷ Object-representation
▷ Affect linking the two
▶ During the growth of an infant, many units of such triads form, these being units of object relations. In time, the various object relations fuse to make an overall object-image and cohesive self-image

Phallic stage

▶ The third of Sigmund Freud's five psychodynamic developmental stages
▶ Age 3–5 years
▶ This stage has the most colorful psychodynamic description, including the famous Oedipus complex, castration anxiety, and penis envy

Preoperational stage

▶ A stage in Jean Piaget's cognitive development theory
▶ Characteristic features
  ▷ Symbolic functions
  ▷ Egocentric thinking
  ▷ Magical thinking
  ▷ Basic moral thought

Puberty development in boys

▶ Stage 1
  ▷ No pubic hair
  ▷ Testes, scrotum, and penis are same as of the childhood
▶ Stage 2
  ▷ Sparse growth of yellowish hair
  ▷ Scrotum and testes are slightly enlarged; scrotal skin is reddened
  ▷ No enlargement of penis
▶ Stage 3
  ▷ Pubic hair becomes darker, coarser, and more curled, but is still sparse
  ▷ Penis starts to grow in length
▶ Stage 4
  ▷ Adult-type pubic hair with smaller covering area
  ▷ Penis grows in breadth; development of glans
  ▷ Testes and scrotum are larger; scrotal skin is darker
▶ Stage 5
  ▷ Adult distribution of pubic hair
  ▷ Mature genitals

Puberty development in girls

▶ Stage 1
  ▷ No pubic hair
  ▷ Elevation of papillae
▶ Stage 2
  ▷ Sparse growth of yellowish hair
  ▷ Budding of breasts
▶ Stage 3
  ▷ Pubic hair becomes darker, coarser, and more curled, but is still sparse
  ▷ Breasts grow in size
▶ Stage 4
  ▷ Adult-type pubic hair with smaller covering area
  ▷ Breasts continue to grow

▶ Stage 5
  ▷ Adult distribution of pubic hair
  ▷ Mature breasts

Rapprochement

This French word means "reconciliation."

▶ The fifth developmental stage in Margaret Mahler's separation-individuation theory
▶ Children constantly are concerned about the actual physical location of their mothers, and have great need for maternal love
▶ Lack of maternal love or absence of the mother during the rapprochement stage may lead to
  ▷ The child's anger, temper tantrums, whining behavior, moodiness
  ▷ Possible linkage to the pathogenesis of borderline personality disorder

Sensorimotor stage

▶ The first of Jean Piaget's four stages for cognitive development
▶ Age 0–2 years
▶ Stereotyped reaction to stimuli
▶ Object permanency (8–9 months)

Separation-individuation

▶ Developmental theory by Margaret Mahler
▶ Theoretical stages for young children acquire a sense of identity apart from mothers
  ▷ Normal autism (birth to 2 months)
  ▷ Symbiosis (2–5 months)
  ▷ Differentiation (5–10 months)
  ▷ Practicing (10–18 months)
  ▷ Rapprochement (18–24 months)
  ▷ Object constancy (2–5 years)

Sigmund Freud's developmental stages (Figure 4–1)

▶ Oral stage (0–1 year)
  ▷ Focusing on feeding
▶ Anal stage (1–3 years)
  ▷ Focusing on bowel functioning
▶ Phallic stage (3–5 years)
  ▷ Focusing on the genitalia
  ▷ Oedipal complex
  ▷ Castration anxiety
  ▷ Penis envy
▶ Latency (6–11 years)
  ▷ Sexual development is stagnant
▶ Adolescence (12–18 years)
  ▷ Sexual development approaches mature stage

Stranger anxiety

▶ First noted at 6 months of age
▶ Fully developed at 8 months

Understanding of the permanency of death

▶ At the age of 7 years, children start to understand that death is permanent

Transitional object

▶ A "not-me" possession, e.g., a blanket or toy, usually soft, furry, and comfortable to hold
▶ The object may be reassuring to an infant and preserve the illusion of the mother even in her absence
▶ A concept in object relations psychotherapy, the term was originally used by Donald W. Winnicott

5 Psychosocial Theories

The understanding of human behavior by psychiatric professionals has benefited significantly from psychosocial theories, which cover a wide range of humane studies, including such fields as sociology, psychology, anthropology, ethology, and epidemiology. Sigmund Freud's and Ivan Pavlov's prudent contributions may arguably be the most fundamental. Important names to be remembered also include Gregory Bateson, Martin Seligman, Lawrence Kohlberg, Carol Gilligan, Heinz Kohut, among a list of others. It is certainly worth mentioning the two cardiologists, Meyer Friedman and Ray Rosenman, who developed a popular theory of personality traits. Selected theories clinically relevant and frequently tested are reviewed in this chapter. Ego defense mechanisms and other elements of Sigmund Freud's theory are given more detailed description, due mainly to the conventional interest in psychiatric practice.

Anal fixation

- ▶ A behavioral regression to anal stage characterized by obsession to details and orderliness often becomes annoyance to others
- ▶ The anal stage is the second stage of Sigmund Freud's psychosexual development, in which a child's pleasure and conflict centers are in the anal area, i.e., the pleasure in controlling his or her bowels
- ▶ Freud theorized that children who experience conflicts during this period of time (castration anxiety) may become victims of their harsh superego, and develop "anal" personality traits
  - ▷ Stubbornness
  - ▷ Compulsion for control
  - ▷ Emotional constriction
  - ▷ Intellectualization
  - ▷ Indecisiveness
  - ▷ Procrastination
- ▶ It is believed to be associated with obsessive-compulsive personality disorder

Abreaction

- ▶ A psychoanalytical term referring to the process of recovering repressed memory that usually associated with painful experience
- ▶ The process is accompanied with significant affective response
- ▶ Hypnosis and other psychological techniques may be used to assist abreaction
- ▶ The process may be therapeutic in posttraumatic stress disorder (PTSD); however, there were reports of psychologically harmful abreaction induced by psychotherapy, and had led to legal dispute

Attribution theory

▶ A theory concerns the cognitive perception to the causes of behavior
▶ Common trend in attribution
  ▷ My behavior is caused by external situation
  ▷ Others' behaviors are caused by their personality traits
▶ The attributed causes may influence the subsequent feelings and behavior

Bonding vs. attachment

▶ Bonding is loosely defined as any form of emotional connection
▶ Sometimes used synonymously to "attachment"
▶ While bond is not necessarily associated with resource and security, attachment is
▶ Attachment refers to the child's feeling toward the mother
▶ Bonding refers usually to the mother's feeling toward the child
▶ The term "attachment bond" is used as equivalence of attachment

Classical conditioning

Ivan Pavlov (1849–1936) was a Russian physiologist and psychologist, Nobel Prize laureate in Physiology or Medicine in 1904.

▶ A form of associative learning, first demonstrated by Ivan Pavlov
▶ A conditioned response (CR) can be established by the paired presentation of a neutral stimulus (conditioned stimulus [CS]) and a stimulus of significance (unconditioned stimulus, UCS)
▶ Example – an organism (e.g., a lab animal) usually salivates when served with food; after repeated exposure to bell sound paired with food, the organism may salivate upon bell sound alone without food
  ▷ UCS – food
  ▷ Unconditional response (UCR) – salivation
  ▷ CS – bell sound
  ▷ CR – salivation

Classical conditioning: discrimination

▶ The ability of an organism to discriminate between two different CS and respond differently
▶ Discrimination can be established through repeated training
  ▷ Two CSs are presented alternatively (e.g., two different bell sounds)
  ▷ Associate one of the two CSs with UCS consistently (e.g., bell sound A is associated with food, bell sound B is not)
▶ Reversal conditioning
  ▷ If the two CSs are switched after the establishment of discrimination, the organism may learn to suppress the CR

Classical conditioning: extinction

▶ An established CR may diminish when the CS is presented repeatedly in the absence of UCS
▶ To prevent extinction, the UCS should present periodically, in a variable-ratio schedule

Classical conditioning: generalization

▷ A CR may be induced by stimuli other than the CS
▷ Example – the sound of foot steps of the animal trainer may induce the same response as the bell sound

Cognitive dissonance

Leon Festinger (1919–1989) was a U.S. social psychologist.

▷ A theory proposed by Leon Festinger
▷ The holding of two conflicting thoughts at the same time, in other words, the perception of incompatibility between two cognitions
▷ Responses to contradicting cognitions
  ▷ Raising uncomfortable tension and anxiety
  ▷ Resisting information that is not already familiar and believed therefore to avoid the tension of cognitive dissonance
  ▷ Motivating the modification of the cognitions through learning, so as to reduce the amount of dissonance between cognitions

Countertransference

▷ Expectations and emotional responses that a doctor brings to the patient–doctor relationship
▷ The influence of countertransference to doctor–patient relationship
  ▷ Can be negative or disproportionately positive, idealizing, and eroticized
  ▷ Can be disruptive to the patient–doctor relationship
  ▷ If recognized and analyzed, may help the doctor better understand the patient who has stimulated the feelings

Defense mechanisms (Figure 5–1)

▷ Ego strategies to cope with anxiety and stress caused by conflict inside id, between id and superego, or from the environment

Defense mechanism: acting out

▷ Unconscious impulses are expressed through behavior to avoid emotional pain
▷ Often impulse with little or no superego intervenes

Defense mechanism: altruism

▷ Unconscious pain is translated into behavior to benefit others

Defense mechanism: blocking

▷ Refusing to allow unacceptable ideas or memories getting into conscious

Defense mechanism: controlling

▷ Unconscious manipulation of people or environment to reduce anxiety and pain

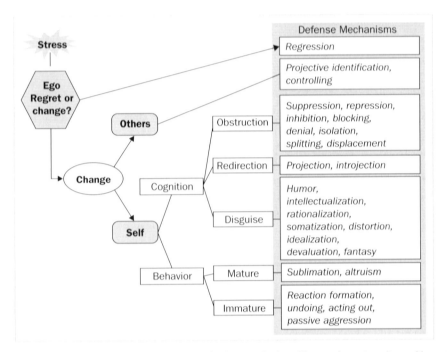

Figure 5-1 Suggested mnemonic categorization of defense mechanisms. When ego faces stress, it may either regress or adjust its cognition and behavior to manage the stress.

Defense mechanism: denial

▶ Refusal to accept the painful conflict by rejecting its existence

Defense mechanism: devaluation

▶ Rejecting unacceptable stressor by attributing exceeding negative qualities to the environment or other people

Defense mechanism: displacement

▶ Transferring feelings and emotions to another object, usually less threatening or more acceptable

Defense mechanism: introjection

▶ An immature defense mechanism
▶ To internalize the qualities of an object, the subject replicates behaviors, attributes or other fragments of the external world
▶ According to Freud, the ego and the superego are constructed by introjecting external behavior into the personality
▶ Introjection of a feared object serves to avoid anxiety when the aggressive characteristics of the object are internalized, thus placing the aggression under one's own control
▶ Identification is believed by some to be a presentation of introjection
▶ The most common defense mechanism in depression

Defense mechanism: isolation

▶ Isolate the feeling from the unacceptable ideas or conflict so to reduce anxiety

Defense mechanism: passive aggression

▶ Expressing hostile feeling in a nonconfrontational, yet often non-cooperative, manner

Defense mechanism: projection

▶ A narcissistic defense mechanism
▶ To attribute the undesirable impulses and feelings to another person, therefore the unacceptable inner impulses are perceived as though they were outside of the self
▶ Example – a cheating husband blames his wife of being unfaithful

Defense mechanism: projective identification

Melanie Klein (1882–1960) was an Austrian-born British psychologist.

▶ An unconscious interaction occurs between two persons; first introduced by Melanie Klein
▶ Person A projects undesirable impulses and feelings to person B
▶ Person B unconsciously alters the behavior in a way as if the projected idea was true
▶ Example – a customer unconsciously felt irritable; however, criticized a sales person for being unpleasant; the sales person was annoyed and started to act in a way as if the original criticism was true

Defense mechanism: rationalization

▶ Providing self-serving logic to explain unacceptable motivation

Defense mechanism: reaction formation

▶ Unacceptable wishes and motivations are transformed into the opposite direction

Defense mechanism: regression

▶ Returning to earlier, less mature developmental stage to deal with conflict

Defense mechanism: repression

▶ Both are defense mechanisms to held unwanted or unpleasant memory or thoughts out of conscious mind
▶ Repression is an unconscious act, while suppression is a conscious effort

Defense mechanism: somatization

▶ Psychological pain is translated into apparently more acceptable physical symptoms

Defense mechanism: splitting

▶ The world is divided into simply good and bad
▶ Rapid shifting from one extreme to another

Defense mechanism: sublimation

▶ It is believed to be the healthiest and mature one
▶ Refocusing of psychic energy away from negative outlets to healthy and creative behavior

Defense mechanism: suppression

▶ Consciously avoiding thinking about disturbing experience or wishes
▶ The only defense mechanism that occurs in conscious

Defense mechanism: undoing

▶ Behaving in the direction opposite to unconscious anticipation or impulse

Double bind

Gregory Bateson (1904–1980) was a British anthropologist and social scientist.

▶ A concept formulated by Gregory Bateson
▶ Contradictory parental messages that command children about their behavior
▶ Originally proposed as a cause of schizophrenia
  ▷ Children who found it impossible to satisfy both parent's demands may become withdrawn into a psychotic state to escape the confusion and tension
  ▷ The causal relationship has not been validated; the original family studies were found methodologically flawed
▶ Current consensus is that double binding is a communication pattern that is negative and harmful to growing up children.
▶ The concept is also applied to any other communication where contradictory message is presented; example
  ▷ Message – "You have to love me"
  ▷ Contradiction – if true love is genuine, then a demanded love must not be true

Downward drift hypothesis

▶ A hypothetic theory offered explanation for the finding that schizophrenic victims, differing from normal patterns, have a lower socioeconomic status than their parents
▶ It proposes that the functional impairment due to the illness leads to a downward drift in socioeconomic status

Dreams: psychoanalytic interpretation

▶ A foundational work for ego psychology originated by Sigmund Freud
▶ Basic concepts
  ▷ Dreams have meanings
  ▷ The meanings of dreams are often hidden or disguised

▷ The contents of dreams are often repressed unconscious memories, fantasies, and impulses

▷ Ego acts as a censor to disguise the unacceptable unconscious contents and to preserve sleep status while dreaming

▶ Two layers of dream content

▷ The manifest content can be recalled when awake

▷ The latent content are inappropriate or unsafe, and therefore not recalled when awake

Dreams: methods of disguise according to Freud's theory

▶ Using defense mechanisms

▷ Displacement

▷ Projection

▶ Condensation

▷ Several unconscious entities are combined into a single image

▶ Symbolic representation

▶ Secondary revision

▷ Ego works to reorganize the dreams and makes dreams more rational

▷ This process is also called secondary process

▶ Altered affect

▷ Affect in dreams may be changed from what would be in wakeful status, often milder in extent and even be opposite

Ego psychology

▶ Prominent features

▷ The tripartite structural model – Id, ego, and superego

▶ Id

▷ The collection of instinctual drives

▷ Dominated by primary process

▷ Unorganized, lacks the capacity to delay or modify the instinctual drives

▷ Largely unconscious

▶ Ego

▷ The executive organ of the psyche

▷ Dictates what is appropriate to do according to internalized values

▷ Delays and modulates instinctual drives

▷ Span over unconscious, preconscious, and conscious

▷ Abstract thinking and verbal expression are conscious or preconscious

▷ Defense mechanisms are unconscious

▶ Superego

▷ Superego dictates moral conscience and value

▷ Proscribes, i.e., dictates what should not do according to moral conscience

▷ Superego is the heir to the Oedipus complex; children internalize parental values and standards during the transition from phallic stage to latency (5–6 years)

▷ Functions largely unconsciously

Learned helplessness

Martin Seligman (1942–) is a U.S. psychologist, known for his classic work on learned helplessness, and more recently his leadership in positive psychology.

▶ An animal model of depression developed by Martin Seligman
▶ The experiment
  ▷ Dogs were exposed to inescapable electric shocks
  ▷ The dogs eventually gave up their attempt to escape
  ▷ The giving up behavior was generalized to other situations, and eventually the dogs became always apathetic
▶ Human application
  ▷ Biochemical change – research subjects under inescapable punishment were found to have release of endogenous opioids, impairment in immunology, and elevation of the tolerance to pain
  ▷ Behavior change – children who repeatedly failed in school may give up their efforts to improve

Learning in negative reinforcement

▶ Negative reinforcement is related to
  ▷ Escape learning
  ▷ Avoidance learning
▶ Escape learning
  ▷ The organism learns to escape geographically from the source of aversive stimuli (punishment)
▶ Avoidance learning
  ▷ A more advanced response than escape learning
  ▷ The organism learns to make anticipatory response to prevent the punishment
  ▷ The behavior terminates the punishment is learned and may be maintained

Moral development

Lawrence Kohlberg (1927–1987) was a U.S. psychologist at the University of Chicago. Carol Gilligan (1936–) is a contemporary U.S. psychologist at the New York University.

▶ Lawrence Kohlberg described three major levels of morality
  ▷ Preconventional – to avoid punishment
  ▷ Conventional – to gain approval from others
  ▷ Principle – to stand for ethical principles
▶ Carol Gilligan's critique
  ▷ Proposed that girls concern more on relationships, and rely more on intuitive sense in decision making, rather than rules and reasoning as in boys
  ▷ She criticized Kohlberg's research, which relied primarily on male participants, and found that the girls had lower level of moral development
  ▷ Kohlberg revised his scoring method, and found that boys and girls scored evenly

Oedipus complex

Oedipus was a Greek mythical king who unknowingly killed his father and married his mother.

Electra was a Greek mythical princess who, after finding her father's murder by her mother, wanted to avenge by killing her mother.

▶ A psychoanalytic concept refers to the children's feeling of tension in competing with father for the exclusive love of their mother
▶ Appears in phallic phase (3–5 years)
▶ Castration anxiety refers to the boys' fear of being castrated by father, the more powerful opponent; it was also assumed that the boys' believe females were from castrated boys
▶ Penis envy refers to the girls' feeling toward males
▶ Jung endorsed the term of Electra complex, the female version of Oedipus complex, refers to the girls' anxiety in competing for the fathers' love
▶ Freud rejected the term of Electra complex, and preferred the term feminine Oedipus complex

Operant conditioning

▶ Also known as "instrumental conditioning"
▶ The form of behavior or the frequency of the behavior can be altered through positive or negative consequences
▶ Distinguished from Pavlovian conditioning in that
  ▷ Pavlovian conditioning seeks the same behavior to occur under new antecedent
  ▷ Operant conditioning modifies the behavior through consequence

Personality development in self-psychology

Heinz Kohut (1913–1981) was an Austrian psychiatrist.

▶ Self-psychology is a school of psychoanalysis, created by Heinz Kohut
▶ Self-object function – individuals (selves) need empathic interaction with their mother and other family members (objects)
▶ Failure of self-object function may lead to developmental arrest and personality disorders

Pleasure and reality principles

▶ Pleasure principle
  ▷ An inborn tendency of the organism to avoid pain and to seek pleasure
  ▷ Dominates id functioning
  ▷ Joins reality principle as two basic tenets of ego functioning
  ▷ Guides the primary process
▶ The reality principle
  ▷ Assesses the reality and modifies the pleasure principle
  ▷ Postpones the immediate gratification
  ▷ A learned function associated with the maturation of ego
  ▷ Guides the primary process

Premack's principle

David Premack is a contemporary U.S. psychologist.

▶ A high frequency behavior (i.e., more desirable) can be used to reinforce a low-frequency behavior (i.e., less desirable)
▶ Also known as "Grandma's rule" – you have to finish the food in dish (low-frequency or less-desirable behavior) before you can eat desert (high frequency or more desirable)
▶ A concept developed by David Premack
▶ This principle may be used in controllable settings for behavior modification

Primary process vs. secondary process

▶ Concepts of psychoanalysis
▶ Primary process is the primitive form of thought that is
  ▷ Associated with id
  ▷ Motivated by the principle of pleasure
▶ Secondary process a mature form of thought guided that is
  ▷ Associated with ego
  ▷ Guided by the principle of reality
  ▷ This process often works to revise dream contents, and termed secondary revision

Priming

▶ A manifestation of implicit memory (nondeclarative memory)
▶ Priming refers to the facilitation of identifying stimuli on the basis of recent experience with the same stimuli
▶ Remembered item is remembered best in the form in which it was originally encountered

Psychic determinism

▶ A concept of psychoanalysis
▶ Adult behavior has its underlined meaning, which is unconscious, and often associated with childhood experience

Sensory deprivation

Donald Hebb (1904–1985) was a Canadian psychologist, arguably the father of neuropsychology.

▶ Prolonged (7 days in Donald Hebb's study) isolation from visual, auditory, and tactile stimulations
▶ Reactions
  ▷ Emotional distress
  ▷ Inability to concentrate or organize thoughts
  ▷ Increased suggestibility
  ▷ Somatic illusions
  ▷ Vivid hallucinations with delusional quality

Strange situation

Mary Ainsworth (1913–1999) was a U.S. psychologist.

▶ Developed by Mary Ainsworth and coauthors
▶ A laboratory procedure designed to assess infant attachment style
   ▷ Parent and infant are alone in the lab when stranger enters and approaches infant
   ▷ First separation episode – parent leaves
   ▷ First reunion episode – parent greets and comforts infant, then leaves again
   ▷ Second separation episode – stranger leaves and infant is alone
   ▷ Continuation of second separation episode – stranger enters and approaches infant
   ▷ Second reunion episode – parent enters stranger leaves

Therapist monkey

Stephen Suomi is a contemporary U.S. psychologist at the National Institute of Health (NIH) in Bethesda, Maryland.

▶ A behavior phenomenon demonstrated in Stephen Suomi's experiment with monkeys
▶ Isolated monkey
   ▷ Monkeys isolated for long may develop depressive symptoms and difficulty in socialization
▶ Therapist monkey
   ▷ Monkeys capable of physical contact without threatening behavior were chosen to be companion to isolated monkeys
   ▷ In 2 weeks the isolates started behavior change toward rehabilitation
▶ The studies served as a model for developing therapeutic treatments for socially retarded and withdrawn children

Transference

▶ Expectations and emotional responses that a patient brings to the patient–doctor relationship
▶ Based on
   ▷ Past experiences with other important authority figures
   ▷ To a lesser degree, how the doctor behaves

Type A and type B personalities

Meyer Friedman (1910–2001) was a U.S. cardiologist.
Ray Rosenman is a U.S. cardiologist and a colleague of Meyer Friedman.

▶ Behavior patterns proposed by Meyer Friedman and Ray Rosenman on the basis of their observation of cardiac patients
▶ Type A personality is
   ▷ Competitive, hard-driving
   ▷ Easily aroused, aggressive, hostile
   ▷ Impatient, with constant feeling of time urgency
▶ Type B is the opposite of type A – calm, relaxed, and easy-going
▶ Type A personality is predisposed to coronary artery disease, and is sometimes called coronary personality
▶ Type B is not susceptible to coronary disease

6 Evaluation of Signs and Symptoms

The language of psychiatry has evolved through the past century into a more precise and intuitive professional lexicon. The ability to precisely describe mental phenomena is a vital skill in clinical practice. Some of the terms may still carry the scent of old time when little scientific evidence was available; however, maintain in active use in accordance with the traditional communication in the profession.

Abulia

▶ Lack of impulse and motivation to act or think spontaneously
▶ Lack of ability to make decisions
▶ Indifference

Acrophobia

▶ Dread of high places
▶ Also known as "high anxiety"

Affect vs. mood

▶ Both are descriptions of emotional status
▶ Affect is the observed outward manifestation
▶ Mood is the subjective inward feeling

Agnosia

▶ Loss of ability to recognize or interpret the significance of sensory stimuli

Agraphia

▶ Loss of ability to write

Akathisia

▶ Subjective feeling of motor restlessness
▶ Feeling the constant need of frequently moving or changing position

Akinesia

▶ Significant decrease or lack of physical movement

Alexithymia

▶ Inability to be aware of or to express one's own mood and feeling

Amaurosis fugax

▶ Transient monocular visual loss
▶ Causes
  ▷ Compromised internal carotid or ophthalmic artery (most common)
  ▷ Optic neuropathies
  ▷ Giant cell arteritis
  ▷ Angle-closure glaucoma
  ▷ Migraine
  ▷ Psychogenic – conversion

Anhedonia

▶ Loss of interest in almost any activity; often seen in depression

Anomia

▶ Loss of ability to tell names of objects

Anosognosia

▶ Loss of ability to recognize physical deficits

Anton's syndrome

▶ Cortically blind patient insists still able to see
▶ Seen in occipital impairment
▶ Often has symptoms of confabulation

Apraxia

▶ Loss of ability to perform purposeful motor activity, such as opening a bottle

Capgras syndrome

Joseph Capgras (1873–1950) was a French psychiatrist.

▶ Delusion of believing someone, usually a close relative or family member, has been replaced by an impostor

Catalepsy

▶ Maintaining the body position as been placed into
▶ Also known as waxy flexibility
▶ Seen in catatonia

Cataplexy

▶ Sudden loss of muscle tone
▶ Seen in narcolepsy

Cathexis and acathexis

▶ Cathexis – paying close attention; investing psychic energy into objects or idea
▶ Acathexis – lack of expected emotional response when facing significant situation or memory

Chorea

▶ Random and involuntary quick, dance-like, purposeless movements

Circumstantiality and tangentiality

▶ Both are thought process disorders
▶ Both present with relatively sequential speech, but cannot direct the conversation toward the goal of discussion
▶ With circumstantiality, the patient eventually gets to the point; circumstantial speech is often overly inclusive in remotely relevant details
▶ With tangentiality, the patient can never get to the point; tangentiality is often seen in demented patients

Confabulation

▶ Creating stories to fill gaps in memory
▶ An unconscious behavior seen in patients with memory impairment
▶ Not intentional lying

Coprolalia

▶ Uncontrollable recurrent use of vulgar or obscene language

Cotard's syndrome

▶ A form of nihilistic delusion

Déjà pense

▶ A completely new thought that sounds familiar to the subject as if he/she had the same thought before

Déjà vu

▶ An illusion in which a new situation is regarded as a previously experienced situation
▶ No pathognomic meaning
▶ May appear in seizure disorders, dissociative disorders, or people with no mental disorders

Dysprosody

▶ Loss of emotionally expressive component of speech, such as normal speech melody, emphasis, and gesture

Eidetic images

▶ Vivid visual memories
▶ Eidetic memory is an unverified human talent that is believed to be possessed by some with extreme ability of memory; the absolute existence of such talent is controversial

Erotomania

Gaëtan de Clérambault (1872–1934) was a French psychiatrist.

▶ A type of delusion where the individual falsely but firmly believed being deeply loved by another person
▶ Also known as Clérambault syndrome

Executive function

▶ Exact elements are not well defined; the generally accepted descriptions are
  ▷ The capacity of purposefully applying one's mental skills
▶ Most mentioned specific executive functions include
  ▷ Working memory
  ▷ Attention
  ▷ Control of emotion and impulse
  ▷ Planning
  ▷ Analysis and problem solving

Folie à deux

▶ From French words meaning "madness shared by two"
▶ The individual develops a delusion similar to another individual who already established a delusion; usually the two individual have a close relationship and a strong connection
▶ In DSM-IV-TR, it is termed as Shared Psychotic Disorder
▶ The same condition may involve more than two persons, hence the alternative terms
  ▷ Folie à trios – madness shared by three
  ▷ Folie à quatre – madness shared by four
  ▷ Folie à famille – madness shared by the family
  ▷ Folie à plusieurs – madness shared by many

Formication

▶ Feeling of insects crawling on the skin

Hyperacusis

▶ Increased sensitivity to sound

Hypnagogic and hypnopompic hallucinations

Mnemonic: hypnagogic contains "ago"–before the sleep

▶ Hallucinations occurring while falling asleep (hypnagogic) and awakening from sleep (hypnopompic)
▶ The hallucinations are associated with a cloudy conscious status, therefore not usually considered pathological

Infantile amnesia

▶ Events happened before the age of 5 years are mostly not remembered
▶ This phenomenon is probably caused by the lack of language-based retrieval of prelinguistic memory

Jamais vu

▶ A familiar situation is not recognized by the person as if he/she sees the situation the first time
▶ May appear in amnesia, epilepsy, and migraine aura

La belle indifference

▶ Inappropriately lack of concern about the deficit or disability
▶ Typically appears in conversion disorders

Lethologica

Carl Jung (1875–1961) was a Swiss psychiatrist, and the founder of Analytical Psychology.

▶ Inability to articulate the individual's thoughts by forgetting key words, phrases, or names in conversation
▶ According to Carl Jung, it is a temporary condition, in contrast to permanent memory condition such as dementia

Neologism

▶ Creation and use of new word or phrase in a bizarre way, which could not be understood given the situation and cultural background
▶ Usually a psychotic symptom

Neurosis

William Cullen (1710–1790) was a Scottish physician and chemist.

▶ Historically refers to disorders affecting the nervous system; originally coined by William Cullen
▶ According to psychoanalytic theory, the etiology of neurotic symptom is associated with impaired ego function, and failure of repression
▶ DSM-III redefined it as symptoms that are ego-dystonic and with intact reality testing
▶ Not used in DSM-IV and DSM-IV-TR, due mainly to its impreciseness in describing clinical entities
▶ Still used in ICD-10, where it refers mainly to anxiety disorders

Nihilism

▶ Firm belief of the nonexistence of the self
▶ A form of delusion

Nymphomania

▶ Pathologically increased sexual desire in a woman

Paramnesia

▶ False memory usually because of the distortion of recall; commonly mentioned ones are
  ▷ Jamais vu – unfamiliarity with a situation that the person has experienced
  ▷ Déjà vu – familiarity with a situation that the person has NOT experienced

Passive aggression

▶ Anger and aggression are expressed through passive behavior
▶ Example
  ▷ Upon demand of doing something, the subject does not do anything that is opposite to the demand, but instead does the job extremely slowly, or overdoes what is appropriate to do

Peduncular hallucinosis

▶ Visual hallucination associated with damage at midbrain or pons

Perseveration

▶ A formal thought disorder
▶ Often associated with cognitive disorders
▶ The patient exhibits a persisting response to a previous stimulus after a new stimulus has been presented
▶ Example – the patient may draw a square when asked to do so, but continues to draw squares even when asked to draw circles

Precox feeling

▶ The ability of quickly sensing the mental pathology without in-depth evaluation
▶ Presumably developed from extensive clinical experience
▶ Usually refers to the difficulty of emotional rapport in schizophrenic patients
▶ The reliability of precox feeling has not been validated by any data

Synesthesia

▶ Stimulation of one sensory pathway leads to the experience of another sensory pathway; such as to hear a picture, or see a sound
▶ Hallucinogen induced synesthesia is particularly mentioned in DSM-IV-TR
▶ Synesthesia may also appear after stroke
▶ Nonpathological synesthesia is seen as a talent among some people

Thought blocking

▶ Also known as thought deprivation
▶ Abrupt interruption in the train of thought; the individual is not able to recall what was being said

Trismus

▶ Tonic contraction of the muscles of mastication
▶ The term is also used to describe any restriction to mouth opening
▶ It is observed as a form of extrapyramidal side effects

Verbigeration

▶ Also known as cataphasia
▶ Meaningless repetition of words or phrases
▶ Usually seen in schizophrenia

7 Classification and Diagnosis

The idea of how to formulate a working definition for mental illness has evolved since the asylum era. The goal of establishing diagnostic criteria is not to provide final words in illness and healing, but to distinguish clinical conditions with the available information and knowledge, to facilitate treatment and communication among health-care professionals. In the early stage of developing a system of diagnostic criteria, there were polarized debates concerning the rational concepts of psychiatric illness. Psychoanalysts, along with members of other psychological schools, challenged the biomedical model in that the latter's reductionistic approach omitted the humane nature of mental disorders. However, the lack of testable evidence to support the asserted etiology also made psychoanalytical claims dubious. In 1977, George L. Engel (1913–1999), a New York psychiatrist, proposed biopsychosocial model. This holistic, tri-dimensional model set the foundation of psychiatric work in the late part of the twenty-first century, and is still widely applied in fields within and beyond psychiatry. At the same time, scientific research started to put all the theoretical models, including psychoanalytic ones, under the test of evidence. In the past decade, evidence-based medicine met with plaudits from the professional circle and general public. It is now clear that evidence-based medicine will set the precept for future versions of diagnostic system in psychiatry and the rest of the medical world.

The two most important psychiatric classifications are Diagnostic and Statistical Manual of Mental Disorders (DSM) developed by the American Psychiatric Association (APA), and International Classification of Diseases (ICD), developed by the World Health Organization (WHO).

DSM: the original version

▶ *Diagnostic and Statistical Manual of Mental Disorders* published in 1952
▶ Adopted from earlier classification system used by the military
▶ Confirmed in a survey of the views of 10% of APA members

DSM-II

▶ Published in 1968
▶ Reflected the then dominating psychodynamic theories
▶ It was criticized for claiming assumed etiology with no evidence

DSM-III and DSM-III-R

▶ DSM-III was published in 1980
▶ A historical major revision known as "neo-Kraepelinian," focused on improving the scientific reliability of psychiatric diagnosis

▶ Psychodynamic view was marginalized in favor of a biomedical model
▶ Categorization was based on description rather than assumptions of etiology
▶ Field trials supported by National Institute of Mental Health (NIMH) were conducted to test the reliability of the new diagnoses
▶ Nomenclature was made consistent with ICD
▶ Started to use the multiaxial system
▶ DSM-III-R was published in 1987
  ▷ Significant changes in criteria were made on the basis of new research data

DSM-IV

▶ Published in 1994
▶ Work model
  ▷ Designated work groups on each category to conduct extensive review of published literature
  ▷ Reanalysis of the research data
  ▷ Issue-focused field trials
▶ New criterion on clinical significance
  ▷ A major improvement in DSM-IV was the inclusion of a clinical significance criterion
  ▷ Requires significant distress or functioning impairment for the majority of diagnoses

DSM-IV-TR

▶ Published in 2000
▶ The current version of official U.S. psychiatric nomenclature and coding system
▶ No significant change in categories and diagnostic criteria from DSM-IV
▶ Text revision provided updated information
▶ Designed to correspond to ICD-10, to
  ▷ Ensure uniform reporting of health statistics
  ▷ Satisfy Medicare's requirement in billing codes
▶ All categories used in DSM-IV-TR are found in ICD-10, but not all ICD-10 categories are in DSM-IV-TR

ICD

Jacques Bertillon (1851–1922) was a French physician and statistician.

▶ Abbreviation for International Statistical Classification of Diseases and Related Health Problems
▶ A classification and coding system widely adopted worldwide as a standard tool in medical statistics and record keeping. Some countries have their own modified version (extensions) of ICD
▶ ICD-1 was evolved from Bertillon Classification of Causes of Death, introduced by Jacques Bertillon in 1893
▶ The responsibility of revision and publication was assumed by the WHO in 1948. WHO published its first ICD, ICD-7, in 1949
▶ The current version is ICD-10, published in 1992
▶ Clinical modifications (CM) were published since ICD-9, which provide clinical pictures and diagnostic procedures for coded conditions
▶ Since 1990s, APA and WHO have been working on bringing the mental disorder section of ICD and DSM into concordance

Multiaxial system

▶ Axis I – mental disorders and other conditions that may be a focus of clinical attention
▶ Axis II – personality disorders and mental retardation
▶ Axis III – physical conditions
▶ Axis IV – psychosocial problems
▶ Axis V – GAF (1–100)
▶ Note – DSM allows clinicians to record diagnoses in nonaxial manner

Specifiers in DSM diagnosis

▶ Provisional diagnosis
  ▷ Strong presumption on a diagnosis but clinical information is not sufficient to meet full criteria of the diagnosis
▶ Severity
  ▷ Mild – minimal symptoms in excess of diagnostic criteria and minor functioning impairment
  ▷ Moderate – between mild and severe
  ▷ Severe – many symptoms in excess of diagnostic criteria and marked dysfunctioning
▶ Course specifiers
  ▷ Partial remission
  ▷ Full remission
  ▷ Prior history – no active symptoms for the diagnosis

Validity of psychiatric diagnosis

Eli Robins (1921–1995) and Samuel Guze (1923–2000) were U.S. psychiatrists at Washington University in St. Louis.

▶ Essential criteria to validate a psychiatric diagnosis
▶ Proposed by Eli Robins and Samuel Guze, known for their advocacy for scientific research and evidence-based approach on mental illness
▶ Adapted in the process of formulating DSM system since DSM-III; however, not all DSM diagnoses are validated
▶ A psychiatric diagnosis is considered valid if it satisfied the following requirements:
  ▷ Content validity – a diagnosis should have replicable clinical description
  ▷ Criterion-related validity – a diagnosis should be supported by reliable clinical tests, i.e., laboratory or psychometric tests
  ▷ Construct validity – a diagnosis should be differentiable from other disorders

8 Psychometrics

Mental faculties were once seemed not measurable in the era of classic physics. However, around the transition of the nineteenth and twentieth centuries, when Charles Darwin's theory of natural selection became popularized, there was a growing desire for an objective tool to measure the ability of species and individuals. It was Francis Galton (1822–1911), Darwin's cousin, an English scholar with encyclopedic knowledge in many fields, who started his effort in measuring intelligence. Galton was often referred to as the father of the science of psychometrics. Another discipline of psychology, psychophysics, born around the same time, also contributed to the study of psychometrics. Psychophysics studies the correlation between physical stimuli and biological responses. Some psychophysical studies described in this book are the changes of evoked potentials in patients with schizophrenia and other mental disorders.

In the past century, a vast number of psychometric tests were invented, and a portion of it remains in active use. With the assistance of biostatistics and information technology, many psychometric instruments have been tested for validity and reliability, and standardized against normal population. The available psychometric instruments can measure a wide range of neurological, mental, and behavioral symptoms and functions including general intelligence, specific abilities, attitudes, academic potentials, personality traits, developmental delays, coping and adaptive skills, social functioning, severity and change of symptoms, and adverse effects of treatments.

The following is a list of selected psychometric tools frequently mentioned and used in clinical settings

- ▶ Projective test
  - ▷ Draw-a-Person Test
  - ▷ Rorschach Test
  - ▷ Thematic apperception test (TAT)
  - ▷ Wisconsin Card Sorting Test
  - ▷ Word-association
- ▶ Neuropsychological functioning tests
  - ▷ Bender Gestalt Test
  - ▷ Halstead-Reitan Neuropsychological Battery
  - ▷ Wada test
  - ▷ Wechsler Intelligence Scales
- ▶ Rating scale for symptom severity and change – clinician-administered
  - ▷ Brief psychotic rating scale (BPRS)
  - ▷ Clinical global improvement scale (CGI)
  - ▷ Hamilton Rating Scale for Depression (HAM-D)
  - ▷ Positive and Negative Syndrome Scale (PANSS)
  - ▷ Yale-Brown Obsessive-Compulsive Scale (Y-BOCS)

▶ Rating scale for symptom severity and change – self-administered
  ▷ Beck Depression Inventory (BDI)
  ▷ Zung Self-Rating Depression Scale
▶ Diagnostic test
  ▷ Structured Clinical Interview for the DSM-IV (SCID)
▶ Personality assessment
  ▷ Defensive Functioning Scale (DFS)
  ▷ Minnesota Multiphasic Personality Inventory (MMPI)
  ▷ Millon Clinical Multiaxial Inventory
▶ Side-effect assessment
  ▷ Abnormal Involuntary Movement Scale (AIMS)
▶ Functional assessment
  ▷ Global Assessment of Functioning (GAF)
  ▷ Global Assessment of Relational Functioning (GARF)
  ▷ Social and Occupational Functioning Assessment Scale (SOFAS)

Psychometrics provided powerful tools in clinical practice and in research. It standardizes the information across time and observers, establishes a baseline for individual follow-up of the progress of illness, and establishes a normative database for the population. However, the quality of the instruments, the training required to administer the tests, and the testee's cooperativeness may cause difficulties and limitations in the interpretation of the results. The decision of using formal assessment tool in clinical practice should rely on the clinical setting and goal, and the potential contribution of the instrument to the diagnosis and treatment.

Abnormal involuntary movement scale

▶ Measures late onset movement disorders, such as tardive dyskinesia
▶ Observes movements of the head, trunk, and extremities
▶ Rates each item on a scale of 1–5

Beck depression inventory

Aaron Beck (1921–) is a U.S. psychiatrist, founder of cognitive therapy.

▶ Measures severity of depression
▶ Contains 21 questions
▶ Can be graded in two subscales
  ▷ Cognitive (psychological)
  ▷ Somatic
▶ Self-rating by patients
▶ Correlates well with HAM-D score
▶ The most recent version is BDI-II, published in 1996

Bender Gestalt test

Lauretta Bender (1897–1987) was a U.S. child neuropsychologist. Gestalt psychology is a German school of psychology and psychotherapy, which proposed that the configuration of brain is organized by its physical and psychological elements, and that the whole is greater than the sum of its elements.

▶ Also known as Bender Visual Motor Gestalt test
▶ Designed for children aged 3 and older, and adults

▶ Evaluate
  ▷ Visual-motor functioning and maturity
  ▷ Visual-perceptual skills
  ▷ Developmental delays
  ▷ Emotional disturbances
  ▷ Neurological impairment
▶ May be used to assess the extent of damage after a traumatic brain injury; common signs of brain damage include
  ▷ Visual neglect
  ▷ Perseveration
  ▷ Rotated or distorted designs

Brief psychotic rating scale

▶ A scale designed as an outcome measure in treatment studies of schizophrenia
▶ Provides quantitative severity of psychotic symptoms
▶ Best used for patients with significant impairment

Clinical global improvement scale

▶ A two-item instrument
  ▷ CGI-S (severity) – the current condition on a scale of 1–7
  ▷ CGI-I (improvement) – the extent of improvement since the start of treatment on a scale of 1–7
▶ Used as an assessment in the treatment of psychiatric disorders

Defensive functioning scale

▶ A rating scale designed to evaluate the patient's coping strategies
▶ A list of defense mechanisms categorized into seven levels
  ▷ High adaptive level
  ▷ Mental inhibitions level
  ▷ Minor image-distorting level
  ▷ Disavowal level
  ▷ Major image-distorting level
  ▷ Action level
  ▷ Defense dysregulation level

Draw-a-person test

▶ A projective test
▶ Techniques
  ▷ The testee is requested to draw a person at his/her best ability
  ▷ Then to draw a person of the opposite sex to the initial draw
  ▷ The testee is questioned about the meaning and assumed behavior of the drawn persons
▶ Modifications
  ▷ Adding a house, tree, animal, and family members to the initial drawing
▶ Assumption and interpretation
  ▷ The drawing of a person represents the expression of the self in the environment

   ▷ Interpretation relies mainly on the functional significance of each body part
   ▷ Detail is correlated with intelligence and developmental level
▶ Application
   ▷ Screening for brain damage
   ▷ Intelligence in children and adults

Construct validity

▶ Refers to whether a test measures the unobservable that it purports to measure
▶ The evaluation of construct validity is based on the following facts
   ▷ Theoretical grounds
   ▷ Correlations from numerous studies using the test
   ▷ Correlations that fit the expected pattern contribute
   ▷ Correlation of the measure with variables that are known to be related to the construct purpose

Global assessment of functioning

▶ A rating scale used in axis V of the multiaxial diagnostic system in DSM-IV-TR
▶ Combination of symptomatic severity and function impairment
▶ Based on the clinician's judgment

Global assessment of relational functioning

▶ A rating scale designed to evaluate the family environment and other relationships
▶ Provides a score in a continuum ranging from 100 to 1
▶ Analogous to Axis V (GAF scale) in DSM-IV-TR
▶ Assessment in the following areas
   ▷ Problem solving
   ▷ Organization
   ▷ Emotional climate

Halstead-Reitan neuropsychological battery

Ward Halstead (1908–1968) was a U.S. psychologist.
Ralph M. Reitan is a contemporary U.S. psychologist.

▶ Assess the location and effects of specific brain lesions
▶ Ten tests to measure
   ▷ Tactile performance
   ▷ Perception of rhythm
   ▷ Finger oscillation
   ▷ Perception of speech-sounds
   ▷ Trail-making
   ▷ Perception of critical flicker frequency
   ▷ Time sense
   ▷ Aphasia screening
   ▷ Sensory perceptual function
▶ May differentiate among early dementia, mild delirium, and depression

Hamilton rating scale for depression

Max Hamilton (1912–1988) was a German-born English psychiatrist.

▶ One of the most commonly used scales for measuring depressive symptoms
▶ The original 17-item scale rates severity of low mood, insomnia, agitation, anxiety, weight loss, and other depressive symptoms
▶ Several modified versions added questions on diurnal variation, paranoia, and other symptoms

Millon clinical multiaxial inventory

Theodore Millon is a contemporary U.S. psychologist.

▶ A psychological test invented by Theodore Millon, intended to provide information on adult psychopathology
▶ 175 true/false questions
▶ Has personality scales, clinical syndrome scales, correction scales, and Grossman personality facet scales
▶ Normed on large samples
▶ The most recent published version is MCMI-III

Mini-international neuropsychiatric interview (MINI)

▶ A semistructured interview for the diagnoses of DSM-IV
▶ Similar to SCID, however, is less comprehensive and requires only qualitative answers (yes or no); some considered MINI a compact version of SCID

Minnesota multiphasic personality inventory

▶ Developed and copyrighted by the University of Minnesota
▶ Designed to help identify personal, social, and behavioral problems in psychiatric patients
▶ A self-report test with more than 500 statements requiring true or false answers. The most recent version, MMPI-2, includes 10 clinical scales and 4 validity scales
▶ Clinical scales
  ▷ Hypochondriasis
  ▷ Depression
  ▷ Hysteria
  ▷ Psychopathic deviation
  ▷ Masculinity–femininity
  ▷ Paranoia
  ▷ Schizophrenia
  ▷ Hypomania
  ▷ Social introversion
▶ Validity scales
  ▷ Cannot say – frequency of the omitted items
  ▷ L – lie assessment
  ▷ F – infrequency scale, to assess the frequency of items rarely endorsed by normal people
  ▷ K – distortion of response, to assess particularly defensive response
▶ It was used by companies to assess employees' potential of performance; this has subjected to criticism the ethics and validity of such use

Positive and negative syndrome scale

▶ A rating instrument designed for the assessment of schizophrenia
▶ Contains 30 items with 7 severity grades for each item
▶ Assess symptoms in the past 1 week
▶ It usually takes 30 minutes to complete the interview
▶ It is applied mostly in research setting

Reliability vs. validity

▶ Reliability
  ▷ Whether the test gives consistent result when used at different time and by different raters; reproducibility
▶ Validity
  ▷ Whether the test measures what it purports to measure

Rorschach test

Hermann Rorschach (1884–1922) was a Swiss psychiatrist and psychoanalyst.

▶ A projective test commonly used to examine the personality characteristics and emotional functioning
▶ It is believed useful in diagnosing underlying subtle thought processes, bizarre ideation, particularly psychotic thought disorders
▶ It comprises a standard card set of 10 inkblots that serve as stimuli for thought associations; five cards are black and white, five are colored
▶ The interpretation of the test is based on detailed records of the patient's verbatim responses, the initial reaction times, the total time spent on each card, etc.
▶ The value of the test is controversial

Social and occupational functioning assessment scale

▶ A rating scale independent of the psychological symptoms
▶ Recommended by DSM-IV-TR
▶ Used to track the patient's progress in social and occupational functioning

Structured clinical interview for the DSM-IV

▶ SCID-I – for Axis I diagnoses, takes 1–2 hours
▶ SCID-II – for Axis II diagnoses, takes 0.5 to 1 hour
▶ A semistructured interview that should be administered by trained clinicians who should also be experienced in nonstructured interview
▶ Answers are recorded on a numerical scale
▶ Is considered time-consuming, and usually used only in research; however, some argued that this might be the most reliable instrument for psychiatric diagnoses

Thematic apperception test

▶ The testee is to tell a story after viewing each of a series of ambiguous pictures showing one or more people in various settings
▶ The tester is to analyze the answer and to reveal the trait of personality
▶ Designed by Murray and Morgan to test normal personality

Wada test

Juhn Wada (1924–) is a Japanese-Canadian neurosurgeon. He invented Wada test when he was a resident in Japan.

▶ Designed to confirm cerebral dominance to help decision on destructive brain surgery
▶ Infusion of a barbiturate (usually amobarbital) into the carotid artery of the dominant side
▶ As the barbiturate infuse across the hemispheres, the step-wise transient aphasia can be observed in seconds to minutes

Wechsler intelligence scales

▶ A global test of intelligence contains seven verbal subtests and seven performance subtests
▶ Verbal subtests
  ▷ Information
  ▷ Comprehension
▶ Provides three scores
  ▷ Verbal intelligence quotient (VIQ)
  ▷ Performance intelligence quotient (PIQ)
  ▷ Full-scale intelligence quotient (FIQ)
▶ The median full-scale intelligence quotient (IQ) score is 100, with a standard deviation of 15
▶ Current version is WAIS-III, while WAIS-IV is undergoing national standardization

Wisconsin card sorting test

▶ It tests the ability to display flexibility in the face of changing schedules of reinforcement; it is used to evaluate mainly the frontal lobe function or executive function
▶ Original version used paper cards; currently a computerized version is available
▶ The following results are analyzed
  ▷ Number of categories achieved
  ▷ Number of trials
  ▷ Number of errors
  ▷ Number and percentage of perseverative errors

Word-association

▶ Developed by Carl Jung
▶ Techniques
  ▷ Initial administration – present a list of stimulus words to the testee, then the testee is requested to respond with the first word that came to mind
  ▷ Modification – repeat the list and request the testee to respond with the same words that he or she used previously
▶ Facts to be considered in interpretation
  ▷ Discrepancies between the two administrations
  ▷ Reaction times
  ▷ Unusual responses
  ▷ Misunderstanding of the word
  ▷ Thought process – blocking, perseveration, clang associations
  ▷ Mannerisms or movements accompanying a response

Yale-brown obsessive-compulsive scale

▶ Extensively used in clinical settings
▶ Measures the severity of obsessive-compulsive symptoms
▶ Monitors the response to treatment

Zung self-rating depression scale

William Zung is a contemporary U.S. psychologist.

▶ A 20-item self-report scale
▶ The score ranges from 25 to 100; each question is scored on a scale of 1–4
▶ The scale provides a global index of the intensity of depression

9 Biostatistics

Biostatics is the application of statistics to biological fields. Using mathematical science to analyze and reason biological phenomena was a critical advance in early twentieth century. Biostatistics since then has become a fundamental instrument in understanding changes and trends that were not qualitatively apparent. Commonly used biostatistic methods are reviewed in this chapter.

Analysis of variance (ANOVA)

▶ A statistical method to compare two or more groups
▶ Designed to determine whether the differences observed are due to chance alone

Case-controlled study

▶ Identify factors that may contribute to a medical condition by comparing subjects who have that condition with subjects that do not
▶ Cost and time effective

Chi-square (χ^2)

▶ Chi-square distribution
  ▷ One of the theoretical probability distribution
▶ Chi-square test
  ▷ To test data against the theoretical chi-square distribution
▶ Assumption – data approximates the chi-square distribution when
  ▷ Sample is large enough
  ▷ Null hypothesis (H_0) is true
▶ Chi-square test is often used for qualitative (categorical) data
▶ Two varieties of chi-square tests are often used in medical research
  ▷ Chi-square goodness of fit – applied to test one set of data against the theoretical expected distribution
  ▷ Chi-square test of independence – applied for two sets of data to test if their relationship is casual or causal

Choosing regression analysis method based on the character of data

▶ Data types
  ▷ Quantitative = continuous
  ▷ Qualitative = catogorical
▶ If the data are all quantitative, use multiple regression

▶ If the data are all qualitative, use ANOVA
▶ If some data are quantitative and some qualitative, use analysis of covariance

Cohort study

▶ A cohort is a group of people who share a common characteristic or experience within a defined time
▶ Prospective cohort
  ▷ The cohort is identified before the appearance of the disease under investigation
  ▷ The study is summarized with the "relative risk"
▶ The cohorts are observed over a period to determine the frequency of new incidence of the studied disease among them
▶ The gold standard of all the medical studies, the double blind randomly controlled study, is a form of prospective cohort study
▶ Retrospective cohort
  ▷ A variety of cohort study, where the cohort is defined after the data is collected
  ▷ The study is summarized with the odds ratio

Confidence interval

▶ The narrower the confidence interval, the closer the estimation to the true measure
▶ Smaller sample sizes yield wider confidence interval
▶ Larger sample sizes diminish confidence interval

Construct validity

▶ Refers to whether a scale measures what it purports to measure

Correlation coefficient

▶ A measurement to test the relation between variables
▶ Ranges between –1 and +1; the sign implies the direction of relation; the absolute value implies the strength of relation
▶ In a positive correlation, when on variable increase (or decreases), the other variable moves in the same direction
▶ In a negative correlation the two variable move in opposite direction
▶ Correlation coefficients indicate only the degree of relationship; they say nothing about cause and effect
▶ Methods
  ▷ Ordinal data – Spearman rank order
  ▷ Nominal data – Pearson correlation

Dependent variable and independent variable

▶ Dependent variable is the value that changes in response to the change of independent variable; it is usually the phenomenon of interest in a research study
▶ Independent variable is the value that can be predicted, set, or manipulated
▶ Example – in a study to observe the symptoms' change in response to medicine dosage
  ▷ The dosage is an independent invariable and can be set or manipulated
  ▷ The change of symptoms is a dependent variable and is the phenomenon to be studied

Descriptive study

▶ Data is collected through objective observation without intervention (i.e., no study medicine is given; no life style change is required)
▶ Through data analysis to describe patterns of condition occurrence in relation to selected variables (e.g., gender, age, time)
▶ Examples include
  ▷ Case report
  ▷ Cross-sectional surveys
  ▷ Correlation study

Errors associated with the null hypothesis

▶ Type I error
  ▷ Also known as α error
  ▷ Rejecting a true null hypothesis and falsely claiming a difference
▶ Type II error
  ▷ Also known as β error
  ▷ Accepting a false null hypothesis while a true difference is not detected

Intervention study

▶ The investigator intervenes, or controls, the experimental conditions of the subjects (e.g., giving medicine, changing life style)
▶ Data analysis includes the comparison of the observation to the intervened group and the control (placebo) group

Kappa

▶ An index that compares the agreement against that which might be expected by chance
▶ Possible value ranges from +1 (perfect agreement) via 0 (no agreement, or completely by chance) to –1 (complete disagreement).
▶ A κ value of –1 or +1 may never happen in reality; absolute κ values greater than 0.6 are considered significant

Meta-analysis

▶ A statistic method that combines the result of several studies that address a set of related research hypotheses
▶ It overcomes the problem of limited statistical power in studies with small sample sizes

Null hypothesis

▶ The hypothesis that the observed difference is solely due to chance (hence the true difference is null)
▶ Researchers try to prove that the difference they found is not due to chance, in another word to reject the H_0, or to accept an alternative hypothesis (H_1)

Positive predictive value and negative predictive value

▶ Two measurements for the quality of diagnostic tests
▶ Positive predictive value (PPV) is the proportion of patients with positive test results who also truly have the tested condition, i.e., correctly diagnosed
▶ Negative predictive value (NPV) is the proportion of patients with negative test results who also truly do not have the tested condition, i.e., correctly ruled out
▶ PPV = True positive / (true positive + false positive)
▶ NPV = True negative / (true negative + false negative)

Prevalence vs. incidence

▶ Prevalence refers to the proportion of existing cases
▶ Incidence refers to new cases
▶ Prevalence is attainable from
  ▷ A specified point in time (point prevalence)
  ▷ A specified interval (period prevalence)
▶ Incidence is attainable only for a specified interval; there is no such thing as "point incidence"

p-value

▶ A measurement for the probability of observing a difference by chance alone
▶ If the *p*-value is smaller than an investigator defined level, the observed difference is believed to be true and not by chance, or in another word, the null hypothesis is rejected
▶ A generally accepted *p*-value is 0.05, which means that the observed difference is equal to or less than 5% likely due to chance

Regression

▶ Methods of predicting the value or behavior of one variable (the dependent variable) on the basis of the value or behavior of another variable (the independent variable)
▶ Example
  ▷ One may predict a student's performance in final exam (Z) on the basis of the student's score on midterm exam (A)
  ▷ A is a known value, therefore is the independent variable
  ▷ Z is unknown but is dependent upon A, and is therefore is the dependent variable
  ▷ The student's frequency of absence (B) also has an impact on the Z; if we predict Z on the basis of both A and B, then there are multiple independent variables
▶ The method of relating dependent variable to two or more independent variables is called multiple regression

Relative risk vs. odds ratio

▶ Relative risk is applied to prospective studies, such as
  ▷ Cohort studies that compare incidence in people with and without certain risks
▶ Odds ratio is applied to retrospective studies, such as
  ▷ Case-controlled studies, comparing risk factors in people with and without a disease

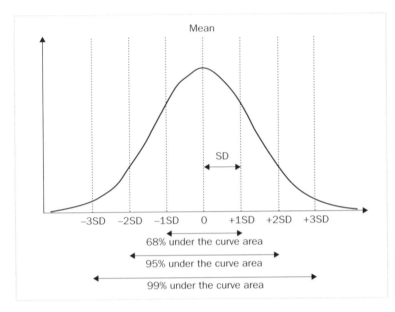

Figure 9-1 Normal distribution and standard deviation (SD) (the bell curve).

Reliability

▶ Reproducibility of a test
▶ May refer to intrarater or interrater reliability

Sensitivity vs. specificity

▶ Sensitivity is the ability of the test to detect disease in diseased people
▶ Specificity is the ability of the test to rule out illness in healthy people
▶ Sensitivity = True positive / (true positive + false negative)
▶ Specificity = True negative / (true negative + false positive)
▶ Highly sensitive tests often falsely claim healthy people sick, i.e., high false positive
▶ Highly specific tests often falsely claim sick people healthy, i.e., high false negative

Standard deviation (SD) (Figure 9-1)

▶ Measurement of the spread (distribution) of the data about the mean
▶ Measured in the same units as the data
▶ In a normal distribution
  ▷ 68% of data points fall in the area from –1SD to +1SD about the mean
  ▷ 95% fall in –2SD to +2SD
  ▷ 99% in –3SD to +3SD

Standard error (SE) vs. standard deviation

▶ Multiple sampling of the same population produces multiple, different standard deviations; SE is a measurement of the spread of the SDs about the mean SD
▶ SE is calculated using the same mathematic equation of calculating SD. However, this time the "data" is a series of SD. SE may be considered as "the standard deviation of standard deviations"

▶ SE is to measure the sampling distribution, but not the data distribution
▶ SE has no unit
▶ The ideal SE is 0, i.e., all the samplings provide the same SD – the true SD of the population
▶ While larger sample sizes diminish SE, SD is not dependent upon sample size

Validity

▶ The accuracy of an instrument in measuring what it seeks to measure
▶ Internal validity – true for the population and conditions tested
▶ External validity – generalizable to other populations and conditions
▶ Construct validity – whether a test measures what it purports to measure

10 Cognitive Disorders

Cognitive impairment of different severity is very common in mental disorders. The shared features of conditions described in this chapter are that the cognitive disturbance starts at a time of life after the birth and is the most prominent symptom of the condition.

The demarcation between cognitive function and noncognitive function may be debatable. However, from the literal meaning of cognition in Latin, "to come to know," we may sense a generally accepted core idea of cognition. It seems that most understandings of cognition are focused on the ability of learning, processing, storing, and retrieving information and knowledge. From a clinical standing point of psychopathology, it may be safe to state that cognition refers to four parts of the brain function

▶ Memory
▶ Language
▶ Attention
▶ Executive function

The cognitive impairment in delirium and dementia is global, while in amnestic disorder it is area specific. DSM-IV-TR categorizes cognitive disorders into four groups with 20 allowed diagnoses

▶ Delirium
  ▷ Due to a general medical condition
  ▷ Due to multiple etiologies
  ▷ Substance intoxication
  ▷ Substance withdrawal
  ▷ Not otherwise specified (NOS)
▶ Dementia
  ▷ Of the Alzheimer's type
  ▷ Owing to Creutzfeldt–Jacob disease
  ▷ Owing to head trauma
  ▷ Owing to Huntington's disease
  ▷ Owing to human immunodeficiency virus (HIV) disease
  ▷ Owing to Parkinson's disease
  ▷ Owing to Pick's disease
  ▷ Substance-induced persisting
  ▷ Vascular
  ▷ Due to other general medical conditions
  ▷ Due to multiple etiologies
  ▷ NOS

▶ Amnestic disorders
  ▷ Due to a general medical condition
  ▷ Substance-induced persisting
  ▷ NOS
▶ Cognitive disorder NOS

Alzheimer's disease: genetic findings

▶ Forty percent of patients have a family history of dementia of the Alzheimer's type
▶ The concordance rate is five times higher for monozygotic twins than for dizygotic twins
▶ Genetic linkage to chromosomes 1, 14, and 21
▶ Amyloid precursor protein (APP) has the gene located on chromosome 21 Mutations in the gene were found to cause excessive deposition of β-amyloid protein
▶ Increased copies of *apolipoprotein E ε4* gene are associated with increased risk; the gene is located on chromosome 19

Alzheimer's disease: neuropathology (Figure 10–1)

Aloysius Alzheimer (1864–1915) was a German psychiatrist and neuropathologist. He worked with Emil Kraepelin.

▶ Gross neuroanatomy
  ▷ Diffuse cortical atrophy involves all cerebral lobes
▶ Microscopic findings
  ▷ Senile plaques – quantitatively correlated with the severity of the dementia; composed of amyloid beta (Aβ), astrocytes, dystrophic neuronal processes, and microglia
  ▷ Neurofibrillary tangles – cytoskeletal elements including phosphorylated tau protein
  ▷ Neuronal loss in the cortex and the hippocampus
  ▷ Synaptic loss

Figure 10–1 Cortical atrophy in dementia of Alzheimer's type. Head CT scans of a 30-year-old healthy male and an 83-year-old male who is demented. Note the prominent culci and significantly enlarged lateral ventricles in the demented patient.
CT, computer tomography.

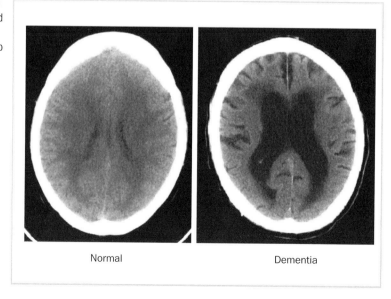

Normal   Dementia

▷ Granulovascular degeneration of the neurons
▷ Decreased neuronal projections from the nucleus basalis of Meynert, and therefore decreased cholinergic transmission

Amnesia: etiology

▶ Core structures
  ▷ Dorsomedial and midline nuclei of the thalamus
  ▷ Hippocampus
  ▷ Mammillary bodies
  ▷ Amygdala
▶ Damage in the left hemisphere is more critical in the development of memory disorders
▶ Frontal lobe impairment may cause accompanying symptoms in amnestic disorders, such as confabulation and apathy

Antipsychotic use in demented or elderly

▶ Mortality increase 1.6% in patients treated with olanzapine or risperidone
▶ Food and Drug Administration (FDA) 2005 black boxed warning
  ▷ Warning to the entire class of atypical antipsychotics for increased death rate, heart attacks, and pneumonia
  ▷ No warning for typical antipsychotics, but safety data lacking
▶ FDA 2008 addition to the 2005 warning
  ▷ Same warning to 11 typical antipsychotics
▶ Clinical consensus – owing to the high probability of tardive dyskinesia induced by typical antipsychotics, atypical antipsychotics remain a viable clinical choice when use is necessary; antidementics and mood stabilizing anticonvulsants are alternative options

Binswanger's disease

Otto Binswanger (1852–1929) was a Swiss psychiatrist.

▶ Also known as subcortical arteriosclerotic encephalopathy
▶ Traditionally considered a rare form of vascular dementia; however, recent findings may reveal that the condition is more common than what was thought
▶ Caused by multiple small infarctions that impair the white matter but spare the cortical regions
▶ Associated with hypertension and atherosclerosis
▶ CT – defused loss of deep hemispheric white matter

Black patch delirium

▶ Delirium because of sensory deprivation in patients wearing eye patches after cataract surgery
▶ Usually in elderly patients
▶ Prevention
  ▷ Pinholes in the patches
  ▷ Occasionally removing one patch at a time

Cognitive impairment

▶ Cognitive function is a loosely defined concept that mainly includes the functional level in
  ▷ Memory
  ▷ Language
  ▷ Attention
  ▷ Executive functions (sequential learning, decision making, calculation, etc.)
▶ Almost all psychiatric disorders may, to some extent, influent the cognitive function
▶ Cognitive impairment is the cardinal symptom in delirium, dementia, and the amnestic disorders

Daily living activities

▶ A functioning assessment for cognitively impaired individuals; mainly include
  ▷ Bathing
  ▷ Dressing
  ▷ Toileting
  ▷ Feeding
  ▷ Ability to escape when facing danger

Delirium: clinical features

▶ Change of consciousness (awareness of the environment, impaired sustained attention)
▶ Change of cognition (memory, orientation, language, new onset illusions or hallucinations)
▶ Symptoms develop quickly and fluctuate
▶ With or without apparent contributing factors, such as substance intoxication or withdrawal, medical conditions

Delirium: course and prognosis

▶ Onset
  ▷ Sudden
  ▷ However, prodromal symptoms may occur a few days before the florid symptoms
▶ The symptoms persist as long as the causative condition is not resolved
▶ After the causative factor is removed, the delirium usually lasts 3–7 days, but residual symptoms may last up to 2 weeks
▶ The older the patient, the longer the delirium takes to resolve
▶ There are anecdotal observations that found delirium progresses to dementia; however, this transition has not been verified by controlled studies

Delirium: epidemiology

▶ In general population
  ▷ Under 55 years – 0.4%
  ▷ Over 55 years – 1.1%
▶ Intensive care unit (ICU) population – 30%
▶ Postsurgery for hip fractures – 40%–50%
▶ Nursing home population over 75 years – 60% has repeated delirium

- ▶ Terminally ill patients – 80%.
- ▶ Postcardiotomy patients – over 90%, the highest prevalence
- ▶ Risk factors
  - ▷ Advanced age
  - ▷ Alcohol dependence
  - ▷ Brain damage
  - ▷ Cancer
  - ▷ Diabetes
  - ▷ Electrolyte imbalances and malnutrition
  - ▷ Fever
  - ▷ History of delirium
  - ▷ Infection
  - ▷ Insomnia
  - ▷ Male gender
  - ▷ Pain and pain medication
  - ▷ Sensory impairment

Delirium: proposed mechanisms

- ▶ Decreased acetylcholine activity in the brain was reported in many studies as delirium-inducing; this often is because of anticholinergic effect of the medicines
- ▶ Hyperactivity of noradrenergic neurons may be attributed and associated with delirium during substance or alcohol withdrawal

Delirium: treatment

- ▶ The primary goal is to treat the underlying cause
- ▶ Nonpharmacotherapy
  - ▷ Physical support to prevent endangering behavior
  - ▷ Environmental support – neither sensory deprived nor overly stimulated; friend, relative, or regular sitter; familiar pictures and decorations; regular orientations (clock and calendar)
- ▶ Pharmacotherapy for anticholinergic toxicity
  - ▷ Physostigmine (Antilirium), 1–2 mg intravenous (IV) or intramuscular (IM), may repeat in 15–30 minutes.
- ▶ Pharmacotherapy for psychosis
  - ▷ Haloperidol 5–40 mg/day
  - ▷ Other antipsychotics – precautions for anticholinergic effects
  - ▷ Patients with Parkinson's disease – clozapine or quetiapine
- ▶ Pharmacotherapy for insomnia
  - ▷ Benzodiazepines with short- or intermediate–half-lives (e.g., lorazepam [Ativan] 1–2 mg at bedtime)
  - ▷ Pain management
- ▶ Electroconvulsive therapy
  - ▷ Rare cases of delirious states caused by intractable medical condition

Dementia with Lewy bodies

Frederic Lewy (1885–1950) was a German-born U.S. neurologist.

- ▶ Second most common cause of dementia, after Alzheimer's disease

- Lewy bodies are eosinophilic neuronal inclusions composed of
  - α-synuclein
  - Ubiquitin
  - Neurofilament protein
  - αB crystallin
- Clinical manifestations
  - Prominent visual hallucinations and delusions
  - Fluctuations in function
  - Sensitivity to extrapyramidal symptoms (EPS) from antipsychotics
- Other diseases associated with Lewy body
  - Parkinson's disease (Lewy bodies confined to the basal ganglia)
  - Lewy body variant of Alzheimer's disease

Dementia: epidemiology

- Prevalence
  - Over 65 years – 5%
  - Over 85 years, 20%–40%
  - In general medical practice – 20%
  - In chronic care facilities – 50%
- Alzheimer's disease
  - Fifty percent of all dementia cases
  - In the United States, 2.3 million are diagnosed with Alzheimer's disease
- Approximately one half of patients with mild to moderate dementia are undiagnosed

Dementia: HIV-related

- Also known as
  - Acquired immunodeficiency syndrome (AIDS) dementia complex
  - HIV dementia
- Diagnosis
  - Laboratory evidence for systemic HIV
  - At least two cognitive deficits
  - Presence of motor abnormalities or personality changes
  - Exclusion of alternative pathology of cognitive impairment
  - Absence of clouding of consciousness

Dementia: infectious etiology

- Neurosyphilis
- HIV
- Creutzfeldt–Jacob disease
- Miliary tuberculosis

Dementia: laboratory work-up

- Basic
  - Complete blood count
  - Complete metabolic panel including hepatic function
  - Urinalysis

▷ Chest x-ray
▷ Electrocardiogram
▶ Recommended
  ▷ Thyroid stimulating hormone (TSH)
  ▷ Serum B12
  ▷ Folate
  ▷ Syphilis serology
▶ Optional
  ▷ Head computer tomography (CT)
  ▷ Neuropsychological test

Dementia: vascular

▶ Also known as multiinfarct dementia
▶ A subcortical dementia, with more motor signs, labile affects, and pseudobulbar signs
▶ Stepwise progression
▶ Risk factors – hypertension, and all risk factors for coronary artery disease

Dementia pugilistica

Pugil is from Latin – "boxer"

▶ Also known as "chronic traumatic encephalopathy"
▶ A neurological decline due to chronic traumatic brain injury
▶ Typically develops over a decade of repeated concussions, such as in professional boxing
▶ Symptoms include
  ▷ Declining memory
  ▷ Parkinsonism
  ▷ Speech problems
  ▷ Unsteady gait
  ▷ Personality change and disinhibition
▶ Treatment – same as Alzheimer's disease and Parkinson's disease
▶ Sufferers may be treated with drugs used for Alzheimer's and parkinsonism

Medicines associated with impaired cognitive function

▶ Anticholinergics
▶ Antihypertensives
▶ Opioids
▶ Benzodiazepines

Mood disorders and dementia

▶ Approximately 30%–50% of patients with dementia of Alzheimer's type develop depression
▶ Approximately 14% of late life depressions have also dementia
▶ Pseudodementia – depression with apparent cognitive decline
▶ Masked depression is common among demented and elderly patients, may present with
  ▷ Somatic complaints
  ▷ Vegetative symptoms
  ▷ Melancholic features

▶ Predispositions
  ▷ Loss
  ▷ Social isolation
  ▷ Medical illness

Normal aging

▶ Minor memory problems
▶ Also known as
  ▷ Benign senescent forgetfulness
  ▷ Age-associated memory impairment
▶ Distinguished from dementia
  ▷ Minor severity
  ▷ No significant impairment in social and occupational functioning

Normal pressure hydrocephalus (NPH)

▶ Chronic communicating hydrocephalus
▶ High normal level of intracranial pressure; the chronic process of the disease allows the brain to equilibrate the elevated intracranial pressure
▶ No classic signs of increased intracranial pressure
▶ Clinical manifestations
  ▷ Gait disturbance and ataxia
  ▷ Dementia
  ▷ Urinary incontinence
▶ Diagnosis
  ▷ Lumber puncture – removal of small volume of cerebrospinal fluid (CSF) may improve the symptoms temporally (Fisher test)
  ▷ CT or magnetic resonance imaging (MRI) scan shows enlarged ventricles without convolutional atrophy
▶ Treatment
  ▷ Ventriculoperitoneal shunt

Pharmacologic treatment for dementia

▶ Cholinesterase inhibitors
▶ NMDA antagonists
▶ Vitamin E
▶ Selegiline
▶ Statins
▶ Moderate alcohol intake

Pick's disease (Figure 10-2)

Arnold Pick (1851–1924) was a Czechoslovakian neurologist and psychiatrist.

▶ Frontotemporal dementia
▶ Epidemiology
  ▷ The second most common cause of dementia under 65 years.
  ▷ The fourth most common above 65 years (after Alzheimer's disease, Lewy body dementia, and vascular dementia)

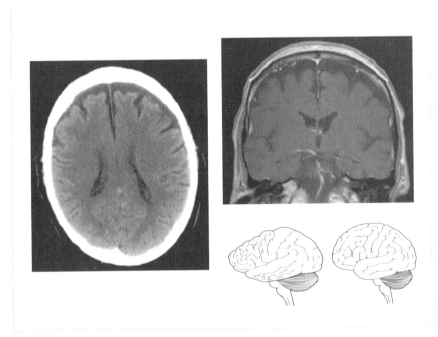

Figure 10-2 Pick's disease has significant lobar atrophy of frontal and temporal lobe with sparing of the posterior and superior temporal gyri, as shown here in CT (left), MRI (right upper) and line-drawn infected brain in comparison to normal brain (right lower).
CT, computer tomography; MRI, magnetic resonance imaging.

▶ Gray matter degeneration in the frontal and anterior temporal lobes
▶ Cellular inclusions
   ▷ Pick bodies – silver-staining, tau protein rich aggregations in neurons
   ▷ Ubiquitin positive – tau negative inclusions
▶ Changes in personality in early stage
▶ Prominent progressive verbal degeneration – aphasia and loss of verbal memory

Pittsburg compound B (PiB)

Produced by researchers in University of Pittsburgh and tested *in vivo* at the Uppsala University in Sweden.

▶ A fluorescent derivative of a histology staining agent
▶ An investigational tool in the diagnosis and progress monitoring of Alzheimer's disease
▶ Binds specifically to the β-sheet structure of Aβ
▶ Used in positron emission tomography to produce image of amyloid β plaques
▶ Potentially other neuronal diseases associated with amyloid β plaques

Sundowning

▶ Elderly patients present with drowsiness, confusion, unsteadiness in gait and fall
▶ Usually occurs or worsens at night
▶ Owing to excessive use of sedative medicines, most often benzodiazepines

Transient global amnesia

▶ Sudden loss of the ability to recall recent events or to remember new information
▶ Often with no insight
▶ Episodes last from 6 to 24 hours
▶ Pathophysiology
  ▷ Unknown
  ▷ Possible ischemic episode of the temporal lobe and the diencephalic brain regions
  ▷ Possible migrainous episodes
▶ Recovery is almost always complete; the rate of recurrence could be up to 20%

11 Addictions: General Consideration

Thomas Sydenham, the renounced English physician of seventeenth century, once said, "Among the remedies which it has pleased Almighty God to give to man to relieve his sufferings, none is so universal and so efficacious as opium." Opium, as one significant example of addictive drugs, was in medicinal use since the Stone Age. Like opium, many other currently illicit substances were once accepted therapeutic agents. Addiction as a self-awarding behavior was first connected to compulsive indulging of habit-forming substance in the early twentieth century. Modern physicians no longer warship opium in the manner Sydenham did, as they understand a quick and powerful relief of suffering alone, without balancing other aspects of health, is not the destination of medicine.

The phenomenon of addiction subjected to extensive scientific investigation. At this time the biological mechanisms of addiction are not yet completely elicited. Key structural elements likely include amygdala, nucleus accumbens, pontine nuclei, arcuate, ventral tegmental area (VTA), prefrontal cortex, thalamus, and pallidum. Neurotransmitters, dopamine, and norepinephrine are most closely involved.

DSM-IV-TR allows fourteen diagnoses of substance-related disorders:

- Substance dependence
- Substance abuse
- Substance intoxication
- Substance withdrawal
- Substance intoxication delirium
- Substance withdrawal delirium
- Substance-induced persisting dementia
- Substance-induced persisting amnestic disorder
- Substance-induced psychotic disorder (including hallucinogen persisting perception disorder)
- Substance-induced mood disorder
- Substance-induced anxiety disorder
- Substance-induced sexual dysfunction
- Substance-induced sleep disorder
- Substance-related disorder not otherwise specified (NOS)

Abuse vs. dependence

- Abuse implies failure to fulfill role – failure of any one of these role meets the criteria of abuse
  - ▷ As a worker (repeated absences, poor work performance)
  - ▷ As a student (suspensions, expulsions from school)
  - ▷ As a responsible family member (neglect, arguments, physical fights)

▷ As a citizen (legal problems)
▷ As a machinery or vehicle operator (driving under influence)
▷ As a conservator to self (physical hazardous to self)
▶ Dependence criteria emphasize loss of control
▷ Loss of control in quantity of substance – desire or need (tolerance) for more, failure to cut, or withdrawal when cut
▷ Loss of control in quantity of time present with extra time spent on substance use and other activities are given up
▷ Loss of control in safety – continued use despite physical or psychological problems
▶ "Dependence" is the more paramount diagnosis
▶ "Abuse" means never have met criteria for substance dependence
▶ Both abuse and dependence count behavior in the past 12 months; both have clinically significant impairment and subjective distress

Acting mechanisms of substances

▶ Lysergic acid diethylamide (LSD): Serotogernic and dopaminergic stimulation
▶ Cocaine – blocks reuptake of dopamine, serotonin, and norepinephrine
▶ Cannabis – cannabinoid receptors
▶ Opioid – opioid receptors
▶ Amphetamine – similar to cocaine
▶ Caffeine – multiple mechanisms
▶ Ecstasy – serotonin reuptake blockade
▶ Nicotine – nicotinic acetylcholine receptors
▶ Phencyclidine (PCP) – binding to N-methyl-D-aspartate (NMDA) receptor blocks the calcium channel

DSM-IV-TR diagnosis: dependence but not abuse

▶ DSM-IV-TR allows diagnoses of nicotine dependence and polysubstance dependence, but not abuse
▶ Polysubstance abuse
▷ The appropriate DSM format is a list of individual substance abuse diagnoses

DSM-IV-TR diagnosis: substances have no withdrawal diagnosis

▶ DSM-IV-TR does not have recognized diagnoses on withdrawal of the listed substances
▷ Caffeine
▷ Cannabis
▷ Hallucinogens
▷ Inhalants
▷ Phencycline
▷ Polysubstance
▶ Not that these substances do not give withdrawal symptoms, but usually not of clinical significance for an independent diagnosis
▶ If a withdrawal diagnosis is clinically appropriate and required, the appropriate DSM format is "-Related Disorder NOS," such as "Caffeine-Related Disorder NOS."

Mental disorders more common amongst drug abusers

▶ Antisocial personality disorder – 44%
▶ Phobic disorders – 39%
▶ Major depressive disorder – 24%
▶ Dysthymia – 12%
▶ Generalized anxiety disorder – 10%
▶ Bipolar disorders – 3%

Remission courses of substance dependence

▶ Remission courses
   ▷ Early full remission
   ▷ Early partial remission
   ▷ Sustained full remission
   ▷ Sustained partial remission
▶ Early – more than 1 month, less than 12 months
▶ Sustained – more than 12 months
▶ Full – no substance use diagnostic criteria are met
▶ Partial – subthreshold diagnosis, still using but no longer meeting full diagnostic criteria
▶ If on agonist therapy, specify so; if in a controlled environment, specify so
▶ If not use for less than 1 month, not counted as remission

The most commonly abused substance

▶ Legal – nicotine
▶ Illegal – marijuana

12 Addictions: Alcohol-Related Disorders

The history of wine production may be traced back to 6000 BC in the Middle East and in China. Around the same time Egyptians and Mesopotamians started making beer. The maximum ethanol level in either wine or beer was set by the biological limit of yeast. With the technical maturation of distillation in the Middle Age, the already problematic behavior of excessive drinking became more widespread. In the eighteenth century, the admiration to ethanol-containing drink led to the birth of the euphemism "alcohol," meant pure spirit of substance. However, just one century later, "alcoholism" became well known as a compelling illness.

Today, alcohol abuse and dependence are costly problems in the United States. Approximately 100,000 Americans die each year from alcohol-related conditions.

DSM-IV-TR allows 14 diagnoses of alcohol-related disorders

- ▶ Alcohol dependence
- ▶ Alcohol abuse
- ▶ Alcohol intoxication
- ▶ Alcohol withdrawal
- ▶ Alcohol intoxication delirium
- ▶ Alcohol withdrawal delirium
- ▶ Alcohol-induced persisting dementia
- ▶ Alcohol-induced persisting amnestic disorder
- ▶ Alcohol-induced psychotic disorder
- ▶ Alcohol-induced mood disorder
- ▶ Alcohol-induced anxiety disorder
- ▶ Alcohol-induced sexual dysfunction
- ▶ Alcohol-induced sleep disorder
- ▶ Alcohol disorder not otherwise specified (NOS)

Alcohol effects on sleep

- ▶ Decreased sleep latency
- ▶ Decreased random eye movement (REM) sleep
- ▶ Decreased stage 4 sleep
- ▶ Increased sleep fragmentation, with prolonged episodes of awakening

Alcohol withdrawal seizures

- ▶ Generalized, tonic-clonic seizures
- ▶ Status epilepticus may occur in less than 3% patients
- ▶ Anticonvulsants are not required

▶ Conditions other than alcohol withdrawal may coexist
  ▷ Head injuries
  ▷ Central nervous system (CNS) infections and tumors
  ▷ Cerebrovascular diseases
  ▷ Electrolyte imbalance – hypoglycemia, hyponatremia, hypomagnesemia

Aspartate aminotransferase and alanine aminotransferase

▶ Less sensitive than gamma-glutamyl peptidase (GGT) for alcohol-related liver disease
▶ Aspartate aminotransferase (AST) more sensitive than alanine aminotransferase (ALT)

CAGE

▶ A simple and popular questionnaire to screen patients for alcoholism
▶ C – cut
  ▷ "Have you ever tried to cut down on your drinking?"
▶ A – annoyed
  ▷ "Have you ever been annoyed by others' criticizing your drinking?"
▶ G – guilty
  ▷ "Have you ever felt guilty about your drinking?"
▶ E – eye-opener
  ▷ "Have you ever had a drink first thing in the morning to steady your nerves or to get rid of a hangover?"

Cloninger types of alcoholism

Robert Cloninger is a contemporary U.S. psychiatrist at Washington University in St. Louis.

▶ An influential theory on personality root of alcoholic behavior by Robert Cloninger
▶ Type 1
  ▷ Onset at older age
  ▷ No gender preference
  ▷ Little family history
  ▷ Low risk-taking behavior
  ▷ Few comorbid with antisocial personality disorder
▶ Type 2
  ▷ Onset at younger age
  ▷ More prevalent in males
  ▷ Strong family history
  ▷ High rate of risk-taking behavior
  ▷ High comorbid rate with antisocial personality disorder

Comorbidity with alcoholism

▶ The majority of alcoholics have at least one other psychiatric disorder
▶ Women are more likely to have comorbid Axis I psychopathology
▶ Common comorbid conditions are
  ▷ Abuse of another substance (most common in both men and women, more common in men)
  ▷ Antisocial personality disorder (more common in men)

  ▷ Anxiety disorders (more common in women)
  ▷ Major depressive disorder (more common in women)

Fetal alcohol syndrome

▶ Facial dysmorphisms
▶ Postnatal growth retardation
▶ Intrauterine growth retardation
▶ Learning difficulties
▶ Change of brain size (micro- or macrocephaly) is significant

Gamma-glutamyl peptidase

▶ Most sensitive test for alcohol abuse
▶ Not specific, may increase in fatty liver and certain medicines
▶ Significant decrease after 2 weeks of abstinence, back to normal in 6–8 weeks

Idiosyncratic alcohol intoxication

▶ A severe behavioral syndrome develops rapidly after a person consumes a small amount of alcohol
▶ Symptoms
  ▷ Confusion
  ▷ Transitory illusions, hallucinations, and delusions
  ▷ Impulsive and aggressive behavior
  ▷ Suicidal ideation and attempts
  ▷ Lasting for a few hours
  ▷ Lack of recall
▶ May be associated with preexisting brain damage, advancing age, sedative drugs, and fatigue
▶ Sometimes used in defense for endangering behavior as the reaction to a minimal amount of alcohol may be argued to be unexpected and unpredictable
▶ Not a DSM-IV-TR diagnosis; the validity of the diagnosis is under debate

Mechanisms of alcohol effects

▶ No single molecular target has been identified
▶ Classic hypothesis
  ▷ Increasing fluidity of the cell membranes with short-term use
  ▷ Decreasing membrane fluidity with long-term use
▶ Recent findings
  ▷ Ion-channel activities enhanced by alcohol – nicotinic acetylcholine, 5-HT3, and gamma-aminobutyric acid (GABA)-A receptors
  ▷ Ion-channel activities inhibited by alcohol – glutamate receptors and voltage-gated calcium channels

Metabolism of alcohol (Figure 12–1)

▶ Ninety percent through oxidation in liver
▶ Ten percent is excreted unchanged by the kidneys and lungs

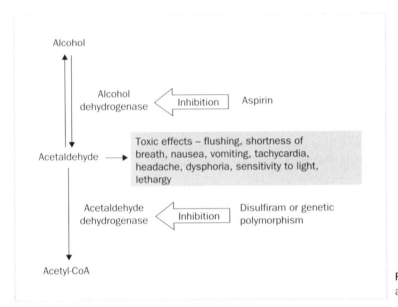

Figure 12-1 Alcohol metabolism and interruptive factors.

▶ Chronic drinkers – upregulation of the hepatic enzymes results in rapid alcohol metabolism
▶ Alcohol is metabolized by alcohol dehydrogenase (ADH) and aldehyde dehydrogenase
▶ ADH catalyzes the conversion of alcohol into acetaldehyde; aldehyde dehydrogenase catalyzes the conversion of acetaldehyde into acetic acid

One drink

▶ Equivalent to 12 g of ethanol
▶ Equivalent to 12 ounces of beer
▶ Equivalent to 4 ounce of wine
▶ Equivalent to 1–1.5 ounces of an 80-proof liquor
▶ May increase the blood alcohol level by 15–20 mg/dL
▶ May be metabolized in 1 hour

Prognosis

▶ Favorable prognostic signs
  ▷ Absence of preexisting antisocial personality disorder
  ▷ Absence of other substance-related problems
  ▷ Having a job
  ▷ Close family contacts
  ▷ Absence of severe legal problems
  ▷ Compliance for the full course of the initial rehabilitation

Psychodynamic theories about alcohol-related disorders

▶ Anxiolytic effect
  ▷ Alcohol is used to decrease the unconscious stress when dealing with a harsh superego

▶ Fixation at the oral stage
  ▷ Alcohol is used to satisfy the desire of mouth when facing frustration

Wernicke's encephalopathy: management

Carl Wernicke (1848–1905) was a German neurologist and psychiatrist.

▶ IV thiamine and glucose
▶ Thiamine must be given first; giving glucose without first replenishing thiamine may further exhaust the body's remaining thiamine and worsen the patient's condition
▶ Supportive treatment and behavior management

Wernicke-Korsakoff syndrome

Sergei Korsakoff (1853–1900) was a Russian neuropsychiatrist. He was once a student of Theodor Meynert.

▶ Alcohol-induced amnestic and cognitive disorder
▶ Symptoms include ataxia, confusion, ophthalmoplegia (horizontal nystagmus, paralysis of the abducens, disconjugate eye movement, and gaze palsy)
▶ Pathophysiology is thiamine deficiency
▶ Wernicke's syndrome, also known as alcoholic encephalopathy, is of acute onset and reversible
▶ Korsakoff's syndrome is chronic and largely (80%) irreversible.
▶ Horizontal nystagmus may appear in
  ▷ Wernicke-Korsakoff syndrome
  ▷ Phencyclidine (PCP) intoxication
  ▷ Opioid withdrawal
  ▷ Cranial nerve (CN) VIII impairment

13 Addictions: Nonalcoholic Substance-Related Disorders

Under the commonality of habit forming, each addictive substance has its own unique mechanism and pattern of abuse. Substance use usually provides apparent reward in short term but has extended risk through chronic use.

Some of the now notorious addictive substances were once legitimate medicinal agents. Amphetamine and its derivative methamphetamine were supplied to the soldiers to combat fatigue in the World War II. The use of cocaine and nicotine through chewing the leaves of coca and tobacco were a practice for many centuries among South Americans. The tax from coca leaf trade was once a source of support for some churches. After the isolation of cocaine alkaloid, it was widely used medicinally as an analgesic agent. The use of caffeine and opiate were found as early as the Stone Age. Even today, opioids still serve as the standard against which pain killing agents are measured. Marijuana's medicinal use has been a long time debation given its prominent effects on appetite stimulation and mood relaxation, under the shadow of its addictive nature. Phencyclidine was once patented and marketed as an anesthesic. Hallucinogen and inhalant are more heterogeneous groups with little known medical usage. The years of 1960s and 1970s witnessed increasingly systemic legal regulation on the use of addictive substances. The pathological substance use, though, continues to be debilitating and costly conditions.

DSM-IV-TR categorized 10 groups of substances other than alcohol

▶ Amphetamine
▶ Caffeine
▶ Cannabis
▶ Cocaine
▶ Hallucinogen
▶ Inhalant
▶ Nicotine
▶ Opioid
▶ Phencyclidine (PCP)
▶ Sedative, hypnotic, or anxiolytic

Amphetamine and cocaine intoxication and withdrawal: signs and symptoms

▶ Both intoxication and withdrawal
  ▷ Psychomotor agitation or retardation
▶ Intoxication
  ▷ Tachy- or bradycardia
  ▷ Pupillary dilation
  ▷ Hyper- or hypotension

▷ Perspiration and chills
▷ Nausea and vomiting
▷ Weight loss
▷ Confusion
▷ Respiratory failure
▶ Withdrawal
▷ Fatigue
▷ Vivid, unpleasant dreams
▷ Insomnia or hypersomnia
▷ Increased appetite

Caffeine: acting mechanism

▶ Antagonist of the adenosine receptors
▶ Adenosine receptors activate inhibitory G-protein and inhibit the formation of the second-messenger cyclic adenosine monophosphate (cAMP)
▶ Caffeine causes an increase in intraneuronal cAMP concentrations in neurons
▶ High-doses caffeine can enhance dopaminergic effects – potentially exacerbates psychosis

Cannabis mechanism of action (Figure 13–1)

▶ Among the over 60 chemical components, delta-9-tetrahydrocannabinol (THC) is the major one causing psychotropic effects
▶ Cannabinoid receptors (CB1, CB2)
▷ G-protein associated receptors
▷ CB1 has been studied in more details; it influences neuronal excitability through various mechanisms
▷ Activation of CB1 causes blockade of voltage-dependent calcium channels, so to reduce calcium influx
▷ CB1 may also modulate potassium channels
▶ Endocannabinoids
▷ Anandamide (AEA) and 2-arachidonoylglycerol (2-AG)
▷ Endogenous arachidonate-based lipids that bind cannabinoid receptors

Cannabis specific signs and symptoms

▶ Intoxication
▷ Conjunctival injection
▷ Increased appetite (may also present in amphetamine withdrawal)
▷ Dry mouth
▷ Tachycardia – may also appear in amphetamine intoxication
▶ No clinically significant withdrawal

Cannabis-induced disorders

▶ Usually during intoxication
▷ Delirium
▷ Psychosis
▷ Anxiety disorder

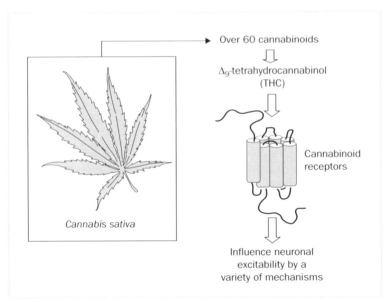

Over 60 cannabinoids

Δ_9-tetrahydrocannabinol
(THC)

Cannabinoid
receptors

Cannabis sativa

Influence neuronal
excitability by a
variety of mechanisms

Figure 13–1 Cannabis mechanism of action.

Club drugs

▶ Drugs associated with dance clubs, bars, and all-night dance parties
▶ A heterogeneous group includes
　▷ Lysergic acid diethylamide (LSD)
　▷ Gamma-hydroxybutyrate (GHB)
　▷ Ketamine
　▷ Methamphetamine
　▷ Methylenedioxymethamphetamine (MDMA) (ecstasy)
　▷ Flunitrazepam (Rohypnol)

Cocaine (See Figure 13–2 on page 92)

▶ Extracted from the plant *Erythroxylum coca*
▶ Preparations include
　▷ Coca leaves
　▷ Cocaine hydrochloride
　▷ Coca paste
　▷ Free base
　▷ Crack
▶ Metabolized to benzoylecgonine
▶ Detected in the urine for up to 36 hours
▶ Binds to the presynaptic transporter of dopamine, serotonin, and norepinephrine

Cocaine: adverse effects

▶ Nasal effects
　▷ Nasal congestion
　▷ Nasal inflammation
　▷ Nasal bleeding

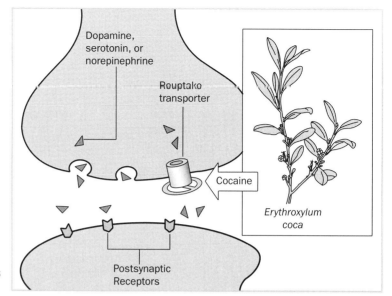

Figure 13–2 Cocaine acting mechanism. This schematic synapse represents either dopaminergic, serotonergic, or adrenergic system. Cocaine blocks the neurotransmitter reuptake transporter, mainly the dopamine transporter, and enhances the downstream effect. The inlet shows the coca plant.

    ▷ Nasal ulceration
    ▷ Perforation of the nasal septa
  ▶ Neurological complications
    ▷ Acute dystonia
    ▷ Tics
    ▷ Migraine-like headaches
  ▶ Cerebrovascular effects – associated with vasoconstriction
    ▷ Nonhemorrhagic cerebral infarctions
    ▷ Transient ischemic attacks
    ▷ Spinal cord hemorrhages, rare
  ▶ Seizures
    ▷ Accounted for 3%–8% of cocaine-related emergency room visits
    ▷ Cocaine is the substance of abuse most commonly associated with seizures (the second is amphetamine)
  ▶ Cardiac effects
    ▷ Myocardial infarctions
    ▷ Arrhythmias
    ▷ Cardiomyopathies
  ▶ Sudden death

Cocaine use during pregnancy

  ▶ Rapid transmission of cocaine across the placenta
  ▶ Potential brain developmental problems secondary to hypoperfusion of the brain
  ▶ Fetal growth retardation
  ▶ Present in breast milk; may increase blood pressure, rapid heart rate, and mydriasis (pupil dilation) in the newborn
  ▶ Decreased birth weight and malformations of the urogenital system of the newborn

Cocaine induced disorders

▶ Both intoxication and/or withdrawal
  ▷ Mood disorder
  ▷ Anxiety disorder
  ▷ Sleep disorder
▶ Usually during intoxication
  ▷ Delirium
  ▷ Psychosis
  ▷ Sexual dysfunction

Date rape drugs

▶ Club drugs that cause disorientation, sedation, and transient amnesia; these drugs might be placed in beverages
▶ Includes
  ▷ GHB
  ▷ Ketamine
  ▷ Flunitrazepam (Rohypnol)

Eye/vision-related specific symptoms of substance intoxication and withdrawal

▶ Conjunctival injection
  ▷ Cannabis intoxication
▶ Diplopia
  ▷ Inhalant intoxication, when the third cranial nerves are impaired
▶ Lacrimation (excessive tearing)
  ▷ Opioid withdrawal – often accompanied by rhinorrhea (excessive nasal discharge)
▶ Pupillary constriction
  ▷ Opioid intoxication
▶ Pupillary dilation
  ▷ Intoxication of cocaine, amphetamine, and hallucinogen
  ▷ Opioid intoxication usually causes papillary constriction, and withdrawal causes dilation; however, when opioid intoxication reaches the stage of coma, the pupils are dilated
▶ Nystagmus
  ▷ Intoxication of alcohol, sedatives, PCP, or inhalant
▶ Visual hallucination
  ▷ Transient visual hallucination is associated with alcohol or sedative withdrawal, and hallucinogen intoxication; usually prominent and vivid, accompanied with mild or no other psychotic symptoms.
  ▷ May be accompanied with tactile hallucination in alcohol or sedative withdrawal, and synesthesia in hallucinogen intoxication

Hallucinogen

▶ Hallucinogen is a loosely defined category of natural and synthetic substances that can induce hallucinations, loss of contact with reality, and an experience of expanded and heightened consciousness

▶ Includes
  ▷ LSD
  ▷ Mescaline
  ▷ Peyote
  ▷ Psilocybin
  ▷ Dimethyltryptamine (DMT)
  ▷ MDMA
▶ Possible tolerance, no clear withdrawal
▶ The neuropharmacologic mechanisms vary and many are not known
▶ Treatment for intoxication
  ▷ Talk down
  ▷ Benzodiazepines
  ▷ Antipsychotics are rarely used

Hallucinogen-induced disorders

▶ Persisting perception disorder (flashbacks)
  ▷ Reexperiencing intoxication symptoms when not using
▶ Intoxication delirium
▶ Psychosis
▶ Mood disorder
▶ Anxiety disorder

Hallucinogens: intoxication signs and symptoms

▶ Perceptual changes
  ▷ Intensified perceptions
  ▷ Dissociative symptoms – depersonalization, derealization
  ▷ Illusions
  ▷ Hallucinations
  ▷ Synesthesia
▶ Other physical signs
  ▷ Pupillary dilation
  ▷ Tachycardia
  ▷ Sweating
  ▷ Palpitations
  ▷ Blurring of vision
  ▷ Tremors
  ▷ Incoordination

Inhalants

▶ Volatile gases and liquids including
  ▷ Solvents
  ▷ Glues
  ▷ Adhesives
  ▷ Paint thinners
  ▷ Fuels
▶ DSM-IV-TR specifically excludes anesthetic gases and short-acting vasodilators from the inhalant-related disorders; these are classified as Other (or Unknown) Substance-Related Disorders

Inhalants: acting mechanisms

▶ Inhalants generally act as a central nervous system (CNS) depressant
▶ Specific pharmacodynamic effects are not well understood
▶ Suggested mechanisms
  ▷ Enhancing the gamma-aminobutyric acid (GABA) system
  ▷ Changing membrane fluidization

Inhalants: pathological effects

▶ Acute effects
  ▷ Respiratory depression
  ▷ Cardiac arrhythmias
  ▷ Aspiration and suffocation
▶ Chronic effects
  ▷ Diffuse cerebral, cerebellar, and brainstem atrophy; leukoencephalopathy; decreased cerebral blood flow
  ▷ Temporal lobe epilepsy
  ▷ Parkinsonism and other motor impairments
  ▷ Memory loss and cognitive deterioration
  ▷ Peripheral neuropathy
  ▷ Hearing loss
  ▷ Hepatic disease
  ▷ Renal damage (tubular acidosis)
  ▷ Muscle damage associated with rhabdomyolysis
  ▷ Possible fetal damage

LAAM

▶ Levo-α acetyl methadol
▶ Long-acting opioid
▶ ↑ QT interval may cause Torsade de pointe

Lysergic acid diethylamide (LSD)

▶ A synthetic hallucinogen
▶ Often taken as the prototype of hallucinogen
▶ It is a partial agonist at postsynaptic serotonin receptors

Methamphetamine and amphetamine

▶ Same mechanism – stimulates dopamine release
▶ Amphetamine is a longer acting version, less addictive, hence used for attention-deficit/hyperactivity disorder (ADHD) treatment

Methylenedioxymethamphetamine (See Figure 13–3 on page 96)

▶ Known on street as ecstasy
▶ A semisynthetic agent closely related to amphetamine-like psychostimulants
▶ The added residuals on the amphetamine core structure are believed to cause hallucinations; it is therefore considered by most as a hallucinogen

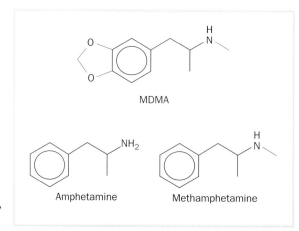

Figure 13-3 Methylenedioxy-methamphetamine (MDMA) is a semisynthetic agent closely related to amphetamine-like psychostimulants. The comparison of the molecular structures of amphetamine, methamphetamine, and MDMA is shown here.

▶ Mechanism
  ▷ Blocks serotonin reuptake
  ▷ Enhance the release of serotonin, norepinephrine, and dopamine
▶ Neural toxicity
▶ Causing feeling of closeness at low dose
▶ Causing intense anxiety and paranoia at high dose
▶ Causing hyperthermia and agitation may be fatal

Nicotine (Figure 13-4)

Jean Nicot (1530–1600) was a French diplomat who brought tobacco from Brazil to France.

▶ The active ingredient of the plant *Nicotiana tabacum*, named after Jean Nicot
▶ Binds to nicotinic acetylcholine receptor, a multiunit ion-channel receptor
▶ Binding of nicotine to nicotinic receptor results in opening of sodium, potassium, and calcium channels
▶ Opening of sodium and potassium channels result in depolarization, which blocks neuronal conduction
▶ Opening of calcium channels causes influx of calcium, which in turn triggers intracellular cascades

Nicotine-related disorders

▶ Nicotine dependence
▶ Nicotine withdrawal
▶ Nicotine-related disorder not otherwise specified (NOS)

Opioids

▶ Natural opioids are alkaloids from the opium poppies
  ▷ Morphine
  ▷ Codeine
▶ Semisynthetic and synthetic opioids are alkaloids
  ▷ Heroin
  ▷ Oxycodone

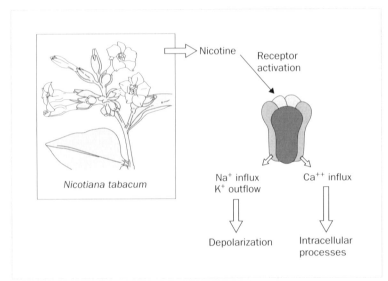

Figure 13–4 Nicotine acting mechanisms.

▷ Fentanyl
▷ Methadone
▶ Endogenous opioids are peptides
   ▷ Endorphins
   ▷ Enkephalins
   ▷ Dynorphins

Opiate dependence: epidemiology

▶ Most common comorbid substance – alcohol, benzodiazepines, cocaine
▶ Eighty to ninety percent carry a life-time psychiatric disorder
▶ Major depression disorder (MDD) and antisocial personality disorder (ASPD) are the two most common comorbid psychiatric disorders
▶ Children and adolescents with conduct disorder are at greater risk of developing substance abuse problems

Opioid detoxification in pregnant women

▶ Methadone maintenance until delivery, then detoxification

Opioid intoxication and withdrawal

▶ Intoxication
   ▷ Nervous – drowsiness, slurred speech, impaired memory and attention; severe intoxication – miosis – pinpoint pupils, seizure, coma
   ▷ Respiratory – pulmonary edema, central respiratory depression
   ▷ Cardiovascular – hypotension
   ▷ With or without perceptual disturbance – illusions and hallucinations
▶ Withdrawal
   ▷ Pupillary dilation
   ▷ Increased secretion – nausea, vomiting, diarrhea, lacrimation, rhinorrhea

▷ Muscle aches
▷ Other – yawning, insomnia, fever

Opioid receptors (Figure 13-5)

▶ Opioid receptors
   ▷ G-protein associated receptors, all with the characteristic seven transmembrane domains
   ▷ Subtypes – δ, κ, μ, ε
▶ Locations
   ▷ Periaqueductal gray matter
   ▷ Spinal cord
   ▷ Peripheral nerves
   ▷ Adrenal medulla
   ▷ Digestive tract

Opioid withdrawal during pregnancy

▶ Acute opioid withdrawal may cause
   ▷ Fetal withdrawal seizure
   ▷ Premature labor
▶ Methadone is recommended in preventing acute withdrawal
▶ Phenobarbital may be used for fetal seizure

PCP: signs and symptoms of intoxication

▶ Ataxia
▶ Diminished pain response

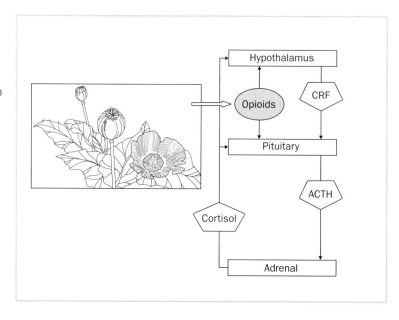

Figure 13-5 The involvement of endogenous opioids in stress regulation. Inlet – the Opium poppy, *Papaver somniferum*, is an annual herb. Opium is the solidified juice from the milky sap of the unripe Ned fruit capsule. ACTH, adrenocorticotropic hormone; CRF, corticotrophin-releasing factor.

▶ Dysarthria
▶ Hypertension
▶ Increased sensitivity to sound (hyperacusis)
▶ Nystagmus
▶ Rigidity
▶ Seizures
▶ Tachycardia
▶ Coma

PCP: receptor mechanism

▶ PCP binds to *N*-methyl-D-aspartate (NMDA) subtype of glutamate receptors
▶ The binding site is probably located in the ion channel
▶ The binding of PCP to NMDA receptor may block the calcium channel hence the calcium influx to the neuron

PCP intoxication: treatment

▶ Benzodiazepines
▶ Antipsychotics, however, avoid drugs with high anticholinergic effect – may cause anticholinergic crisis
▶ Nonstimulating environment
▶ Talk-down is NOT effective (talk-down is used for hallucinogen intoxication)
▶ Acidification of urine

Substance-specific symptoms

▶ Conjunctival injection – cannabis intoxication
▶ Diplopia – inhalant intoxication
▶ Hyperacusis – PCP intoxication
▶ Lacrimation – opioid withdrawal
▶ Piloerection – opioid withdrawal
▶ Pupillary constriction – opioid intoxication
▶ Rhinorrhea – opioid withdrawal
▶ Yawning – opioid withdrawal

14 Psychotic Disorders

The world of psychiatry started from the medical concern of "psyche" – the mind, soul, or spirit in its Greek roots. The only syndrome in psychiatry that remains a linguistic link to psyche, psychosis is one of the most intriguing phenomena of human mind, the most impairing mental deficiencies, and the primary topic of psychiatric research.

The clinical features of psychosis are centered in the impairment of reality test. Psychotic symptoms include disorganized thought, disturbing behavior, and, most memorably, the formation of hallucinations and delusions, which are often peculiar and bizarre.

The DSM-IV-TR allows nine diagnoses of psychotic disorders

▶ Schizophrenia
▶ Schizophreniform disorder
▶ Schizoaffective disorder
▶ Delusional disorder
▶ Brief psychotic disorder
▶ Shared psychotic disorder
▶ Psychotic disorder due to general medical condition
▶ Substance-induced psychotic disorder
▶ Psychotic disorder not otherwise specified (NOS)

The diagnosis of psychosis relies on clinical assessment and exclusion of general medical conditions that may also cause psychotic symptoms. Neurological abnormalities have been reported, primarily in limbic system, basal ganglia, and thalamus; however, these changes are not significant enough to have diagnostic value. Schizophrenia is considered by many the prototype of psychotic disorders, and is subjected to extensive research. The etiology of schizophrenia is not yet completely unveiled. Accumulated evidence traces down the contributing factors of both genetic and environmental nature. Regarding the nature of the process of the disease, there seems to be more evidence to support the assumption of neurodegenerative than neurodevelopmental. Schizophrenia may also be the manifestation of more than one disease process.

Antipsychotic medication is the mainstay of treatment. Electroconvulsive therapy is an alternative option for acute schizophrenia with marked positive symptoms, specific population (such as pregnant women and those who cannot tolerate pharmacotherapy), and those who failed pharmacologic treatment. Psychotherapy and social support, when properly combined with medication, have significant impact on long-term prognosis, particularly the preservation of social functioning.

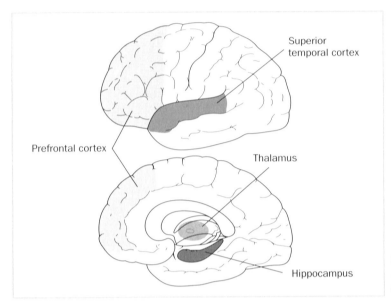

Figure 14–1 Areas of volume reduced in patients with schizophrenia.

Brain volume reduction in schizophrenia (Figure 14–1)

▶ Reduced volume in
  ▷ Prefrontal cortex
  ▷ Thalamus
  ▷ Hippocampus
  ▷ Superior temporal cortex
▶ Presumably result from reduced density of the axons, dendrites, and synapses

Brain volume increase in schizophrenia

▶ Increased volume in
  ▷ Lateral and third ventricles
  ▷ Basal ganglia (only in patients treated with neuroleptics)

Brief psychotic disorder

▶ Same symptoms as schizophrenia
▶ Duration at least 1 day but less than 1 month
▶ Return to baseline function after episode resolves

Delusional disorder

▶ Nonbizarre delusions for at least 1 month
▶ Relative preservation of function
▶ Never met symptomatic criteria for schizophrenia
▶ May have olfactory and tactile hallucinations congruent with delusional theme

- ▶ Subtypes
  - ▷ Erotomanic
  - ▷ Grandiose
  - ▷ Jealous
  - ▷ Persecutory
  - ▷ Somatic
  - ▷ Mixed
  - ▷ Unspecified

Dementia precox

Emil Kraepelin (1856–1926) was a German psychiatrist.
Eugen Bleuler (1857–1939) was a Swiss psychiatrist.

- ▶ The old term for the disease known today as schizophrenia
- ▶ Kraepelin translated a French term "démence précoce" into German "dementia precox"
- ▶ The term emphasized the deterioration in cognition and early onset of the disorder
- ▶ Kraepelin distinguished dementia precox from "manic-depressive psychosis," which has distinct episodes of illness alternating with periods of normal functioning; the latter is resembled most closely by what is now called bipolar disorder
- ▶ Bleuler coined the term schizophrenia, which had replaced dementia precox in the literature since 1920s

Diagnostic criteria for schizophrenia

- ▶ Two or more active symptoms for at least 1 month
  - ▷ Delusions
  - ▷ Hallucinations
  - ▷ Disorganized speech
  - ▷ Disorganized behavior
  - ▷ Negative symptom
- ▶ Only one symptom would be enough for making diagnosis if
  - ▷ Voices with running commentary on the individual's physical or mental activity, or voices conversing with each other
  - ▷ Bizarre delusions
- ▶ Continuous signs of disturbance for at least 6 months
- ▶ Impaired social/occupational function
- ▶ Rule out
  - ▷ Other mental disorders – schizoaffective, mood, and substance-related disorders
  - ▷ Medical etiologies

Dopamine hypothesis

- ▶ A hypothesis of the etiology of schizophrenia, which states the disease results from too much dopaminergic activity
- ▶ The theory evolved from two observations
  - ▷ The efficacy of antipsychotics is correlated with their antagonistic binding to dopamine type 2 (D2) receptor
  - ▷ Agents that increase dopaminergic activity, such as cocaine and amphetamine, are psychotomimetic

Dopamine type 2 receptor: locations of increased density

▶ In individuals with schizophrenia, dopamine D2 receptor density may be increased in
   ▷ Striatum
   ▷ Nucleus accumbens

Epidemiology of schizophrenia

▶ Prevalence: 1%
▶ Male:female = 1:1
▶ Age of onset
   ▷ Males 15–25 years
   ▷ Female 25–35 years
▶ More likely to be born in winter or early spring
▶ Drift assumption – the higher incidence of schizophrenia among the urban poor was believed due to economic drift of chronically disabled toward urban areas
▶ Season of birth – the higher prevalence of schizophrenia among those born in the spring and early winter led to the assumption of exposure to seasonal infections

Evoked potentials P300

▶ A positive evoked potential wave that occurs 300 ms after a sensory stimulus
▶ The structural source is likely in the limbic system
▶ In schizophrenic patients, the P300 appears smaller and later than normal controls
▶ First-degree relatives may have similar defect

Evoked potential P50

▶ In normal controls, P50 waveforms decreases after the first of paired stimuli
▶ In patients with schizophrenia, the decrease is not seen
▶ This indicates impairment of gating auditory input
▶ Approximately half of first-degree relatives have this defect

Expressed emotion

▶ Refers to the emotion expressed among family members and the manner it is expressed
▶ Family's emotion to a person with schizophrenia may be expressed with
   ▷ Overt criticism
   ▷ Hostility
   ▷ Over involvement
▶ High level of expressed emotion is a risk factor to the relapse of schizophrenia

First-rank symptoms

Kurt Schneider (1887–1967) was a German psychiatrist.

▶ Described by Schneider as fundamental symptoms of schizophrenia
   ▷ Audible thoughts (auditorization)
   ▷ Voices arguing or discussing
   ▷ Voices commenting
   ▷ Somatic passivity experiences

▷ Thought withdrawal
▷ Thought broadcasting
▷ Delusional perceptions
▷ Volition, made affects, and made impulses
▶ However, according to Schneider, the diagnosis of schizophrenia can be made with only second-rank symptoms, which include
▷ Non–first-rank hallucinations
▷ Delusions
▷ Perplexity
▷ Emotional impoverishment

Freud's formulation of schizophrenia

▶ Fixation – developmental fixations produce defects in ego development
▶ Regression – ego disintegration represents a regression to the time when the ego was not yet established
▶ Intrapsychic conflict from the developmental fixations and the ego regression result in
▷ Withdrawal of cathexis (psychic charged attention) from the environment
▷ Reconstruction of reality (delusions and hallucinations)

Gamma-aminobutyric acid (GABA) in the pathophysiology of schizophrenia

▶ Loss of GABAergic neurons in the hippocampus was found in schizophrenic patients
▶ GABA is involved in dopamine regulation
▶ Suppression of GABA activity may lead to hyperactivity of dopaminergic neurons

Genetics of schizophrenia

▶ One schizophrenic parent – 12% chance in offspring
▶ Two schizophrenic parents – 40% chance in offspring
▶ Monozygotic twins – 47% concordance
▶ Dizygotic twins – 12% concordance
▶ Nontwin affected sibling – 8% in other siblings

Glutamate receptors: locations of increased density (Figure 14–2)

▶ In patients with schizophrenia, glutamate receptors were found increased in areas of the brain
▷ Frontal cortex
▷ Hippocampus

Glycine treatment for schizophrenia

▶ Glycine is an amino acid neurotransmitter
▶ It has a binding site on N-methyl-D-aspartate (NMDA) type of glutamate receptor
▶ Binding of glycine may enhance glutamate binding and downstream effect
▶ Glycine, when coadministered with antipsychotics, was found to improve both positive and negative symptoms, and cognitive function

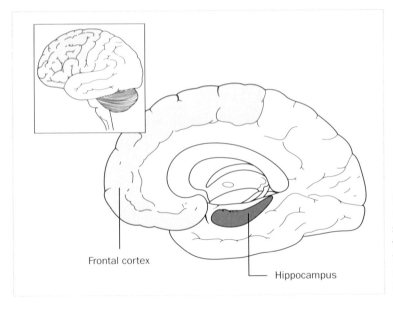

Figure 14-2 Areas of glutamate receptor increased in patients with schizophrenia. Medium cut of brain with brainstem removed; shows frontal cortex and hippocampus areas. The inlet shows the frontal lobe.

Frontal cortex

Hippocampus

Late-onset schizophrenia

▶ Schizophrenia with an onset after age 45
▶ Appears more frequently in women
▶ Often with predominant paranoid symptoms
▶ Responds well to medication
▶ The prognosis is favorable

Limbic system changes in schizophrenia

▶ Decrease in the size of the amygdala, the hippocampus, and the parahippocampal gyrus
▶ Abnormal glutamate transmission in hippocampus
▶ Disorganization of the neurons within the hippocampus

Mahler's formulation of schizophrenia

▶ Distortions in the reciprocal relationship between the infant and the mother, leading to persistent symbiosis
▶ The child is unable to separate from, or is dependent upon, the mother–child relationship
▶ As a result, the person's identity is not secured

Negative symptoms of schizophrenia

▶ Affective flattening
▶ Decreased spontaneous movements
▶ Alogia (poverty of speech)
▶ Avolition (poverty of activity)
▶ Anhedonia
▶ Attentional deficits

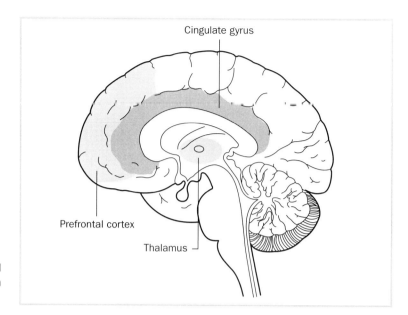

Figure 14–3 Areas of reduced neuronal density in patients with schizophrenia.

Neuronal density: reduction in schizophrenia (Figure 14–3)

▶ Among individuals with schizophrenia, reduced neuronal density was found in the following areas
  ▷ Prefrontal cortex
  ▷ Thalamus
  ▷ Cingulate gyrus

Paraphrenia

▶ A term refers to one of the following
  ▷ Paranoid schizophrenia
  ▷ Schizophrenia with progressively deteriorating course
  ▷ Schizophrenia with a well-systemized delusional system
▶ No longer a preferred term due to being ineffectual in scientific communication

Perinatal risks of developing schizophrenia

▶ Perinatal anoxia
▶ Birth trauma
▶ Second trimester viral infection
▶ Rhesus factor (Rh) incompatibility
▶ Maternal diabetes
▶ Maternal preeclampsia

Positive symptoms

▶ Formal thought disorder
▶ Hallucinations

▶ Bizarre behavior
▶ Delusions
▶ Catatonia

Postpartum psychosis

▶ Prevalence: 1%–2%
▶ Risk of infanticide: 4%
▶ Risk factors
  ▷ History of postpartum psychosis
  ▷ History of bipolar disorders
  ▷ Nonpsychiatric perinatal complications
▶ Medical etiologies
  ▷ Cushing's syndrome
  ▷ Infections
  ▷ Toxemia
  ▷ Medication induced
▶ Treatment
  ▷ Symptom oriented psychotropics
  ▷ Often requires hospitalization

Prognosis of schizophrenia: good prognostic indicators

▶ Female
▶ Later age of onset
▶ Married status
▶ Negative family history of schizophrenia
▶ Absence of perinatal complications
▶ Acute onset
▶ Predominance of positive symptoms
▶ Obvious precipitating factors
▶ Affective symptoms
▶ Confusion or other organic symptoms
▶ Paranoid subtype
▶ Family history of affective disorder
▶ Good premorbid functioning
▶ High intelligence quotient (IQ)

Prognosis of schizophrenia: poor prognostic indicators

▶ Male
▶ Younger age of onset
▶ Never married
▶ Family history of schizophrenia
▶ History of perinatal complications
▶ High expressed emotion
▶ Insidious onset
▶ Negative symptoms
▶ No precipitating factors
▶ Absence of affective symptoms

▶ Clear sensorium
▶ Comorbid substance use
▶ Longer duration of untreated illness

Prognosis of schizophrenia: statistics

▶ In 5–10 year follow-ups after the first psychiatric hospitalization
  ▷ Good outcome with minimal symptoms and near normal functioning: 10%–20%
  ▷ Continue to have moderate symptoms: 20%–30%
  ▷ Poor outcome with repeated hospitalizations: over 50%

Psychoanalytical treatment for psychotic disorders

▶ Long-term follow-up studies show that patients with frank psychotic episodes do not benefit from exploratory/interpretive therapy
▶ Those patients who are able to reintegrate into their lives after an acute psychotic experience may benefit from some insight-oriented approaches

Schizophrenia in females

▶ Later age of onset
▶ Better course than males
▶ Same lifetime prevalence as males

Schizophreniform disorder

▶ Meets symptom requirement for schizophrenia, but not the duration requirement
▶ The total duration of the combination of prodromal phase, active phase, and residual phase is at least 1 month but less than 6 months
▶ Return to baseline function after episode resolves

Schizophrenic reaction

Adolf Meyer (1866–1950) was a U.S. psychiatrist.

▶ A nomenclature of 1950s, referring to schizophrenia
▶ According to Adolf Meyer's view of psychobiology, schizophrenia was a maladaptive reaction to stresses; the condition results from personality dysfunction rather than brain pathology

Smooth pursuit eye movements

▶ Abnormalities of smooth pursuit eye movement is seen in
  ▷ Fifty to eighty-five percent of schizophrenics
  ▷ First-degree relatives of schizophrenic probands
  ▷ People with schizotypal personality disorder
▶ It is independent of drug treatment or clinical status

Sociocultural factors in schizophrenia

▶ Cities vs. rural communities
  ▷ Incidence twice as high in cities
▶ Developed countries vs. underdeveloped countries
  ▷ Prevalence higher in developed countries
  ▷ Course of illness and prognosis are more benign in underdeveloped countries
▶ Prevalence higher in recent immigrants
▶ In industrialized countries, there is a disproportionate prevalence of schizophrenia in low socioeconomic status groups (downward drift hypothesis)

15 Mood Disorders

In his ground-breaking work that set the foundation of scientific psychiatry, Emil Kraepelin grouped mental diseases based on classification of not only common symptoms but also longitudinal courses. He divided insanity or psychosis into two major categories: dementia precox and manic-depression. The latter, as seen today as the combination of all mood disorders, is characterized by prominent mood symptoms, and relatively normal period between symptomatic episodes. Psychotic symptoms may appear during episodes of mood disturbance; however, it should not be the dominating feature and should not appear during periods of normal mood.

This group of diseases was previously called "affective disorders." The term "mood disorders," however, is preferred today. "Mood disorders" refers to disturbance in sustained emotional states rather than external expression of the present emotional state. The DSM-IV-TR provides definition of four types of mood episodes: major depressive episode, manic episode, hypomanic episode, and mixed episode. On the basis of the combination of episodes, longitudinal courses, and the severity of functioning impairment, DSM-IV-TR categorized 10 mood disorders

▶ Major depressive disorder
▶ Dysthymic disorder
▶ Depressive disorder not otherwise specified (NOS)
▶ Bipolar I disorder
▶ Bipolar II disorder
▶ Cyclothymic disorder
▶ Bipolar disorder NOS
▶ Mood disorder due to general medical condition
▶ Substance-induced mood disorder
▶ Mood disorder NOS

The etiology of mood disorders is a complex interplay of multiple factors. Current research has led to the assumption of the existence of an inherited predisposition or susceptibility to the disease. It is associated with functional disturbance in several neurotransmitter systems, in particular, the norepinephrine, serotonin, dopamine, and gamma-amino butyric acid (GABA) systems. Hormonal dysregulation and sleep disturbance are also implicated in the etiology of mood disorders. There are evidences, which implied that genetic, environmental, and psychosocial factors all played crucial roles in the etiology.

Treatment for mood disorders, in accordance to the complexity of etiology, demands the collective strength of a variety of resources, a combination of methodology, and often collaboration of multiple healing professionals.

Atypical depression

▶ Accepted by DSM-IV-TR as a specifier for major depressive disorder, bipolar I and II disorders, and dysthymic disorder
▶ Younger age of onset
▶ More frequent, coexisting with panic disorder, substance-related problems, and somatic symptoms
▶ Clinical features
   ▷ Mood reactivity (as compared to usual depression's lack of response to positive events)
   ▷ Overeating
   ▷ Oversleeping
   ▷ Leaden paralysis
   ▷ Sensitivity to interpersonal rejection
▶ Treatment
   ▷ More likely to respond to monoamine oxidase inhibitors (MAOI)s

Bipolar disorder with rapid cycling

▶ In DSM-IV-TR, rapid cycling is one of the two longitudinal specifiers (another one is with seasonal pattern) for bipolar I and II disorders
▶ Four or more mood episodes in a year
▶ More common in females
▶ Not an inherited pattern
▶ Possible comorbidities
   ▷ Medical conditions
   ▷ Substance-related disorders
▶ Treatment
   ▷ Taper any antidepressants
   ▷ First line is lithium or valproate
   ▷ Lamotrigine is an alternative
   ▷ Often needs combination treatment

Bipolar mania in elderly

▶ Usually relapses from previously diagnosed bipolar
▶ New onset mania is uncommon, requires medical evaluation
▶ Possible precipitants
   ▷ Stroke
   ▷ Thyroid disturbance
   ▷ Vitamin B12 deficiency
   ▷ Corticosteroids
   ▷ Stimulants
   ▷ Dementia
▶ Treatment
   ▷ Same as for younger populations, but with cautious dosing
▶ Caution for valproate
   ▷ Highly protein bound
   ▷ At tested therapeutic level may still be clinically toxic because of depleted albumin in elderly

Brain imaging studies in mood disorders

▶ Subcortical regions – increased frequency of abnormal hyperintensities
  ▷ Seen in depression, bipolar I disorder, and elderly
  ▷ Assumed to be caused by deleterious neurodegenerative effects of recurrent affective episodes
▶ Also were reported in depressive disorders
  ▷ Ventricular enlargement
  ▷ Cortical atrophy
  ▷ Reduced hippocampal and caudate nucleus volumes
▶ Regional metabolism and blood flow associated with mood episodes
  ▷ Depression – left hemisphere reduction; decreased anterior brain metabolism on the life side and relatively increased nondominant hemispheric activity
  ▷ Mania – right hemisphere reductions
  ▷ Antidepressants may partially normalize these changes

Comorbidity in mood disorders

▶ Anxiety disorders: 70%
▶ Alcohol related disorders: 30%–60%

Cyclothymic disorder

▶ A bipolar disorder that is less severe than bipolar I or bipolar II disorders
▶ Recurrent episodes of hypomania and minor depression (depressive symptoms that are not severe enough to meet criteria for major depressive episode)
▶ For at least 2 years, the patient had not been continuously symptom-free for more than 2 months

Depression in older population

▶ Depression is more common in older people than in the general population
▶ Depression in older people is underdiagnosed and undertreated
▶ Correlated factors
  ▷ Low socioeconomic status
  ▷ Loss of a spouse
  ▷ Physical illness
  ▷ Social isolation

Depressive disorder not otherwise specified

▶ Diagnosis
  ▷ DSM-IV-TR allows this diagnosis on conditions that do not meet any specific depression criteria but clinically believed to be a depressive disorder
▶ Examples
  ▷ Premenstrual dysphoric disorder
  ▷ Minor depressive disorder
  ▷ Recurrent brief depressive disorder
  ▷ Postpsychotic depressive disorder

Dexamethasone suppression test

▶ Severe stress may be associated with malfunction of the hypothalamic-adrenal-pituitary axis
▶ Dexamethasone suppression test (DST) may help to confirm the diagnosis of depressive disorders, and follow the response to treatment
▶ Procedure
  ▷ Day 1 – give 1 mg of dexamethasone PO at 11 p.m.
  ▷ Day 2 – measure plasma cortisol at 8 a.m., 4 p.m., and 11 p.m.
▶ Plasma cortisol above 5 mcg/dL at any point is considered abnormal (nonsupressive, or positive)
▶ Rarely used today in psychiatry because of varying reports of sensitivity and specificity

Double depression

▶ Major depressive disorder superimposed on dysthymic disorder
▶ Prevalence – approximately 40% of patients with major depressive disorder
▶ Poor prognosis than those without dysthymia
▶ Chronic functional impairment even with resolution of major depressive episode

Duration of depressive episodes

▶ Untreated depressive episode – 6–13 months
▶ Treated depressive episode – 3 months; the withdrawal of antidepressant treatment before 3 months has elapsed and bears great risk of relapse

Dysthymic disorder

▶ A depressive disorder less severe than major depressive disorder
▶ Chronic depressive symptoms, which are not severe enough to fit the diagnosis of major depressive episode
▶ Lasted at least 2 years

Endocrinological changes in depression

▶ Pituitary size is often enlarged
▶ Cortisol
  ▷ Hypercortisolemia appears in approximately 50% of depressed patients
▶ Thyroid hormone
  ▷ Thyroid disturbances are found in approximately 10% of patients with depression
▶ Growth hormone
  ▷ Depressed patients have a blunted growth hormone release upon stimulation by either sleep or clonidine
▶ Somatostatin
  ▷ Cerebrospinal fluid (CSF) somatostatin levels are lower in depressed patients and higher in manic

Epidemiology of bipolar disorders

▶ Lifetime prevalence: 1%
▶ Annual incidence: <1%
▶ Female:male = 1:1
▶ Age of onset: 5–50 years, mean 30 years

Epidemiology of major depression

▶ Lifetime prevalence: 17%
▶ Annual incidence: 1.6%
▶ Female:male = 2:1
▶ No ethnic differences
▶ Prevalence higher in rural areas
▶ Age of onset: 20–50 years, mean 40 years

Genetics of bipolar disorders

▶ Parental genetics
  ▷ One affected parent: 25% chance in children
  ▷ Two affected parents: 50%–75% in children
▶ Estimated contributing power (nature vs. nurture)
  ▷ Genes: 50%–70%
  ▷ Environment or other noninheritable factors: 30%–50%
▶ Concordance rate from twin studies
  ▷ Monozygotic: 70%–90%
  ▷ Same-sex dizygotic: 16%–35%
▶ Genetic linkage
  ▷ Chromosome 18q – bipolar II
  ▷ Chromosome 22q

Mania

From Greek; insanity, madness, rage

▶ An emotional status characterized with
  ▷ Inflated self-esteem
  ▷ Increased energy and decreased need for sleep
  ▷ Easy to be distracted
  ▷ Over involvement in pleasurable behavior
▶ Manic episode
  ▷ Elevated, expansive, or irritable mood
  ▷ May have psychotic features
  ▷ Lasted for at least 1 week, or less if severe enough to be hospitalized
▶ Hypomanic episode
  ▷ Similar to manic episode but less severe in symptoms
  ▷ Lasted at least 4 days
  ▷ No psychotic features
  ▷ No significant functional impairment

Norepinephrine in mood disorders

▶ Down regulation of postsynaptic β-adrenergic receptors is correlated with positive responses to antidepressant treatment

▶ Increased sensitivity of presynaptic $β_2$-receptors among depressed patients; activation of presynaptic $β_2$-receptors results in decreased release of both norepinephrine and serotonin

Postpartum blues

▶ A mild form of dysphoria
▶ Benign and self-limited
▶ Prevalence: 30%–70%
▶ Peaks in 4–5 days postpartum
▶ Usually resolves by 10 days postpartum

Postpartum depression

▶ Prevalence: 10%–20%
▶ Recurrence: 50%–60%
▶ Onset usually within 1 month, but may occur up to 12 months postpartum
▶ Increased risk if there is history of major depressive disorder
▶ Treatment – consider electroconvulsive therapy (ECT), particularly if complicated by psychosis or suicidality

Pseudodementia

▶ Elderly patients with depression may present with cognitive symptoms and appear as if demented
▶ True dementia takes a deteriorating course while depression is a reversible condition
▶ Depression
    ▷ Relatively quick onset
    ▷ Lack of motivation to answer questions
    ▷ Memory may be improved by coaching and encouragement
    ▷ Diurnal variation in the cognitive symptoms
▶ Dementia
    ▷ Gradual and subtle onset
    ▷ Motivated and may confabulate during interview
    ▷ Memory is not improved by coaching and encouragement
    ▷ Cognitive deficiency has no diurnal variation

Psychodynamic view of depression

Karl Abraham (1877–1925) was a German psychoanalyst.
Edward Bibring (1895–1959) was an Australian psychoanalyst.
Silvano Arieti (1914–1981) was an Italian-born U.S. psychiatrist.

▶ Classic view of depression defined by Sigmund Freud, supported by Karl Abraham and Melanie Klein
    ▷ Childhood predisposition – oral phase difficulty in the infant–mother relationship predisposes to depression

▷ Loss – real or imagined
▷ Introjection – a defense mechanism to deal with the loss
▷ Expression of anger – anger toward the loved one or the loss is expressed as aggression inward at the self
▶ Edward Bibring
▷ Depression may be caused by the discrepancy between goals and the inability to meet goals
▶ Silvano Arieti
▷ The concept of "the dominant other" – many people lived their lives for a principle, an idea, or another person, that were collectively called the dominant other
▷ Depression is associated with the realization of the inability to meet the expectations of the dominant other
▶ Heinz Kohut
▷ Depression as loss of self-esteem, which normally should be given by parents during childhood
▶ John Bowlby
▷ Depression is predisposed to by damaged attachments and traumatic separation in childhood

Psychodynamic factors in mania

▶ Defensive reaction against depression
▶ Intolerable self-criticism from superego may be replaced by euphoric self-satisfaction
▶ Overwhelmed reaction by pleasurable impulses

Serotonin in mood disorders

▶ Depletion of serotonin may precipitate depression
▶ Suicidal patients may have low CSF concentration of serotonin metabolite
▶ Low concentrations of serotonin uptake sites on platelets may be associated with depression and suicide

Sleep disturbance in depression

▶ Delayed sleep onset
▶ Shortened rapid eye movement latency (rapid eye movement [REM] latency)
▶ A longer first REM period
▶ Abnormal delta sleep

Treatment for bipolar depression

▶ First line
▷ Lithium and/or lamotrigine
▶ Alternative
▷ Lithium and an antidepressant
▶ Severe episodes
▷ Consider ECT
▶ Nonresponders
▷ Bupropion
▷ Serotonin-specific reuptake inhibitors (SSRIs)

▷ Serotonin-norepinephrine reuptake inhibitor (SNRIs)
▷ MAOIs
▶ Adjunctive psychotherapy
▷ Cognitive behavior therapy (CBT)
▷ Interpersonal psychotherapy (IPT)
▶ Psychotic features
▷ First line is ECT
▷ May add adjunctive antipsychotics

Treatment for manic or mixed episodes

▶ First line
▷ Lithium
▷ Valproate
▶ Severe episodes
▷ Combine with an antipsychotic, preferably atypical, for more severe episodes or with psychotic features
▶ Alternatives
▷ Carbamazepine or oxcarbazepine are acceptable alternatives
▶ Adjunctive short-term benzodiazepine
▶ For break through episodes, add another first line agent
▶ Refractory cases
▷ Clozapine
▷ ECT

Treatment of bipolar disorders: maintenance

▶ Best supported by evidence
▷ Lithium
▷ Valproate
▶ Alternatives
▷ Lamotrigine
▷ Carbamazepine
▷ ECT
▶ Antipsychotics – need periodical reassessment
▶ Discontinuation of treatment – need to weigh benefit and risk, need periodical reassessment
▶ Psychosocial therapies
▶ Breakthrough episodes – add another maintenance medication

Treatment of depression: factors associated with inadequate response

▶ Inadequate dose/duration of treatment
▶ Medical illness
▶ Poor compliance
▶ Psychosocial issues
▶ Psychotic symptoms
▶ Substance abuse
▶ Undiagnosed bipolar disorders

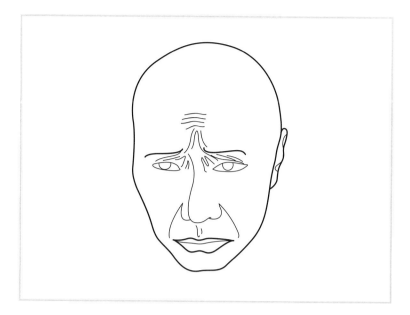

Figure 15–1 Veraguth's fold.

Veraguth's fold (Figure 15–1)

Otto Veraguth (1870–1944) was a Swiss neuropsychiatrist.

▶ A triangle-shaped skin fold that runs obliquely from the lower outside to the upper inside on the upper eyelid

▶ Described by Otto Veraguth, and assumed to be characteristic for depression

16 Anxiety Disorders

Anxiety disorders as a group have the highest prevalence among all the mental disorders. Anxiety is the feeling of fear and apprehension. The fear is usually regarding unsure future events and situations that are potentially stressful or painful. The etymologic connection between "anxiety" and "anger" further implies underlying feeling of hostility. Clinically, anxiety and anger often appear hand in hand, depicting the "fight or flight" response. The feared danger can be nonspecific and ubiquitous, or specific and predictable. It is often not the fear itself but the accompanied emotional disturbance, physical reaction, and behavior adaptation that are the most debilitating.

The complex interplay of biological and psychosocial elements is under continuous investigation. New treatment approaches have been invented, tested, and reported frequently. Its rich history and constantly growing knowledge rendered anxiety among the most fascinating conditions in psychiatry.

DSM-IV-TR allows 12 diagnoses in the category of anxiety disorders

▶ Panic disorder without agoraphobia
▶ Panic disorder with agoraphobia
▶ Agoraphobia without history of panic disorder
▶ Specific phobia
▶ Social phobia
▶ Obsessive-compulsive disorder
▶ Posttraumatic stress disorder (PTSD)
▶ Acute stress disorder
▶ Generalized anxiety disorder
▶ Anxiety disorder due to general medical condition
▶ Substance-induced anxiety disorder
▶ Anxiety disorder not otherwise specified (NOS)

Acute stress disorder

▶ Dissociative symptoms
  ▷ Numbing
  ▷ Reduction of awareness
  ▷ Derealization
  ▷ Depersonalization
  ▷ Dissociated amnesia
▶ Other symptoms similar to PTSD
▶ Symptoms last for 2 days to 4 weeks

Adenosine receptor and panic disorder

▶ Caffeine was known to bind to the adenosine 2A receptor and generate anxiety
▶ Single-nucleotide polymorphisms (SNPs) in DNA sequence in the *adenosine 2A receptor* gene were found with linkage to familial panic disorder
▶ The strength of the linkage increased when agoraphobia was included in the panic disorder phenotype

Agoraphobia

▶ Fear about being in a place where escape may be difficult
▶ With or without panic attacks
▶ Over 95% of individuals presenting with agoraphobia also have panic disorder
▶ Two to three times more frequent in women than men

Agoraphobia vs. specific phobia

▶ In agoraphobia, the focus of fear is the anxiety response
▶ In specific phobia, the focus of fear is the object

Generalized anxiety disorder: treatment

▶ Most effective treatment
  ▷ Combination of psychotherapeutic and psychopharmacological
▶ Psychotherapy
  ▷ Cognitive-behavioral therapy
  ▷ Supportive therapy
  ▷ Insight-oriented therapy
▶ Antidepressants
  ▷ Serotonin-specific reuptake inhibitors (SSRIs)
  ▷ Serotonin-norepinephrine reuptake inhibitors (SNRIs)
▶ Benzodiazepines
  ▷ Brief course in the initial stage for acute symptoms
▶ Buspirone

Neurophysiology of anxiety

▶ Stimulation of locus coeruleus, the major source of central norepinephrine, may generate panic attacks, while blockade of locus coeruleus decreases panic attacks
▶ Structures in the limbic system, particularly amygdale, mediate anxiety response
▶ Serotonin and neuropeptides are involved in modulating noradrenergic and gamma-amino butyric acid (GABA)ergic system
▶ GABAergic system – widely distributed with highest density at the limbic system; binding with benzodiazepines reduces anxiety

Obsession vs. compulsion

▶ Both are time consuming (over 1 hour per day)
▶ Both are repetitive and recognized by the patient to be excessive or unreasonable
▶ Both cause distressing

▶ Both are persistent – more than 6 months
▶ Obsession – intrusive thoughts, ideas, impulses, or images
▶ Compulsion – behaviors and mental acts targeting at reducing distress preventing dreaded event associated with obsession

Obsessive-compulsive disorder: epidemiology

▶ Lifetime prevalence 2.5%
▶ Gender – equal in adulthood, more common in boy than in girls
▶ Age of onset – male 6–15 years, female 20–29 years
▶ Genetics – higher concordance in monozygotic twins than in dizygotic
▶ Ten to twenty-five percent of cases are purely obsessiveness
▶ Comorbidity
  ▷ Major depression
  ▷ Tourette's disorder
  ▷ Learning disorders
  ▷ Disruptive behavioral disorders

Obsessive-compulsive disorder: treatment

▶ SSRI – high dose
▶ Clomipramine – first drug approved for obsessive-compulsive disorder (OCD)
▶ Most effective – combination of pharmacotherapy and behavioral therapy

Panic attack: clinical features

▶ Intense fear or discomfort reaches peak within 10 minutes
▶ At least 4 of 13 symptoms
  ▷ Mind – derealization/depersonalization, fear of losing control, and fear of dying
  ▷ Head – lightheaded/dizzy
  ▷ Neck – choking
  ▷ Chest – palpitation, shortness of breath, chest pain
  ▷ Abdomen – nausea
  ▷ Whole body – sweating, trembling, paresthesias, chills/hot flushes

Panic disorder

▶ Recurrent and unexpected panic attacks followed by at least one month of concern or worry related to future attacks
▶ Rule out substance use or general medical condition

Panic disorder: comorbid conditions

▶ Ninety percent of patients with panic disorder have another psychiatric condition
▶ Sixty percent comorbidity for major depressive disorder
▶ High comorbidity with other anxiety disorders and substance abuse
▶ Conditions of cardiology, respiratory, and neurology

Panic disorder: treatment

▶ SSRIs
  ▷ Preferred treatment
  ▷ Start with low dosage and titrate slowly
▶ Benzodiazepines
  ▷ Useful adjuncts to antidepressants
  ▷ Prolonged treatment can lead to tolerance, abuse, and disinhibition
▶ Tricyclic antidepressants (TCAs)
  ▷ Clomipramine and imipramine were supported by data
▶ Monoamine oxidase inhibitors (MAOIs)
  ▷ Effective but limited by the dietary restrictions
  ▷ Less likely to cause early activation
▶ Buspirone
  ▷ Effective for anxiety but not for panic disorder
▶ Cognitive-behavior therapy
  ▷ Alone or as an adjunct to pharmacotherapy
▶ β-blockers
  ▷ May be used as an adjunct

Phobia: epidemiology

▶ DSM-IV-TR categories – specific phobia and social phobia
▶ The combination of all forms of phobias (specific phobias and social phobia) is the single most common mental disorder, 10%–25% of population
▶ Specific phobia is the most common mental disorder order among women, twice as likely in females then males
▶ Lifetime prevalence
  ▷ Specific phobia: 11%
  ▷ Social phobia: 3%–13%

Phobia: treatment

▶ Specific phobia
  ▷ Behavioral therapy (desensitization and exposure)
  ▷ Benzodiazepines for temporary treatment
▶ Social phobia
  ▷ Cognitive-behavioral therapy
  ▷ SSRIs and other antidepressants except Bupropion
  ▷ Temporary treatment with benzodiazepines for less generalized and infrequently encountered phobic symptoms
▶ Performance anxiety (usually considered a form of social phobia)
  ▷ Adrenergic receptor antagonists, such as propranolol

Posttraumatic stress disorder: biological changes

▶ Physiological arousal after exposure to cues in individuals with PTSD – increase in heart rate, skin conduction, blood pressure, and electromyography (EMG) activity
▶ Increase in norepinephrine turnover in the locus coeruleus, limbic regions, and cerebral cortex

▶ Abnormalities of hypothalamus-pituitary-adrenal (HPA) axis
▶ Hyper-reactive in limbic/paralimbic structures – amygdala, hippocampus, anterior cingulated cortex.

Posttraumatic stress disorder: clinical features

▶ Exposure to traumatic stressors
▶ Reexperiencing – intrusive thoughts and perceptions
▶ Avoidance – avoidance of thoughts and situations, withdrawal, detachment
▶ Arousal – poor sleep, hypervigilance
▶ Acute PTSD – symptoms present for less than 3 months
▶ Chronic PTSD – symptoms for more than 3 months
▶ Delayed PTSD – onset delayed for more than 6 months following the stressor
▶ More common in
  ▷ Women
  ▷ Immigrants from areas with social unrest or combat
  ▷ Individuals reluctant to divulge symptoms (cultural consensus)

Posttraumatic stress disorder: comorbidity

▶ Depressive disorders
▶ Substance-related disorders
▶ Anxiety disorders
▶ Bipolar disorders
▶ Two-thirds of patients with PTSD suffer from two additional psychiatric disorders

Posttraumatic stress disorder: pharmacotherapy

▶ Combination of medication, psychotherapy, and education/supportive treatment
▶ SSRIs – first line supported by randomized trials
▶ TCAs – may be useful for male combat veterans
▶ Benzodiazepines – no evidence in efficacy against core symptoms; may worsen the outcome
▶ Antipsychotics – comorbid psychosis, augmentation for refractory core symptoms

Posttraumatic stress disorder: psychotherapies

▶ Cognitive-behavioral therapy – desensitization, relaxation
▶ Eye movement desensitization and reprocessing (EMDR)
▶ Psychodynamic therapy
▶ Psychological debriefing
▶ Psychoeducation

Posttraumatic stress disorder: stages

▶ Stage 1 – immediate response to traumas, 4–6 weeks
▶ Stage 2 – acute stage, helplessness, loss of control
▶ Stage 3 – chronic stage, demoralization, disability

Prevalence of anxiety disorders

▶ Anxiety disorders are the most prevalent psychiatric disorders; lifetime prevalence of any anxiety – 25%

▶ Among anxiety disorders, social phobia is the most prevalent, with simple phobia the close second; lifetime prevalence of social phobia and simple phobia: 11%–13%

▶ Lifetime prevalence of panic disorder, agoraphobia, and generalized anxiety disorder: 3%–5%

▶ First-degree relatives of patients with anxiety disorders have up to eight-fold risk for anxiety disorders

Primary anxiety disorders vs. organic anxiety syndrome

▶ Clinical factors associated with organic anxiety
  ▷ Onset of symptoms after the age of 35 years
  ▷ No anticipatory anxiety
  ▷ Lack of avoidance behavior
  ▷ Lack of personal or family history of anxiety disorders
  ▷ Poor response to anxiolytic agents
▶ Medical work-up focus on
  ▷ Endocrine dysfunction – pheochromocytoma, thyroid disturbance, hyper-parathyroidism
  ▷ Drug intoxication or withdrawal – caffeine, alcohol, benzodiazepines, cocaine, corticosteroids, sympathomimetics
  ▷ Hypoxia – cardiovascular, respiratory, or cerebral anoxia
  ▷ Electrolyte abnormalities, acidosis
  ▷ Temporal lobe seizures

17 Somatoform Disorders

Somatoform disorders are psychiatric conditions with manifestation of physical symptoms. The symptoms of somatoform disorders often suggest, on the surface, the existence of related general medical conditions. The diagnosis relies on findings of inconsistent connection between symptoms and the apparent medical conditions, negative medical work-up, and the underlying psychological conflict. Comorbidity with mood and anxiety disorders is high.

DSM-IV-TR recognizes seven somatoform disorders

- ▶ Somatization disorder
- ▶ Undifferentiated somatoform disorder
- ▶ Conversion disorder
- ▶ Pain disorder
- ▶ Hypochondriasis
- ▶ Body dysmorphic disorder
- ▶ Somatoform disorder not otherwise specified (NOS)

The challenge of treatment is the patient's resentment toward the suggestion of a psychological source of the physical symptoms. Unnecessary medical work-up and procedures are often difficult to avoid, and may cause worsening of the symptoms. The primary treatment role, in spite of the condition's psychiatric nature, is best assumed by a primary care physician.

Body dysmorphic disorder

- ▶ Formerly known as dysmorphophobia as described by Emil Kraepelin
- ▶ Preoccupation with an imagined or psychological exaggerated defect in appearance
- ▶ Causes clinically significant distress and impairment

Body dysmorphic disorder: treatment

- ▶ Reported useful pharmacotherapy
    - ▷ Tricyclic antidepressants
    - ▷ Monoamine oxidase inhibitors (MAOIs)
    - ▷ Pimozide (Orap)
    - ▷ Serotonin-specific reuptake inhibitors
    - ▷ Clomipramine (Tofranil)
- ▶ Augmentation
    - ▷ Buspirone (BuSpar)
    - ▷ Lithium (Eskalith)
    - ▷ Methylphenidate (Ritalin)
    - ▷ Antipsychotics

▶ Psychotherapy for coexisting mental disorders, particularly depression
▶ Medical procedures addressing the perceived defects are mostly unsuccessful
▶ Prognosis is guarded

Briquet's syndrome

Paul Briquet (1796–1881) was a French physician.

▶ The syndrome with symptoms involving multiple organs, chronic in course, yet no apparent physical causes
▶ The condition was referred as Briquet's syndrome, which was later renamed as somatization disorder

Conversion disorder

▶ Historical terms
  ▷ Hysteria
  ▷ Conversion reaction
  ▷ Dissociative reaction
▶ Symptoms affect voluntary motor or sensory functions
▶ Common symptoms
  ▷ Paralysis
  ▷ Blindness
  ▷ Mutism
  ▷ Pseudoseizure
  ▷ La Belle indifférence
▶ Clinically judged to be caused by psychological factors, often associated with psychological gain
▶ Symptoms are not intentionally produced
▶ Symptoms are not caused by substance use
▶ Symptoms are not limited to pain or sexual symptoms

Conversion disorder: treatment

▶ The most important issue of the therapy
  ▷ Therapeutic relationship between the patient and the therapist
▶ Interview with assistance of amobarbital or lorazepam may be helpful in obtaining information, but not always reliable
▶ Psychotherapy
  ▷ Insight-oriented supportive therapy
  ▷ Behavior therapy
  ▷ Brief psychotherapy
  ▷ Focus on stress and coping
▶ Hypnosis may be effective in some cases
▶ Anxiolytics may be effective in some cases
▶ Spontaneous resolution is not unusual

Hypochondriasis: course of the disease and prognosis

▶ The course is usually episodic with months to years of interims
▶ Episodes may be triggered by psychosocial stressors

▶ Prognosis – no well-conducted outcome studies have been reported; however, generally estimated as fair to good
▶ A good prognosis is associated with
  ▷ High socioeconomic status
  ▷ Treatment-responsive mood or anxiety disorders
  ▷ Sudden onset of symptoms
  ▷ Relatively adaptive personality
  ▷ The absence of a related general medical condition

Hypochondriasis: diagnosis

▶ For at least 6 months, the patient
  ▷ Is preoccupied with the concern of having a serious disease
  ▷ Misinterprets physical signs or sensations
▶ No findings from medical examinations reasonably support the concern
▶ Differential diagnoses
  ▷ Delusional disorder – if symptoms reach the intensity of a delusion
  ▷ Body dysmorphic disorder – if symptoms restricted to distress about appearance
▶ Causes emotional distress and functional impairment
▶ The patient may have poor insight

Hypochondriasis: epidemiology

▶ Reported 4%–15% inpatients visiting general medical clinic
▶ Prevalence is not affected by
  ▷ Gender
  ▷ Socioeconomic status
  ▷ Marital status
▶ Onset usually between 20 and 30 years of age
▶ Transient hypochondriacal complaints were reported in 3% of junior medical students

Hypochondriasis: theories of etiology

▶ The mainstay theory (DSM-IV-TR) – misinterpretation of physical symptoms
  ▷ Preoccupied with amplified somatic sensations
  ▷ Decreased tolerance of physical discomfort
  ▷ Misinterpret the meaning of the symptoms with a faulty cognitive scheme
▶ Social learning model – assumption of sick role to
  ▷ Avoid obligations
  ▷ Postpone challenges
  ▷ Be excused from usual duties
▶ A variant (somatizing) form of other mental disorders
  ▷ Depressive disorders
  ▷ Anxiety disorders
  ▷ Comorbidity of depressive or anxiety disorders reaches 80%
▶ The psychodynamic theory
  ▷ Defense mechanisms – repression, displacement, and undoing
  ▷ Repressed anger from past loss is expressed toward self – distress is transferred into physical complaints

▷ Repressed anger from past loss is expressed toward others – solicited help is rejected as ineffective

▷ Physical symptoms may also be used as a punishment for innate badness, such as perceived past wrongdoing, sense of guilt and sinfulness

Obsession de la honte du corps

▶ French – obsession with shame of the body
▶ Pierre Janet's term referring to body dysmorphic disorder

Pain disorder

▶ Diagnosis
  ▷ Pain – true and not feigned, and severe enough to warrant clinical attention
  ▷ Pain – functional impairment
  ▷ Pain – judged to be associated with psychological factors (e.g., unconscious stress or developmental trauma)
▶ Epidemiology
  ▷ Female:male = 2:1
  ▷ Age – fourth or fifth decade
▶ Comorbidity
  ▷ Depressive disorders
  ▷ Alcohol and other substance abuse
  ▷ Personality traits – dependent or histrionic
▶ Treatment
  ▷ Therapeutic alliance
  ▷ Antidepressant medications

Pseudocyesis

▶ Categorized in Somatoform Disorder NOS in DSM-IV-TR
▶ Rare condition in which a nonpregnant patient has the signs and symptoms of pregnancy, such as abdominal distention, breast enlargement, pigmentation, cessation of menses, and morning sickness

Pseudoseizure

▶ A symptom of conversion disorder
▶ Approximately one-third of cases have a coexisting seizure disorder
▶ Differentiation from seizure
  ▷ Tongue-biting, urinary incontinence, and injuries after falling are rare in pseudoseizure
  ▷ Pupillary and gag reflexes are intact after pseudoseizure, but suppressed after seizure
  ▷ Postictal prolactin elevation is not usually seen in pseudoseizure; however, other factors may cause elevated prolactin level, such as cocaine withdrawal and antipsychotic use

Somatization disorder vs. hypochondriasis

▶ Symptoms
  ▷ Hypochondriasis is about the concern of a disease
  ▷ Somatization disorder is about many symptoms
▶ Age of onset
  ▷ Somatization disorder has an onset before age 30
  ▷ Hypochondriasis has no specific age of onset
▶ Gender
  ▷ Somatization disorder is more common in women
  ▷ Hypochondriasis is not affected by gender

Somatization disorder: diagnosis

▶ Symptoms at any time during the course of the disease
  ▷ Four pain symptoms
  ▷ Two gastrointestinal symptoms
  ▷ One sexual symptom
  ▷ One pseudoneurological symptom
▶ No organic base for the symptoms, or excessive symptoms related to medical conditions
▶ Onset before 30 years
▶ Symptoms cause
  ▷ Treatment seeking or
  ▷ Functional impairment

Somatization disorder: psychopharmacological treatment

▶ No data supporting psychotropic treatment for somatization disorder
▶ Medicines are prescribed to treat the coexisting psychiatric conditions
▶ Due to the usually erratic pattern of medical compliance, medication should be closely monitored

Somatization disorder: psychotherapy

▶ Individual and group therapies
▶ Focus on
  ▷ Coping with physical symptoms
  ▷ Developing the appropriate ways of emotional expression
▶ Data showed 50% decrease in health-care expenditures for patients receiving psychotherapy

Somatoform disorders: principle of treatment

▶ One physician strategy
  ▷ Best to have a single identified physician as primary caretaker
▶ Regular visit
  ▷ Visits should be regularly scheduled, brief, and straightforward
▶ Medical work-up

▷ Once somatization disorder is diagnosed, additional tests and procedures should be avoided unless necessary

▷ It is a judgment call about what symptoms require work-up and to what extent

▶ Patient education

▷ The symptoms are not faked (differentiated from factitious disorder)

▷ Slowly and tactfully increase the patient's awareness of probable role of psychological factors

▶ Psychiatric consult

▷ Focus on distress and mood symptoms

▷ Suggestion of psychiatric consult in early stage may cause patient's resentment

18 Dissociative Disorders

Dissociation is one of the most controversial, yet poorly understood, conditions in psychiatry.

Dissociation refers to the disruption (or "split," in Pierre Janet's word) of the usually integrated consciousness. The symptoms of dissociation have been recorded from the time of antiquity. Many historical cases of spirit or demon possession seemed very much like dissociative disorders in modern eyes. In a mild level of severity, many people can consciously experience brief derealization and depersonalization. Severe dissociative symptoms are usually unconscious and pathological. Among the conditions with dissociation, the most dramatic is dissociative identity disorder, formerly termed multiple personality disorder. The claim that multiple minds can exist within one body had faced challenges from scientific researches due to short of empirical data. Rare in reality, the theatrical inlay of multiple personality disorder, along with other dissociative disorders, attracted waxing and waning public enthusiasm.

Over the past century, surmounting volume of literature has been published in the study of dissociative disorders. However, little conclusion was drawn from well-designed, controlled studies. Historically, dissociation was considered to be part of hysteria (somatoform disorders in DSM nomenclature) due to its lack of physical findings. In recent years, formation of dissociation has been attributed to traumatic experience in childhood. The theory of dissociation being a posttraumatic spectrum disorder has gained some acceptance. There are also neurobiological changes found in dissociative disorders.

DSM-IV-TR allows five diagnoses in the category of dissociative disorders

- ▶ Dissociative amnesia
- ▶ Depersonalization disorder
- ▶ Dissociative fugue
- ▶ Dissociative identity disorder
- ▶ Dissociative disorder not otherwise specified (NOS)

Betrayal trauma

Jennifer Freyd is a contemporary U.S. psychologist.

- ▶ A concept introduced by Jennifer Freyd in 1991
- ▶ Refers to the traumatic effect of being betrayed, i.e., violated by the people or institutions the individual depends on for survival
- ▶ Betrayal trauma is thought to cause dissociative amnesia toward childhood abuse experience, through blocking the painful memory from the mental mechanism of attachment

Depersonalization disorder

▶ Persistent or recurrent episodes of detachment or estrangement from one's self
▶ Reality testing is intact
▶ A rare disorder, more often occurs in women
▶ Episodes last from a few hours to a few weeks
▶ Treatment – treating accompanying psychiatric conditions; supportive psychotherapy

Dissociative amnesia

▶ Inability to recall important personal information that is usually of a traumatic nature
▶ Global or episodic
▶ A common short-term reaction in both genders
▶ Prevalence peaks in the third and fourth decades
▶ Recovery is usually quick and prognosis is usually benign

Dissociative fugue

▶ The rarest of the dissociative disorders
▶ Traveling away from place of daily activities
▶ Inability to recall relevant personal information
▶ The onset is usually sudden and unexpected
▶ Prevalence is more common during wartime or after natural disasters
▶ Most episodes last from a few days to a few months
▶ Treatment – restore memory through
　▷ Psychotherapy with free association
　▷ Hypnosis
　▷ Amytal interview
▶ Prognosis – varies; most episodes tend to resolve spontaneously, but some may become chronic and intractable

Dissociative identity disorder

▶ Formerly known as "multiple personality disorder"
▶ Two or more distinct personality states
▶ At least two of these identities periodically take control of the person's behavior; the mean number of personality states is 13
▶ Variable degree of amnesia for alternate personalities
▶ Coconsciousness – simultaneous experience of multiple personalities at the same time
▶ Common comorbid symptoms – depression, auditory hallucinations
▶ More common in women than in men
▶ Treatment – extended psychotherapy, may combine with psychopharmacologic treatments

Proposed etiology of dissociative disorders

▶ Internal conflicts
　▷ Ego's defense against painful experience

    ▷ Dissociative amnesia and dissociative fugue may serve as an unconscious escape from intolerable emotions

    ▷ The underlined emotion often results from unacceptable urges or impulses that are in conflict with the patient's conscience or ego ideals

▶ Traumatic experience

    ▷ History of traumatic experience is commonly seen in all forms of dissociation

    ▷ Traditional psychodynamic formulations have emphasized the disintegration of the ego or defense of ego, both associated with past trauma

    ▷ Military studies find that depersonalization and derealization are commonly evoked by stress and fatigue

    ▷ Dissociative identity disorder is particularly linked to early childhood trauma or maltreatment

    ▷ Endangering environment may lead to an altered state of consciousness dominated by a wish to flee, hence the fugue

▶ Neurobiological factors were found in depersonalization

▶ Complex partial seizure is also a proposed etiology in some cases

Neurobiological researches on dissociative disorders

▶ Depersonalization is primary dissociative symptom that has been found associated with neurobiological change

▶ Serotoninergic system

    ▷ Depersonalization appears in migraines and marijuana, and is often responsive to serotonin-selective reuptake inhibitors (SSRIs)

    ▷ Depletion of L-tryptophan, a serotonin precursor, can worsen the depersonalization symptoms

▶ Glutaminergic system

    ▷ Studies found involvement of the N-Methyl-D-aspartate (NMDA) receptor in the genesis of depersonalization symptoms

Recovered memory syndrome

▶ A syndrome of emotional stress associated with the process of recovering the memory of painful experience

    ▷ Usually under hypnosis or during psychotherapy

    ▷ Accompanied by the trauma appropriate, often strong, affective response (abreaction)

    ▷ May induce false memory

▶ Recovered memory therapy is a controversial form of psychotherapy focusing on facilitating memory recovery

Central concept of dissociation

▶ Disintegrated consciousness

▶ Alteration in perception

▶ Alteration in mood and impulse regulation

▶ Incongruent self-referential experience

Treatment for dissociative amnesia

▶ Psychotherapy
  ▷ Dynamic style with free association to help recover memory
  ▷ Cognitive therapy – to identify the specific cognitive distortions in the trauma
▶ Hypnosis
  ▷ Symptom modulation and containment
  ▷ Self-hypnosis may help crises outside of sessions
  ▷ Requires informed consent – controversial over the accuracy of recollection and impact on patient
▶ Somatic therapies
  ▷ Pharmacologically facilitated interviews – amobarbital, thiopental (Pentothal), benzodiazepines, and amphetamines

19 Sexual and Gender Identity Disorders

Human sexuality is a complicated phenomenon with convoluted science and myths. Besides its biological foundation, psychological and cultural influences are paramount. Many destructive, compulsive, and distressful sexual behaviors have been observed and recorded since ancient times. The pathology behind some of the sexual abnormalities is still not fully unveiled. Our understanding of paraphilia, in particular, is in large descriptive. For a long period in history, homosexuality was believed to be pathological. However, there has been no scientific evidence to support that view. The current consensus regarding homosexuality is that it is a preferred lifestyle belongs to a significant minority. The differentiation between sex and gender is yet another often misunderstood and misused concept. Gender identity disorder was previously referred to as transsexualism, though it concerns a broader sense of social behavior and self-perception rather than just a disturbance of sexual orientation.

DSM-IV-TR allows 23 diagnoses in the category of sexual and gender identity disorders

▶ Sexual desire disorders
　▷ Sexual aversion disorder
　▷ Hypoactive sexual desire disorder
▶ Sexual arousal disorders
　▷ Female sexual arousal disorder
　▷ Male erectile disorder
▶ Orgasmic disorders
　▷ Female orgasmic disorder
　▷ Male orgasmic disorder
　▷ Premature ejaculation
▶ Sexual pain disorders
　▷ Dyspareunia (not due to a general medical condition)
　▷ Vaginismus (not due to a general medical condition)
▶ Sexual disorder due to a general medical condition
▶ Substance-induced sexual dysfunction
▶ Paraphilias
　▷ Exhibitionism
　▷ Fetishism
　▷ Frotteurism
　▷ Pedophilia
　▷ Masochism
　▷ Sadism
　▷ Transvestic fetishism
　▷ Voyeurism
　▷ Paraphilia not otherwise specified (NOS)

- ▶ Sexual disorder NOS
- ▶ Gender identity disorders
  - ▷ Gender identity disorder in children
  - ▷ Gender identity disorder in adolescents or adults

Dyspareunia

- ▶ A sexual pain disorder
- ▶ Physical pain in sexual intercourse
- ▶ Usually emotionally caused
- ▶ More common in females than in males
- ▶ Physical causes
  - ▷ Cystitis
  - ▷ Urethritis
  - ▷ Other medical conditions

Exhibitionism

- ▶ Recurrent fantasies and/or actions of exposing genitals to unsuspecting strangers
- ▶ Six month duration, with marked distress and/or interpersonal difficulty

Female orgasmic disorder

- ▶ Lack of orgasm though with normal sexual excitement phase
- ▶ Diagnosis is based on the clinician's judgment considering the facts of age, sexual experience, and the adequacy of sexual stimulation

Female sexual arousal disorder

- ▶ Inability to reach or maintain adequate physical response during sexual activity, such as lubrication and swelling of vagina
- ▶ The condition is persistent or recurrent and causes significant distress and difficulty
- ▶ Not due exclusively to physiological condition or another mental disorder

Fetishism

- ▶ Sexually arousing fantasies and/or behaviors of using nonliving objects
- ▶ Six month duration, with marked distress and/or interpersonal difficulty

Frotteurism

Frott, "to rub," from French

- ▶ Sexually arousing fantasies, urges, and/or behaviors of rubbing against a nonconsenting person
- ▶ Six month duration, with marked distress and/or interpersonal difficulty

Gender identity disorder

- ▶ Strong cross-gender identification
- ▶ Persistent discomfort with current sex

▶ Not because of an underlying physical condition, e.g., pseudohermaphroditism
▶ Most commonly presents in childhood; however, adulthood is possible
▶ A rare condition
▶ May have comorbidity with cluster B personality traits, and substance abuse

Gender identity disorder: differential diagnoses

Harry Klinefelter (1912–) was a U.S. internist.

▶ Schizophrenia with delusion of belonging to the other sex
▶ Paraphilia – transvestic fetishism refers to impulse and behavior of cross-dressing, not the gender identity
▶ Borderline personality disorder with transient sexual identity diffusion
▶ Homosexual individuals seeking to become more attractive to the same sex partners
▶ Testicular feminization – XY chromosome pattern with resistance to testosterone at the androgen receptor
▶ Klinefelter's syndrome – 47 XXY
▶ Congenital adrenal hyperplasia (CAH) – 21- or 11-hydroxylase deficiency, adrenal enzymatic defect in cortisol synthesis

Gender identity, gender role, and sexual orientation

▶ Gender identity
  ▷ Internal self-perception, developed by age 3 years
▶ Gender role
  ▷ External manifestation or social role
▶ Sexual orientation
  ▷ Erotic attractions

Hypoactive sexual desire disorder

▶ Lack of sexual desire and fantasies
▶ Marked distress or interpersonal difficulty
▶ Diagnosis is based on the clinician's judgment

Hypoactive sexual desire disorder: medical evaluation

▶ Renal disease
▶ Liver disease
▶ Chronic infection – HIV, other sexually transmitted diseases (STDs)
▶ Endocrinopathy – low testosterone, high prolactin, thyroid disturbance, adrenal insufficiency
▶ Medicines – serotonin-selective reuptake inhibitor (SSRI), corticosteroids, estrogen

Hypoactive sexual desire disorder: treatment

▶ Treatment for correctable medical conditions
▶ Couples therapy
▶ Behavioral therapy – sensation focusing exercises
▶ Androgenic agent

Hypoxyphilia

▶ Sexual gratification is associated with oxygen deprivation that causes an altered state of consciousness
▶ A paraphilia that is a deviated form of masochism
▶ Can be fatal

Male erectile disorder

▶ Inability to attain or maintain erection through sexual activity
▶ Not due exclusively to effects of drugs, medical conditions, or another mental disorder

Male orgasmic disorder

▶ Lack of orgasm following a normal sexual excitement phase
▶ Clinical judgment based on age and situation
▶ Not due exclusively to physical conditions, drugs, or another mental disorder (except another sexual disorder)

Orgasmic disorder

Arnold Kegel (1894–1981) was a U.S. gynecologist

▶ Medical evaluation on medication side effects and neurologic impairments
▶ Psychiatric evaluation on anxiety and relationship problems
▶ Couples therapy
▶ For females – pubococcygeal exercise, also known as Kegel exercises; the exercise is focused on strengthening the pelvic diaphragm
▶ Behavioral strategies
  ▷ Masturbation
  ▷ Vibrator
  ▷ Sensate focus exercises
▶ Possible role for bupropion and PE5 inhibitors

Paraphilia NOS

▶ Telephone scatologia
  ▷ Making unsolicited telephone calls with sexual language
  ▷ May be associated with exhibitionism
  ▷ Legally considered a harassment and misdemeanor
  ▷ Not to include mutually consented phone sex
▶ Necrophilia
  ▷ Sexual attraction to corpses
▶ Partialism
  ▷ Sexual gratification is concentrated exclusively on one part of the body
  ▷ Sexual contacts with other parts of the body are refused
▶ Zoophilia
  ▷ Sexual attraction to nonhuman animals
▶ Coprophilia
  ▷ Sexual pleasure from activities involving feces

▶ Klismaphilia
  ▷ Sexual pleasure from introducing enema into anus and rectum
▶ Urophilia
  ▷ Sexual pleasure from activities involving urine or urination

Pedophilia

▶ Sexual urges and fantasies involving children ≤13 years
▶ Patients should be ≥16 years and at least 5 years older than the child
▶ Consistent symptoms over at least 6 months
▶ Marked distress and interpersonal difficulty

Pedophilia: risk factors

▶ History of sexual abuse in childhood
▶ Male:female = 8:1
▶ Comorbid depression, anxiety, personality – prevalence uncertain

Pedophilia: treatment

▶ Cognitive-behavioral group therapy
▶ SSRIs-targeting obsessive symptoms, depression, impulse control, and decreasing libido
▶ Testosterone regulating medicine
  ▷ Medroxyprogesterone (MPA, depo-provera)
  ▷ Cyproterone
  ▷ Leuprolide
  ▷ Triptorelin
▶ Naltrexone – possible effect

Phases of sexual response

▶ Four phases
  ▷ Desire
  ▷ Excitement/arousal
  ▷ Orgasm
  ▷ Resolution

Phosphodiesterase type 5 (PE5) inhibitors

▶ Trade names and dosages
  ▷ Sildenafil – Viagra, maximum 100 mg/day; Revatio is indicated for pulmonary arterial hypertension, dosage – 20 mg tid
  ▷ Vardenafil – Levitra, maximum 20 mg/day
  ▷ Tadalafil – Cialis, maximum 20 mg/day
▶ Side effects and cautions – mainly associated with general vessel dilation, e.g., severe hypotension, myocardial infarction (MI), stroke, arrhythmia, organ hemorrhage, vision loss, seizure, and possible sudden death
▶ P450 – all primarily substrates of 3A4
▶ Pregnancy – all class B

▶ Half-life
  ▷ Sildenafil and vardenafil – 4 hours
  ▷ Tadalafil – 17.5 hours

Premature ejaculation

▶ Ejaculation happens before or shortly after penetration and with only minimal stimulation

Sexual arousal disorder: medical evaluation

▶ Renal conditions
▶ Liver conditions
▶ Vascular diseases
  ▷ Hypertension
  ▷ Diabetes vascular condition
▶ Diabetes
  ▷ Vascular
  ▷ Neuropathic influences
▶ Endocrinopathy
  ▷ Low testosterone
  ▷ High prolactin
  ▷ Thyroid disturbance
  ▷ Pituitary tumor
▶ Medications
  ▷ Tricyclic antidepressant (TCAs)
  ▷ SSRIs
  ▷ β-blockers
  ▷ Clonidine
  ▷ Antipsychotics
  ▷ Corticosteroids
  ▷ Estrogens
▶ Sleep disorders
▶ Local nerve injury
  ▷ Spinal injury
  ▷ Pudendal nerve
  ▷ Sacral plexus

Sexual arousal disorder: treatment

▶ Couples therapy
▶ Sensate focus exercises
▶ Medications are only indicated for males; however, there are positive trials on sildenafil used in women
▶ PE5 inhibitors
  ▷ Sildenafil
  ▷ Tadalafil
  ▷ Vardenafil
▶ Yohimbine, an adrenergic α-2 antagonist
▶ Intraurethral or intracavernous alprostadil, a prostaglandin E2 agonist

Sexual arousal disorders: psychiatric evaluation for

▶ Depression, particularly in older men
▶ Anxiety, particularly in younger men
▶ Substance and alcohol abuse, at any age
▶ Combination of psychiatric and medical etiologies most common
▶ Nocturnal penile tumescence test (NPT) – popular but may have false negatives and false positives

Sexual aversion disorder

▶ Differential diagnoses – panic disorder, obsessive-compulsive disorder (OCD), post-traumatic stress (PTSD)
▶ Treatment – behavioral desensitization, psychotherapy, treatment for comorbid psychiatric conditions

Sexual dysfunction associated with antidepressants

▶ Likely to cause sexual dysfunction – SSRIs, Venlafaxine, and monoamine oxidase inhibitors (MAOIs)
▶ Less likely – bupropion, nefazodone, and mirtazapine

Sexual masochism and sadism

Marquis de Sade (1740–1874) was a French novelist notorious for his paraphilia. Leopold von Sacher-Masoch (1836–1895) was an Austrian journalist who first described symptoms of masochism.

▶ Sadism
  ▷ Sexual gratification gained through causing pain or degradation to others
  ▷ A felony when acted on nonconsenting partner
▶ Masochism
  ▷ Sexual gratification depends on suffering, physical pain, and humiliation
▶ Diagnosis
  ▷ Six-month duration
  ▷ With marked distress and/or interpersonal difficulty

Transvestic fetishism

▶ Heterosexual person with fantasies and/or behaviors of cross-dressing
▶ Diagnosis
  ▷ Six-month duration
  ▷ With marked distress and/or interpersonal difficulty

Vaginismus

▶ Involuntary spasm of the outer third of the vagina
▶ Significantly interferes with intercourse
▶ DSM-IV-TR specified "not due to a general medical condition"
▶ May be lifelong or acquired
▶ May be generalized or situational

Voyeurism

Compare "voyeur" to "vision" – both from Latin "videre," meaning "to see"

▶ Sexual gratification gained from observing an unsuspecting person, often naked or involved in sexual activities
▶ Diagnosis
  ▷ Six-month duration
  ▷ With marked distress and/or interpersonal difficulty

Yohimbine

▶ Brand name – Yocon
▶ Dosage – 5.4 mg tid
▶ Mechanism – antagonizes α-2-adrenergic receptors
▶ Indication – erectile dysfunction
▶ Safety caution and adverse effect
  ▷ Pregnancy – no category assigned
  ▷ Headache
  ▷ Urinary retention
  ▷ Tachycardia.
  ▷ Respiratory depression (rare)
▶ Metabolism
  ▷ CYP450 – unknown
  ▷ Half-life – approximately 36 hours

20 Eating Disorders and Weight Issues

The central concern of eating disorders is not about eating, but controlling over physical image. The existence of eating disorders reflects the emotional impact of social pressure to mental condition. Voluntary starvation was reported from ancient times in many cultures. One of the early reports happened around the sixth century BC in China. King Ling of Chu was notorious for his obsession with slim-waisted servants. When King Ling's subordinates realized that thinness was linked to potential of political promotion, starvation quickly became zeal in the court. The kingdom finally crashed out of King Ling's erratic rule, and the King himself committed suicide. Regulating body image with extreme measures was also seen in Victoria era, when obesity was seen as a characteristic of poverty. The phenomenon of voluntary starvation by itself was not viewed as a medical condition until the nineteenth century, when published medical description of anorexia started to appear in France and England. Contemporary societal trend of thinness contributed to escalated prevalence of anorexia nervosa since 1950s, prominently in industrialized countries. Forms of binge eating was also reported for thousands of years, and believed to be more prevalent than anorexia. However, some cases of simple greed for gourmet food may well be slipped in before the establishment of diagnostic criteria.

DSM-IV-TR allows three diagnoses of eating disorders

▶ Anorexia nervosa
▶ Bulimia nervosa
▶ Eating disorder not otherwise specified (NOS)

Obesity is a common and chronic medical condition, but not a psychiatric disorder by itself. It, however, imposes significant emotional distress and often comorbid with mood disturbances. The etiology of obesity is not fully understood and is presumed to be multifactorial. In spite of the wide variety of proposed remedies, obesity endures or relapses in majority of cases. Cynically, the capitalized desire to be thin has been long known as a commercial success for entrepreneurs. The clinical concern is further raised by the fact that many medicines designed for weight loss, sometimes termed anorexiants, tend to be inappropriately used and abused by those who suffer from eating disorders.

Anorexia nervosa

▶ Two subtypes
  ▷ Restricting type
  ▷ Binge eating/purging type
▶ Clinical features
  ▷ Refusal to maintain a minimally normal weight (85% of the expected body weight)
  ▷ Extreme fear of weight gaining
  ▷ Distorted perception of body image
  ▷ Amenorrhea as a result of malnutrition, for at least three consecutive menstrual cycles

Anorexia nervosa: prognosis

▶ Ten year outcome
  ▷ Approximately one-fourth recover completely
  ▷ About half improved markedly
  ▷ About one-fourth become chronic and functions poorly
  ▷ Mortality: 5%–18%
▶ Possible prognosis
  ▷ Spontaneous recovery
  ▷ Recovery after treatments
  ▷ Fluctuating course of weight gains/relapses
  ▷ Deteriorating course leading to complications of starvation and death
▶ Prognosis of binge eating-purging type better than restricting-type
▶ Positive factors
  ▷ Admission of hunger
  ▷ Lessening of denial
  ▷ Mature self-esteem
▶ Negative factors
  ▷ Parental conflict
  ▷ Laxative abuse
  ▷ Comorbid behavioral and mood conditions

Binge eating disorder

▶ Binge eating, at least twice weekly for at least 6 months
▶ No regular use of pathological compensatory behaviors
▶ Clinical features
  ▷ Eating abnormally rapidly
  ▷ Eating when not hungry and eating until uncomfortably full
  ▷ Eating alone because of embarrassment
  ▷ Disgusted and guilty after bingeing
  ▷ Not meeting criteria of anorexia nervosa or bulimia nervosa
▶ Belongs to "Eating Disorder NOS" in DSM-IV-TR

Bulimia nervosa: clinical features

▶ Two subtypes
  ▷ Purging type
  ▷ Nonpurging type
▶ Clinical features
  ▷ Binge eating, at least twice weekly for at least 3 months
  ▷ Compensatory behaviors to prevent weight gain, at least twice weekly for at least 3 months; inappropriate compensatory behaviors include – self-induced vomiting; use of laxatives, enemas, diuretics, stimulants, diet pill abuse, restrictive eating, and exercise
  ▷ Distorted body image

Bulimia nervosa: pharmacological treatment

▶ Fluoxetine
  ▷ The only Food and Drug Administration (FDA)-approved medication for bulimia nervosa

▷ Higher dosages (60–80 mg/day) are needed for the treatment of bulimia nervosa
▶ Other medicines may be helpful
  ▷ Antidepressants
  ▷ Ondansetron (Zofran)
  ▷ Naltrexone (ReVia)
▶ Augmentation to antidepressants
  ▷ Levothyroxine (Synthroid)
  ▷ Topiramate (Topamax)
▶ Genera medical care for
  ▷ Dehydration
  ▷ Dental erosion
  ▷ Electrolyte disturbances
  ▷ Mallory-Weiss syndrome

Developmental traits of adipocytes

▶ The number and size of adipocytes are established in early life and susceptible to no significant change through life
▶ Juvenile-onset obesity – increased number and size of adipocytes
▶ Adult-onset obesity – increased only size of adipocytes

Epidemiology of eating disorder

▶ The least prevalent eating disorder – anorexia nervosa.
▶ The most prevalent eating disorder – binge eating disorder

Fat distribution

▶ Areas of active metabolism – waist, flanks, and abdomen
▶ Areas of inactive metabolism – thighs and buttocks
▶ Accumulation of fat in areas of active metabolism is associated with cardiovascular risks
▶ Accumulation of fat in areas of inactive metabolism is associated with cosmetic problems such as nostrums (cellulite)

Ipecac syrup

▶ An over-the-counter agent popularly used for inducing vomiting
▶ Made from extracts of a plant ipecacuanha
▶ Often abused by patients with eating disorder
▶ Usual dosage is 15–30 mL of the 70 mg/mL syrup
▶ Mechanism – alkaloids from the plant stimulate the gastric mucosa and the medullary chemoreceptor to induce vomiting
▶ Indication – emesis induction above age 1 year
▶ Safety caution and adverse effect
  ▷ Pregnancy – C
  ▷ Diarrhea
  ▷ Cough
  ▷ Lethargy and central nervous system (CNS) suppression
  ▷ Long-term use may cause cardiotoxicity – cardiomyopathy, arrhythmias, and prolonged QTc interval

▶ Metabolism
  ▷ CYP450 – unknown
  ▷ Half-life – very long, probably weeks

Laboratory changes in eating disorders

▶ Both anorexia and bulimia
  ▷ Hypokalemic alkalosis
  ▷ Elevated serum salivary amylase, in patients purge
▶ More prominent in anorexia
  ▷ Leukopenia with relative lymphocytosis
  ▷ Hypoglycemia
  ▷ Hypothyroidism
  ▷ Hypersecretion of corticotrophin-releasing hormone (CRH)
  ▷ Elevated β-carotene
▶ Tests usually normal
  ▷ Protein and albumin
  ▷ Erythrocyte sedimentation rate (ESR)

Leptin: the regulatory hormone for fatty tissue

▶ Leptin, a hormone produced by adipocytes, acts as a fat thermostat
▶ Low blood level of leptin demands more fat consumption
▶ High blood level of leptin demands less fat consumption

Anorexia nervosa: medical treatment

▶ Primary medical goal is weight restoration
▶ Correction of electrolyte disturbance, particularly hypokalemia
▶ Vitamin supplementation
▶ Avoid pregnancy until the illness is stabilized
▶ Dental care
▶ Indications for inpatient medical treatment
  ▷ Severe hypokalemia or dehydration
  ▷ Less than 75% expected body weight or rapid weight loss
  ▷ Growth arrest (in adolescents)

Orlistat

▶ Brand names and dosages
  ▷ Alli – PO 60 mg tid
  ▷ Xenical – PO 120 mg tid
▶ Indication – obesity
▶ Mechanism – inhibitor to gastric and pancreatic lipase
▶ Safety caution and adverse effect
  ▷ Over the counter medicine
  ▷ Pregnancy – B
  ▷ Weight change – expected weight loss
  ▷ Diarrhea
  ▷ Fatty stool
  ▷ Flatulence

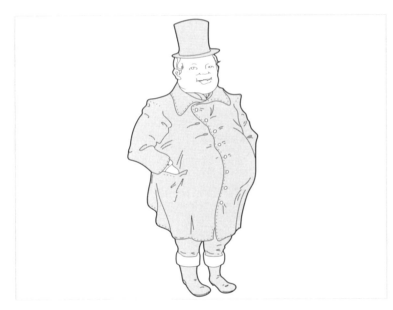

Figure 20–1 Joe as commonly depicted on stage. This original prototype of Pickwickian syndrome was a fictional role in Charles Dickens's novel "*The Posthumous Paper of the Pickwick Club.*"

▶ Metabolism
  ▷ Minimal systemic absorption
  ▷ CYP450 – unknown
  ▷ Half-life – approximately 1–2 hours

Pickwickian syndrome (Figure 20–1)

▶ Also known as
  ▷ Obesity hypoventilation syndrome
▶ Combination of
  ▷ Severe obesity
  ▷ Daytime somnolence
  ▷ Obstructive sleep apnea
  ▷ Chronic respiratory acidosis

Psychiatric treatment for eating disorders

▶ Psychotherapy is the treatment of choice
  ▷ Cognitive-behavioral therapy – the best-studied treatment for bulimia nervosa and binge eating disorder
  ▷ Interpersonal psychotherapy – effective for bulimia and binge eating disorder
  ▷ Family therapy – effective for anorexia nervosa and as adjunctive therapy for other eating disorders
  ▷ Group therapy – adjunctive therapy
  ▷ Psychodynamic psychotherapy
  ▷ Dialectical behavioral therapy
  ▷ Motivational enhancement therapy
▶ Pharmacotherapy
  ▷ As adjunctive treatment, not replacement for psychotherapy

> ▷ No medication is useful for the primary symptoms of anorexia nervosa.
> ▷ Bulimic symptoms are moderately responsive to antidepressants, but not as robust as cognitive-behavioral therapy
▶ Indications for psychiatric inpatient treatment
> ▷ Risk of self-harm or psychosis
> ▷ Failure of outpatient management

Recommended tests for eating disorder work-up

▶ Blood chemistry
▶ Complete blood count (CBC)
▶ Electrocardiogram (ECG)
▶ ESR (for differential purpose; usually normal)
▶ LFT
▶ Thyroid stimulating hormone (TSH)
▶ Urinalysis

21 Sleep Disorders

Sleep is essential for the survival of the organism. The phenomenon of sleep has been observed in every animal species. From ancient times people noticed the restorative power of sleep. Through religion, art, and literature, people often expressed their wishes that the loved ones' death was a long sleep, and the enemies' sleep connected to death. Ancient civilizations often worshiped gods of sleep (e.g., Greek gods Hypnus and Morpheus) or dream (e.g., Celtic god Angus), but rarely any god of wakefulness. The exact purpose of sleep, and dream as part of sleep, however, are not yet fully understood. Proposed functions of sleep include restorative function, homeostatic function, thermoregulation, energy conservation, and metabolic function.

There has been debate regarding the necessary amount of sleep for human being. Variety from person to person exists. In general, most adult people need 7–8 hours of good quality sleep every day. Younger adults and children need longer sleep to maintain health. Sleep disorders are conditions that disturb the quantity and quality of sleep to the extent that the restorative function is impaired and often caused emotional distress.

DSM-IV-TR categorizes sleep disorders in three groups

▶ Primary sleep disorders
  ▷ Dyssomnias
  ▷ Parasomnias
▶ Sleep disorders related to another mental disorder
▶ Other sleep disorders

There are six DSM-IV-TR allowed diagnoses of dyssomnias

▶ Primary insomnia
▶ Primary hypersomnia
▶ Narcolepsy
▶ Breathing-related sleep disorder
▶ Circadian rhythm sleep disorder
▶ Dyssomnia not otherwise specified (NOS)

There are four DSM-IV-TR allowed diagnoses of parasomnias

▶ Nightmare disorder
▶ Sleep terror disorder
▶ Sleepwalking disorder
▶ Parasomnia NOS

Hypnotics and sedative antidepressants or antipsychotics are often used as sleep aids. Selected medicines indicated for sleep-related disorders are reviewed here. It is important to remember that good sleep hygiene is the best proven strategy for all types of sleep disorders.

Alcohol: effects on sleep

▶ Individuals without chronic consumption
  ▷ Temporal decrease of sleep latency
  ▷ Alcohol consumed within 6 hours before bed time may disrupt sleep structure, such as increase of rapid eye movement (REM) that may be associated with unpleasant dreams
▶ Individuals with chronic consumption
  ▷ Sleep latency – increased
  ▷ Slow wave sleep – increased early in night, but overall decreased
  ▷ Total sleep time – decreased
  ▷ REM – increased in the early morning, but overall decreased
  ▷ Sleep fragmentation
  ▷ Reduction of restful sleep, day time fatigue
  ▷ Sleep disturbances may continue even with prolonged abstinence
  ▷ Relapse may temporally reduce the sleep disturbances

Alpha wave (Figure 21–1)

▶ An electroencephalogram (EEG) pattern of people being awake, relaxed with eyes closed
▶ Frequency: 8–12 Hz
▶ Mildly higher amplitude on dominant side

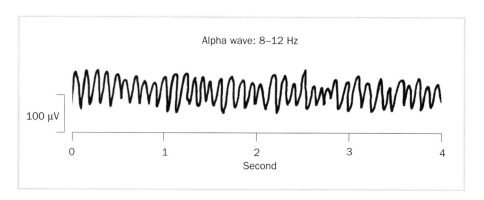

Figure 21–1 Alpha waves.

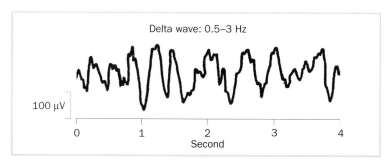

Figure 21–2 Delta waves.

Chronic excessive daytime sleepiness: causes

▶ Sleep apnea
▶ Narcolepsy
▶ Restless leg syndrome
▶ Occupational or social schedules
▶ Medication
▶ Drug or alcohol use
▶ Depression

Delta wave (Figure 21–2)

▶ Stages 3 and 4 sleep, also known as slow wave sleep
▶ Highest in amplitude and lowest in frequency
▶ Frequency – up to 3 Hz

Depression: associated changes in sleep

▶ Shortened REM latency
▶ Increased REM density
▶ Low sleep efficiency
▶ Early morning awakening

Dreams

▶ Occur in both REM and nonrapid eye movement (NREM) periods
▶ REM dreams are often abstract and surreal
▶ NREM dreams are likely to be lucid and purposeful

Melatonin (Figure 21–3)

▶ An indolamine synthesized from tryptophan

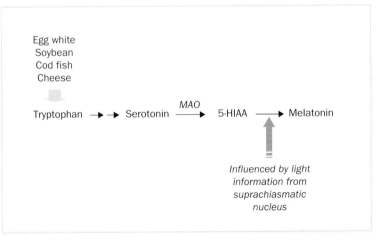

Figure 21-3 Biosynthesis of melatonin.

Egg white
Soybean
Cod fish
Cheese

Tryptophan → → Serotonin —MAO→ 5-HIAA ——→ Melatonin

Influenced by light information from suprachiasmatic nucleus

▶ Anatomy
  ▷ Synthesized in the pineal gland
  ▷ Synapses and receptors at suprachiasmatic nucleus (SCN) of the hypothalamus
▶ Synthesis
  ▷ Precursors – tryptophan, serotonin
  ▷ Synthesis is stimulated by the darkness, and suppresses by the daylight
▶ Physiological role
  ▷ Acts as a hypnotic that increases REM
  ▷ Important role in circadian regulation
▶ Regulation of synthesis
  ▷ Receives positive feedback from increased sleep drive in the evening
  ▷ Receives negative feedback from the retinohypothalamic tract
  ▷ Increased by serotonin-selective reuptake inhibitors (SSRIs), norepinephrine reuptake inhibitors, and neuroleptics

Modafinil

▶ Brand name – Provigil
▶ Dosage – 100 mg/day to 400 mg/day
▶ Mechanism
  ▷ Activates orexin neurons
  ▷ Increases histaminergic tone in the hypothalamus
▶ Indication
  ▷ Narcolepsy
  ▷ Obstructive sleep apnea
  ▷ Shift work sleep disorder
▶ Safety caution and adverse effect
  ▷ Pregnancy – C
  ▷ Schedule IV
▶ Metabolism
  ▷ CYP450 – 3A4 substrate, 1A2, 3A4 inducer
  ▷ Half-life – approximately 15 hours

Narcolepsy

▶ Sleep attacks with a REM onset
▶ Closely associated with certain human leukocyte antigen (HLA) types
▶ Orexin A and B (hypocretin 1 and 2) promote wakefulness and inhibit REM sleep
▶ Narcolepsy patients have
  ▷ Very few orexin cells in the hypothalamus
  ▷ Very low level orexin in cerebrospinal fluid (CSF)
▶ Treatment
  ▷ Modafinil
  ▷ Gamma-hydroxybutyrate (GHB)

Nonrapid eye movement sleep

▶ Stages 1 through 4
▶ Physiological functions
  ▷ Generally lower than in wakefulness
  ▷ Pulse rate slowed 5–10 per minute

Orexins

▶ A group of highly excitatory neuropeptides
▶ Also known as hypocretins
▶ Produced by a small group of neurons in hypothalamus
▶ Orexin receptors are G-protein coupled receptors, with wide distribution in the brain
▶ Medical use is under investigation

Parasomnias

▶ All arise in stages 3 and 4 NREM sleeps, also known as slow wave sleeps (SWS)
▶ Sleep walking, bed wetting, and night terrors

Pramipexole

▶ Brand name – Mirapex
▶ Dosage – PO 0.125 mg tid up to 4.5 mg/day
▶ Mechanism – dopamine agonist
▶ Indicated for Parkinson's disease and restless leg syndrome
▶ Safety caution and adverse effect
  ▷ Pregnancy risk category
  ▷ Weight change
  ▷ Sudden sleep episodes
  ▷ Syncope
  ▷ Hypotension
  ▷ Dyskinesia
▶ Metabolism
  ▷ No hepatic metabolism; excreted unchanged through active tubular secretion
  ▷ CYP450 – none
  ▷ Half-life – 8 hour

Rapid eye movement sleep (Figure 21–4)

▶ Also know as paradoxical sleep
▶ High level of
  ▷ Brain activity
  ▷ Physiological activity
  ▷ Physiological variability – pulse, respiration, blood pressure

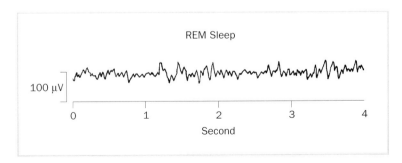

Figure 21–4 REM sleep – low voltage, random, fast, with sawtooth waves.

- ▶ Low level of
  - ▷ Temperature regulation; body temperature in REM sleep varies with the changes in the surrounding temperature; this is known as poikilothermia
  - ▷ Muscle tone; near-total paralysis
- ▶ EEG
  - ▷ Low voltage, random, fast activity
  - ▷ Sawtooth waves
- ▶ Male penile erections

REM latency

- ▶ The time lag between the times of sleep onset to the first REM episode

Restless leg syndrome

- ▶ Unpleasant aching and drawing sensations
- ▶ The urge to move the legs can be suppressed voluntarily for a brief period
- ▶ Associated with
  - ▷ Peripheral neuropathy
  - ▷ Pregnancy
  - ▷ Anemia with low ferritin
- ▶ Causes insomnia and excessive daytime sleepiness
- ▶ May be familial

Restless leg syndrome: pharmacologic treatment

- ▶ Dopaminergic agents
  - ▷ Pergolide (Permax)
  - ▷ Carbidopa/levodopa (Sinemet)
  - ▷ Bromocriptine (Parlodel)
  - ▷ Ropinirole hydrochloride (Requip)
  - ▷ Pramipexole (Mirapex)
- ▶ Benzodiazepines
  - ▷ Clonazepam (Klonopin)
- ▶ Opioids
  - ▷ Codeine
- ▶ Anticonvulsants
  - ▷ Gabapentin (Neurontin)
- ▶ Presynaptic α-2-adrenergic agonists
  - ▷ Clonidine (Catapres)

Restless leg syndrome: work up

- ▶ Primarily a subjective disease
- ▶ Rating scale
  - ▷ International RLS study group (IRLSSG)
- ▶ Polysomnography
- ▶ Tests to rule out secondary causes
  - ▷ Blood count and chemistry
  - ▷ Thyroid function

▷ Vitamin B-12 and folate
▷ Venereal Disease Research Laboratory (VDRL) test
▶ If polyneuropathy is suspected
▷ Needle electromyography and nerve conduction studies

Ropinirole

▶ Brand name and dosage
▷ Requip – PO 0.25 mg tid up to 24 mg/day
▷ Requip XL – PO 2 mg qd up to 24 mg/day
▶ Mechanism – dopamine agonist
▶ Indicated for Parkinson's disease and restless leg syndrome
▶ Safety caution and adverse effect
▷ Pregnancy risk category – C
▷ Sudden sleep episodes
▷ Orthostatic hypotension
▷ Nausea
▷ Somnolence
▷ Avoid abrupt withdrawal

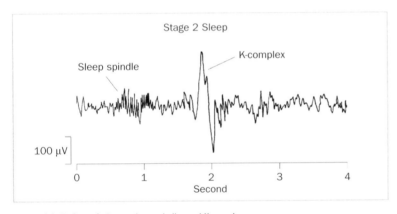

Figure 21-5 Stage 2 sleep – sleep spindles and K-complexes.

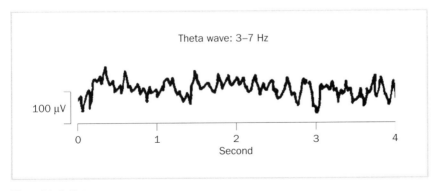

Figure 21-6 Theta waves.

▶ Metabolism
  ▷ CYP450 – substrate of 1A2
  ▷ Extensive liver metabolism
  ▷ Half-life – 6 hour

Sleep spindles and K-complexes (See Figure 21–5 on page 155)

▶ Stage 2 sleep
▶ Sleep spindles: 12–16 Hz
▶ K-complexes – brief high voltage peaks

Theta wave (See Figure 21–6 on page 155)

▶ Drowsy, stage 1 sleep, meditation
▶ Frequency: 3–7 Hz

22 Factitious Disorders and Malingering

Factitious disorders and malingering share the common feature of false or grossly exaggerated symptoms that are intentionally produced. The conscious goals are either the pleasure of being in sick role, or external incentives. While malingering is not considered a mental disorder, DSM-IV-TR allows four diagnoses in the category of factitious disorders

▶ Factitious disorder with predominantly psychological signs and symptoms
▶ Factitious disorder with predominantly physical signs and symptoms
▶ Factitious disorder with combined psychological and physical signs and symptoms
▶ Factitious disorder not otherwise specified (NOS)

Faking symptoms does not preclude coexistence of genuine medical and mental disorders. A patient with schizophrenia may fake hallucinations sometimes. The challenge of diagnosis lays in the difficulty in differentiating genuine and faked symptoms. Commonly believed signs of deception that have been proved inaccurate in detection include decreased gaze, shifting posture, longer pause before answering questions, feigned smile. These signs usually are manifest of anxiety. Anxiety often appears when an inexperienced person is making an unpremeditated lie, but it is not difficult to overcome through experience and premeditation. This chapter also provides some study-proven detective strategies and treatment principles.

Factitious disorder: clinical features

▶ Conscientiously produced symptoms that mimic medical or mental disorders
▶ The symptoms are under voluntary control
▶ The underline motivation of factitious behavior is to assume the patient role
▶ Lack of external incentives such as economic gain or avoidance of legal responsibility
▶ Often induce negative countertransference
▶ Subtypes
  ▷ Predominantly psychological symptoms
  ▷ Predominantly physical symptoms
  ▷ Combined type
  ▷ NOS

Factitious disorders: defense mechanisms

▶ Identification (with the aggressor)
▶ Regression
▶ Repression
▶ Symbolization

Factitious disorders: treatment principles

▶ Focus on management, not cure
▶ Avoid unnecessary tests and procedures
▶ Avoid aggressive and direct confrontation
▶ Regular interdisciplinary communication to coordinate the care
▶ No specific psychiatric therapy besides treating comorbid psychiatric conditions
▶ Designate a primary care provider as a gatekeeper
▶ Possible requirement for guardianship in treatment decision making
▶ Legal intervention for factitious disorder by proxy that involves children

Ganser syndrome

Sigbert Ganser (1853–1931) was a German psychiatrist who is known as the first described factitious disorder in prisoners.

▶ The anchor symptom is approximate answers; e.g., $4 + 5 = 8$
▶ True Ganser syndrome, as proposed by some, should also include clouding of consciousness, hallucinations, and somatic conversion symptoms
▶ Usually has a time-limited course, sudden remission, and amnesia for events
▶ May occur
   ▷ As a dissociative symptom (classified as Dissociative Disorder NOS)
   ▷ In malingering
   ▷ In factitious disorder

Hallucination: genuine vs. faked

▶ Auditory hallucination is the most common malingered psychotic symptom
▶ Faked hallucination is generally more dramatic and attention-catching, yet lack of realistic richness
▶ Signs point to genuine hallucination
   ▷ Associate the contents of delusions or some psychic purpose
   ▷ Unpleasant and offensive in nature, but to some degree comfortably accepted
   ▷ Somehow predictable
   ▷ May be reduced to some degree, usually by increasing background noise (turning on radio) or distracting (involving in activity)
   ▷ Clear to perception (audible, visible, etc.)
   ▷ Rich in volunteered details (gender, tone, accent, direction, etc.)
   ▷ Plain language by the voices
   ▷ Visual – normal-sized with color (except alcohol withdrawal hallucinosis with small sizes figures)
▶ Signs point to faked hallucination
   ▷ Not associated with delusions; less context-dependent
   ▷ Dramatically frightening and abusive, unbearably distressing
   ▷ Unpredictable
   ▷ Uncontrollable
   ▷ Lack of a strategy to diminish the hallucinated voices
   ▷ Vague
   ▷ Lack of details
   ▷ Use of stilted language by the voices
   ▷ Visual – black and white, giant or miniature figures

Malingering

▶ Not considered a mental illness
▶ Most common goals are to obtain
  ▷ Drugs
  ▷ Shelter
  ▷ Financial compensation
▶ Suspicious history
  ▷ Medicolegal issues
  ▷ Discrepancy between the claimed distress and the objective findings.
  ▷ Antisocial personality disorder (ASPD).

Malingering: assessment

▶ The most effective differentiation between real and malingered psychosis relies on
  ▷ Thorough, prolonged examination and observation
  ▷ Reliable collateral information
▶ The most difficult, hence the rarest symptom to be malingered, is thought process disturbance
▶ Suspicious behavior
  ▷ Lack of cooperation
  ▷ Inconsistency in claimed distress
  ▷ Lack of knowledge of the nuances of the feigned disorder
  ▷ Contradictory responses in interview
  ▷ Easy to endorse improbable symptoms
  ▷ Vague or evasive complaints
  ▷ Improbable anatomical distributions of symptoms
▶ Tests
  ▷ Minnesota Multiphasic Personality Inventory (MMPI), atypical response patterns tested in F scale and F-K index
  ▷ Structured Interview of Reported Symptoms (SIRS)

Malingering: differential diagnoses

▶ Factitious disorder
  ▷ Consciously produced symptoms
  ▷ Goal is to assume patient role
▶ Somatoform disorders
  ▷ Conversion disorder
  ▷ Somatization disorder
  ▷ Symptoms are produced unconsciously
▶ Dissociative disorders
▶ True medical or psychiatric conditions

Malingering: psychiatric management

▶ Maintain clinical neutrality during evaluation
▶ If the diagnosis of malingering is of significant clinical certainty, the patient should be appropriately confronted
▶ Discuss with the patient

  ▷ The consequence of malingering
  ▷ The possible reasons of malingering
  ▷ Alternative pathways to the desired outcome
▶ Comorbid psychiatric disorders
  ▷ Should be properly evaluated and treated
  ▷ For patients unwilling to interact with the psychiatrist under any terms other than manipulation, the evaluation can be abandoned

Münchausen syndrome

Karl Münchausen (1720–1797) was a German cavalry officer who was known to tell fantasized adventurous stories as if he personally experienced them.

▶ A syndrome of chronic fabricating medical conditions to get hospital admission; some called it hospital addiction syndrome
▶ The patients are usually knowledgeable in medicine, and are able to do a decent job in faking; this makes the diagnosis difficult
▶ Often results in numerous unnecessary surgical procedures
▶ It is a form of factitious disorder, with prominent physical symptoms and chronicity

23 Personality Disorders

The word "personality" originates from the Latin "personalitas," which in its early use referred to the fact and quality of existence as a person. The modern sense of the totality of character and temperament probably started with Carl Jung, who stated, "Personality is the supreme realization of the innate idiosyncrasy of a living being." According to DSM-IV-TR, personality refers to the enduring pattern of inner experience and behavior.

Several terms are often interchangeably used in nonpsychiatric writing, including temperament, character, and persona. However, only "personality" pertains more to the wholeness of emotional and behavioral appeal. Temperament refers more to the inner and inherited aspect of personality. Character refers to both the inner experience and the outward behavior, which is less of the heritable pattern and more influenced by social and cultural learning. Persona refers to the outward, social image of personality. Among all these terms, only "character" suggests a sense of morality. Therefore suggestions of unhealthy temperament and deviated personality are usually more acceptable than character flaw.

Personality is generally assumed to be formed in early adulthood and relatively consistent throughout the life. However, personality modification and continuous maturation in adult life have been observed under the influence from environment, life events, learning ability, personal motivation, and many other factors. Long-term, insight-oriented psychotherapy is traditionally believed to be effective for personality modification. Personality change may also be caused by general medical conditions, which is coded in Axis I in the multiaxial diagnostic formulation.

Personality disorder refers to the deviation of personality from social and cultural expectations. It is manifested in pathological patterns of cognition, affectivity, interpersonal functioning, and impulse control. Abnormal personalities are usually inflexible, poorly adaptive, and lead to significant distress or impairment in social and occupational functioning.

DSM-IV-TR allows diagnoses of 11 personality disorders in three clusters and one residual category

▶ Cluster A
  ▷ Paranoid personality disorder
  ▷ Schizoid personality disorder
  ▷ Schizotypal personality disorder
▶ Cluster B
  ▷ Antisocial personality disorder
  ▷ Borderline personality disorder
  ▷ Histrionic personality disorder
  ▷ Narcissistic personality disorder

- ▶ Cluster C
  - ▷ Avoidant personality disorder
  - ▷ Dependent personality disorder
  - ▷ Obsessive-compulsive personality disorder
- ▶ Personality disorder not otherwise specified (NOS)

Some authors argued that the categorical diagnosis imposed qualitative judgment and produced not enough precision. Robert Cloninger and his colleagues suggested a dimensional or quantitative diagnostic system. Two components of personality, character, and temperament, were studied and analyzed. The following are the seven personality dimensions that were identified in Cloninger's configurations

- ▶ Temperament dimensions
  - ▷ Harm avoidance
  - ▷ Novelty seeking
  - ▷ Reward dependence
  - ▷ Persistence
- ▶ Character dimensions
  - ▷ Self-directedness
  - ▷ Cooperativeness
  - ▷ Self-transcendence

Antisocial personality disorder

- ▶ Disrespectful to laws and rules
- ▶ Deceitful
- ▶ Impulsive and reckless
- ▶ Irritable and aggressive
- ▶ Irresponsibility
- ▶ Lack of remorse
- ▶ A pattern of disregard for and violation of other people's rights started from age 15 years, usually also met criteria for conduct disorder

Antisocial personality disorder: treatment

- ▶ Often resistant to treatment
- ▶ Behavioral therapies and self-help groups in a confined setting yield best results
- ▶ Pharmacotherapy
  - ▷ Targeting incapacitating symptoms such as anxiety, rage, and depression
  - ▷ Treatment for ADHA and other comorbid Axis I pathology
  - ▷ Antiepileptic drugs and β-blockers may be tried

Avoidant personality disorder

- ▶ Has chronic feelings of inadequacy
- ▶ Is sensitive to other's evaluation
- ▶ Avoids interpersonal contact because of fears of disapproval and rejection
- ▶ Shows restraint and inhibition in relationships
- ▶ Is reluctant to engage in new activities

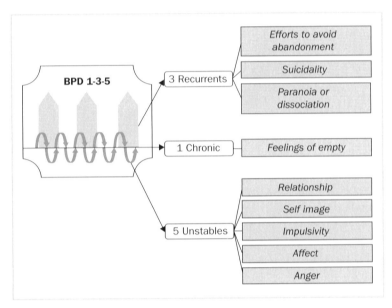

Figure 23–1 Visual mnemonics for borderline personality disorder (BPD). The diagnosis requires five of the listed nine symptoms, including one symptom that's chronic, represented by a straight baseline; three symptoms that are episodic, represented by three high peaks, and five symptoms that are unstable and frequently changing, represented by a wave line with five cycles of wave.

Borderline personality disorder (Figure 23–1)

▶ Recurrent, frantic efforts to avoid abandonment
▶ Recurrent suicidal behavior
▶ Recurrent, transient, stress-related paranoia and dissociative symptoms
▶ Chronic feelings of emptiness
▶ Unstable relationship, unstable self image, unstable affect, unstable anger control, and impulsiveness

Borderline personality disorder: alternative terminology

▶ Emotionally unstable personality disorder (ICD-10)
▶ Ambulatory schizophrenia
▶ As-if personality (Deutsch)
▶ Pseudoneurotic schizophrenia (Hoch and Politan)
▶ Psychotic character disorder (Frosch)

Borderline personality disorder: treatment

▶ Psychotherapy is the treatment of choice
▶ Dialectical behavior therapy (DBT) is designed for borderline personality disorder. DBT focuses on
  ▷ Mood regulation
  ▷ Reduction of suicidality
▶ Pharmacotherapy
  ▷ Antipsychotics for anger, hostility, and brief psychotic episodes

▷ Benzodiazepines may help anxiety and depression but may induce disinhibition

▷ Anticonvulsants and serotonin-selective reuptake inhibitors (SSRIs) may be helpful

Cluster A personality disorders

▶ Common characters

▷ Social isolation

▷ Detachment

▷ Suspiciousness

▶ Types

▷ Paranoid personality disorder

▷ Schizoid personality disorder

▷ Schizotypal personality disorder

▶ Schizotypal, but not schizoid personality disorder, most closely resembles schizophrenia

Defense mechanisms characteristic for personality disorders

▶ Paranoid personality disorder

▷ Projection

▶ Schizoid and schizotypal personality disorders

▷ Fantasy

▶ Borderline personality disorder

▷ Splitting

▷ Projective identification

▷ Passive aggression

▶ Histrionic personality disorder

▷ Repression

▷ Denial

▷ Dissociation

▶ Narcissistic personality disorder

▷ Idealization

▶ Obsessive-compulsive personality disorder

▷ Isolation

▶ Antisocial personality disorder

▷ Acting out

Dependent personality disorder

▶ Is difficult in

▷ Making decisions or assume responsibility

▷ Expressing disagreement

▷ Initiating projects or activities

▶ Goes to excessive lengths to

▷ Please others or seek new relationship as a source of support

▶ Fears of being unable to obtain support to take care of self

Dependent personality disorder: psychotherapies

▶ Group therapy

▶ Social skill training

▶ Assertiveness training
▶ Cognitive therapy

Dependent vs. avoidant personality disorder

▶ Both are associated with
  ▷ Anxiety symptoms
  ▷ Fears of abandonment
▶ Individuals with dependent personality disorder tend to
  ▷ Embrace relationships, often unselectively
  ▷ Have greater fear of abandonment than those with avoidant personality disorder

Epidemiology of personality disorders

▶ Onset in adolescence or early adulthood
▶ Causing distress or impairment
▶ Prevalence
  ▷ 10%–20% in general population
  ▷ 30%–50% in outpatient psychiatric population

Family history of personality disorders

▶ Cluster A
  ▷ Paranoid, schizoid, and schizotypal
  ▷ First-degree relatives present a greater prevalence of schizophrenia than general population
▶ Cluster B
  ▷ Antisocial, borderline, histrionic, and narcissistic
  ▷ Families have higher rates of impulse control difficulties and mood disorders
▶ Cluster C
  ▷ Avoidant, dependent, and obsessive-compulsive
  ▷ Family members have higher rates of anxiety disorders

Harm avoidance

▶ One of the four identified temperament dimensions
▶ Gene expression of the serotonin transporter may be correlated with the variation of harm avoidance
▶ High harm avoidance
  ▷ Pessimistic, fear of uncertainty, shy, lack of energy
  ▷ Increased activity in the anterior paralimbic circuit
▶ Low harm avoidance
  ▷ Optimistic, daring, outgoing, energetic
  ▷ High gamma aminobutyric acid (GABA) concentrations

Histrionic personality disorder

▶ Is suggestible and has frequent mood swing
▶ Seeks attention by
  ▷ Seductive or provocative behavior

▷ Physical appearance
▷ Exaggerated expression of emotions

ICD-10 vs. DSM-IV-TR: similar or equivalent diagnoses in personality disorders

▶ Dissocial personality disorder (ICD-10)
  ▷ Antisocial personality disorder (DSM-IV-TR)
▶ Emotionally unstable personality (ICD-10)
  ▷ Borderline personality disorder (DSM-IV-TR)
▶ Anankastic personality disorder (ICD-10)
  ▷ Obsessive-compulsive personality disorder (DSM-IV-TR)
▶ Anxious personality disorder (ICD-10)
  ▷ Avoidant personality disorder (DSM-IV-TR)

Narcissistic personality disorder

▶ Is grandiose
  ▷ Exaggerates achievements
  ▷ Fantasizes success
  ▷ Feels entitled and special
  ▷ Requires unrealistic admiration
▶ Takes advantage of others
▶ Lacks empathy
▶ Envies others

Novelty seeking

▶ One of the four identified temperament dimensions
▶ High novelty seeking
  ▷ Curious, impulsive, irritable, easily bored
  ▷ Increased reuptake of dopamine at presynaptic terminals
  ▷ High pleasure-seeking behaviors, such as smoking
▶ Low-novelty seeking
  ▷ Reserved, deliberate, slow tempered, frugal

Obsession vs. compulsion

▶ Obsessions are
  ▷ Thoughts
  ▷ Impulses
  ▷ Images
▶ Compulsions are
  ▷ Behaviors
  ▷ Mental acts
▶ Both obsessions and compulsions are recurrent and repetitive
▶ Obsessions are intrusive, inappropriate, and therefore undesired to the individual
▶ Compulsions are aimed at preventing or reducing distress and anxiety that often associated with obsessions
▶ Obsessions cause marked anxiety or distress
▶ The excessiveness and debilitating nature of compulsions cause even more distress

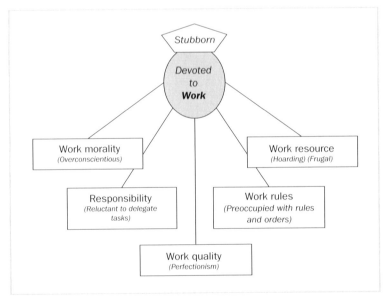

Figure 23-2 Mnemonic diagram for obsessive-compulsive personality disorder (OCPD). Imagine OCPD as a stubborn workaholic who cares a lot about work morality, work rules, work responsibility, work quality, and work resource. The diagnosis requires four of the eight elements in italic font.

Obsessive-compulsive disorder vs. obsessive-compulsive personality disorder

▶ Obsessive-compulsive disorder (OCD)
  ▷ Refers to distinct symptoms of recurrent or persistent obsessions and compulsions
  ▷ Symptoms may fluctuate through life
▶ Obsessive-compulsive personality disorder (OCPD)
  ▷ Refers to patterns of feeling, response, and behavior, usually consistent through out much of life
  ▷ Characterized by perfectionism, inflexibility, emotional constriction, and indecisiveness

Obsessive-compulsive personality disorder (Figure 23–2)

▶ Is stubborn and hard working
▶ Is preoccupied with morality, ethics, rules, order
▶ Is perfectionistic
▶ Has habits of hoarding and being frugal
▶ Is reluctant to delegate work with others

Paranoid personality disorder

▶ Is suspicious, and doubtful about others' trustworthiness and loyalty
▶ Is fearful of other's being hostile and harmful
▶ Is reluctant to share information
▶ Is unforgiving and counterattacks quickly to perceived attacks

Persistence

▶ One of the four identified temperament dimensions
▶ High persistence
  ▷ Hard working, determined, enthusiastic
  ▷ Individuals with high persistence tend to respond to reward positively

▶ Low persistence
  ▷ Indolent, spoiled, underachieving, erratic
  ▷ Individuals with low persistence tend to be lazy and rarely strive for higher accomplishments
▶ Persistence may be enhanced by psychostimulants

Personality change due to general medical condition

▶ Not counted as a personality disorder, which is defined as enduring pattern of behavior and cognition started before the age of 18 years
▶ Significant personality in adult life indicates possible organic cause
▶ Usually associated with cortical or subcortical structural change
▶ DSM-IV-TR subtypes
  ▷ Labile
  ▷ Disinhibited
  ▷ Aggressive
  ▷ Apathetic
  ▷ Paranoid
  ▷ Other
  ▷ Combined
  ▷ Unspecified

Quality of life associated with personality disorders

▶ Schizotypal, borderline, and avoidant have the most reduction in quality of life
▶ Obsessive-compulsive and histrionic have the least reduction in quality of life

Reward dependence

▶ One of the four identified temperament dimensions
▶ High reward dependence
  ▷ Sentimental, warm, affectionate, socially dependent
  ▷ Associated with increased activity in the thalamus
  ▷ Low level of 3-methoxy-4-hydroxyphenylglycol (MHPG)
▶ Low novelty seeking
  ▷ Detached, aloof, tough minded, independent

Schizoid personality disorder

▶ Is odd and eccentric in having
  ▷ Ideas of reference
  ▷ Unusual perceptions and beliefs
  ▷ Vague and metaphorical speech
  ▷ Inappropriate affect
  ▷ Behavior and appearance
▶ Is suspicious and paranoid
▶ Socially isolated and anxious due to paranoid fears

Schizotypal personality disorder

▶ Is aloof, indifferent and emotionally detached
▶ Desires no close relationship or sexual intimacy
▶ Prefers to work and live alone

Schizotypal personality disorder: biological abnormalities

▶ Most of the biological changes resemble schizophrenia
▶ Morphologic change
  ▷ Ventricular enlargement
  ▷ Reduction of volume in the temporal lobe and striatal volume
▶ Functional abnormality
  ▷ Functional hypoactivity in the dorsal prefrontal cortex in response to learning or executive tasks
  ▷ Elevated plasma homovanillic acid – a metabolite of dopamine
  ▷ Abnormalities of smooth pursuit eye movements

Twin studies: personality and behavior patterns

▶ Similarities in Minnesota Multiphasic Personality Inventory (MMPI) test scores
  ▷ Strong genetic influence through all MMPI scales
▶ Similarities in behavior traits
  ▷ Alcohol use
  ▷ Substance abuse
  ▷ Antisocial behavior
  ▷ Visuomotor skills
  ▷ Religious interests
  ▷ Job satisfaction
  ▷ Social attitudes
  ▷ Vocational interests
  ▷ Work values
▶ Similarities in electroencephalogram (EEG) pattern and skin conductance in response to
  ▷ Music, voices, and sudden noises
  ▷ Other perceptional stimulations

24 Child and Adolescent Psychiatric Disorders

The disorders discussed in this chapter are usually first diagnosed before the age of 18 years. This provision does not imply that these disorders appear only in childhood. Rather, it merely states the fact that most individuals with these disorders present for clinical attention first during childhood. Many of the disorders persist through adult life, and some are diagnosed during adulthood.

Psychiatric evaluation of children has its own preferred approach that is different from adult evaluation. It usually requires more nonverbal observation, more collateral information (particularly from parents), assessment of the children's academic functioning, and behavior in different settings. Many symptoms have different presentation in children and in adults. Children often have limited skill in articulation and verbal expression of their thoughts and feelings. The continuous treatment and follow-up are accompanied with children's growth and continuous change of physical status. Treatment is heavily relying on the cooperation and supervision from parents, teachers, and other adults in the children's life.

The following are disorders included in the section of "Disorders Usually First Diagnosed in Infancy, Childhood, or Adolescence" in DSM-IV-TR

- ▶ Mental retardation (MR)
  - ▷ Mild MR
  - ▷ Moderate MR
  - ▷ Severe MR
  - ▷ Profound MR
  - ▷ MR, severity unspecified
- ▶ Learning disorders
  - ▷ Reading disorder
  - ▷ Mathematics disorder
  - ▷ Disorder of written expression
  - ▷ Learning disorder not otherwise specified (NOS)
- ▶ Communication disorders
  - ▷ Expressive language disorder
  - ▷ Mixed receptive-expressive language disorder
  - ▷ Phonological disorder
  - ▷ Stuttering
  - ▷ Communication disorder NOS
- ▶ Pervasive developmental disorders
  - ▷ Autistic disorder
  - ▷ Rett's disorder
  - ▷ Childhood disintegrative disorder
  - ▷ Asperger's disorder

▷ Pervasive developmental disorder NOS
▶ Attention deficit and disruptive behavior disorders
  ▷ Attention-deficit/hyperactivity disorder
  ▷ Attention-deficit/hyperactivity disorder NOS
  ▷ Conduct disorder
  ▷ Oppositional defiant disorder
  ▷ Disruptive behavior disorder NOS
▶ Feeding and eating disorders
  ▷ Pica
  ▷ Rumination disorder
  ▷ Feeding disorder of infancy or early childhood
▶ Tic disorders
  ▷ Tourette's disorder
  ▷ Chronic motor or vocal tic disorder
  ▷ Transient tic disorder
  ▷ Tic disorder NOS
▶ Elimination disorders
  ▷ Encores
  ▷ Enuresis
▶ Other disorders of infancy, childhood, or adolescence
  ▷ Separation anxiety disorder
  ▷ Selective mutism
  ▷ Reactive attachment disorder of infancy or early childhood
  ▷ Stereotypic movement disorder
  ▷ Disorder of infancy, childhood, or adolescence NOS

Antipsychotics approved for children and adolescents

▶ Risperidone
  ▷ Autistic disorder: 5–16-year-olds
  ▷ Schizophrenia: 13–17-year-olds
  ▷ Bipolar disorder: 10–17-year-olds
▶ Aripiprazole
  ▷ Schizophrenia: 13–17-year-olds
  ▷ Bipolar disorder: 10–17-year-olds

Antidepressants approved for children and adolescents: serotonin-selective reuptake inhibitors (SSRIs)

▶ Fluoxetine
  ▷ Major depressive disorder: 8–17-year-olds
  ▷ Obsessive-compulsive disorder: 7–17-year-olds
▶ Sertraline
  ▷ Obsessive-compulsive disorder: 6–17-year-olds
▶ Paroxetine
  ▷ Obsessive-compulsive disorder: 7–17-year-olds
▶ Escitalopram
  ▷ Major depressive disorder: 12–17-year-olds

Antidepressants approved for children and adolescents: tricyclics

▶ Amitriptyline
  ▷ Depression: 9–12-year-olds
  ▷ Chronic pain: 6-year old
▶ Nortriptyline
  ▷ Nocturnal enuresis and depression: >6-year old
▶ Clomipramine
  ▷ Obsessive-compulsive disorder: >10-year old
▶ Imipramine
  ▷ Nocturnal enuresis, depression, and chronic pain: >6-year old

Asperger's disorder

Hans Asperger (1906–1980) was an Austrian pediatrician.

▶ Originally described by Asperger in 1940 as "autistic psychopathy"
▶ Inadequacy of social interaction
  ▷ Impairment in the use of eye contact, facial expression, body language
  ▷ Inability to develop and maintain peer relationships
  ▷ Lack of spontaneous social and emotional response
▶ Restricted interest and stereotypic behavior
▶ No significant delays in language and cognitive development
▶ Etiology
  ▷ Global impairment of brain development
  ▷ Impairment occurs soon after conception
  ▷ Some hypothesized abnormal migration of embryonic cells during fetal development
▶ Differential diagnosis
  ▷ Autistic disorder – language delay is a core feature in autistic disorder; children with Asperger's disorder are also more likely to look for social interaction
  ▷ Schizoid personality disorder
▶ Treatment
  ▷ Supportive treatment
  ▷ Promoting social relationships
  ▷ Fostering good habits to facilitate rule adaption
  ▷ Developing problem-solving skills
▶ Prognosis
  ▷ No long-term study
  ▷ Anecdotal positive prognostic factors – normal intelligence quotient (IQ), less impairment in social skills

Attention deficit/hyperactivity disorder

▶ The most common psychiatric disorder in children
▶ Prominent symptoms of inattention, hyperactivity, and impulsivity
▶ Symptoms present before the age of 7 years
▶ Often persists into adulthood
▶ Impairment in functioning must occur in more than one setting
▶ Stimulants are the first line of treatment

Autistic disorder

Leo Kanner (1894–1981) was an Austria-born U.S. psychiatrist.

▶ Also known as Kanner's syndrome
▶ Prevalence – about 1–2/1,000
▶ Usually can be detected at the age of 3 years; however, onset is before 3
▶ Impairment with
  ▷ Social interactions – inability to interact appropriately, lack of emotional reciprocity and spontaneity
  ▷ Communications – delay or lack of speech, inability to sustain conversations
  ▷ Behavior – restricted, repetitive, and stereotyped patterns of behavior and interests

Childhood disintegrative disorder

▶ Regression in areas of functioning following at least 2 years (typical age 3–4 years) of normal development
▶ Etiology unknown
▶ Boys:girls = 8:1
▶ Often associated with seizure disorder

Children with deceased parents: tasks of bereavement

▶ Accepting the reality of loss
▶ Experiencing the pain or emotional aspects of loss
▶ Adjusting to an environment in which the deceased is missing
▶ Relocating the deceased within the child's life
  ▷ Finding ways to memorialize the deceased
  ▷ The apparent difficult task is to deal with a prior conflictual relationship between the child and the deceased parent

Chronic motor or vocal tic disorder

▶ Motor or vocal tics (if both, consider Tourette's disorder)
▶ More than 1 year in course, without more than 3 months of tic-free period
▶ Onset before age 18 years

Clonidine

▶ Brand name
  ▷ Catapres, Catapres TTS (transdermal)
▶ Dosage
  ▷ PO 0.1 mg BID up to 2.4 mg/day
  ▷ Transdermal – one patch per week, 0.1 mg/24 hrs to 0.6 mg/24 hrs
▶ Mechanism
  ▷ Antagonist on α-2 adrenergic receptors
▶ Indication
  ▷ Hypertension
  ▷ Off-label use for ADHD, Tourette's syndrome, opioid withdrawal, and other behavior disturbances

▶ Safety caution and adverse effect
  ▷ Pregnancy risk category – C
  ▷ Weight change – not expected
  ▷ Hypotension
  ▷ Rebound hypertension
  ▷ Drowsiness
  ▷ Dizziness
▶ Metabolism
  ▷ CYP450: unknown
  ▷ Half-life: 13 hours

Conduct disorder

▶ Aggression
  ▷ Bullying, threatening, intimidating, and fighting
  ▷ Using weapon
  ▷ Being cruel to people and animals
  ▷ Enforcing sexual activity
▶ Destruction
  ▷ Setting fire
  ▷ Destroying property
▶ Deceitfulness
  ▷ Stealing
  ▷ Lying
▶ Violations of rules
  ▷ Staying out at night without parental consent
  ▷ Truanting
  ▷ Running away

Depression in children

▶ The diagnostic criteria for a major depressive episode are modified from that of adults
▶ Mood change can present as irritable mood instead of depressed mood; prepubertal children have more frequent episodes of irritable mood than do adult depressive patients
▶ Instead of significant weight loss, children with depression may present failure to make expected weight gains

Developmental coordination disorder

▶ Motor coordination is below the expected level given the age and intelligence
▶ Not due to cerebral palsy, muscular dystrophy, and other general medical condition

Diagnosis for mental retardation

▶ The diagnosis of mental retardation (MR) requires
  ▷ Subaverage intelligence quotient (IQ) (lower than 70)
  ▷ Significant dysfunction in skill areas including communication, self-care, home living, social skills, work, leisure, health, and safety
▶ Onset must occur before 18 years of age

▶ IQ range
  ▷ Mild MR 50: 55–70
  ▷ Moderate MR 35: 40–50
  ▷ Severe MR 20: 25–40
  ▷ Profound MR below 20–25
▶ IQ 71–84 is known as borderline intellectual functioning, a V code for Axis II

Disorder of written expression

▶ Writing skills are below expected level given the age, intelligence, education, and sensory ability

Down's syndrome

John Langdon Down (1828–1896) was a British physician.

▶ Prevalence – about 1/1,000
▶ Trisomy 21
▶ Physical features
  ▷ Single transverse palmar crease
  ▷ Epicanthic fold of the eyelid
  ▷ Shorter limbs
  ▷ Poor muscle tone
  ▷ Larger than normal space between the big and second toes
  ▷ Protruding tongue
▶ Higher risk for
  ▷ Congenital heart defects
  ▷ Gastroesophageal reflux disease
  ▷ Recurrent ear infections
  ▷ Obstructive sleep apnea
  ▷ Thyroid dysfunctions
▶ High incidence of Alzheimer's dementia

Drug metabolism in children

▶ Metabolism is more efficient, and often requires two-fold greater weight-corrected doses
▶ Higher peak plasma concentrations and lower trough plasma concentration

Encores

▶ Beyond age 4 years, making feces onto inappropriate places, at least once a month for at least 3 months
▶ May be involuntary or intentional
▶ Not due to physical deficit or medicine
▶ With or without constipation and overflow incontinence

Enuresis

▶ Beyond age 5 years, making urine in inappropriate places, at least twice a week for at least 3 months.
▶ Not due to a general medical condition.

Expressive language disorder

▶ Expressive language development is below expected level given the age and intelligence
▶ Has limited vocabulary and difficulty in tense
▶ Has academic or occupational impairment

Fetal alcohol syndrome

▶ Prevalence – about 1 per 1,000 live births
▶ Clinical features
   ▷ MR
   ▷ Abnormal facial features
   ▷ Growth delay
   ▷ Vision or hearing defects
   ▷ Behavior problems

Kleine-Levin syndrome

Willi Kleine was a German psychiatrist.
Max Levin (born 1901) was an American neurologist.

▶ A periodic, episodic condition
▶ Etiology is not clear
▶ Clinical features
   ▷ Hypersomnolence
   ▷ Hyperphagia
   ▷ Aggressive behavior
   ▷ Sexual disinhibition
▶ Treatment
   ▷ No definitive treatment
   ▷ Trials of stimulants, mood stabilizers, and hormonal (for teenage girls) had limited success

Landau-Kleffner syndrome

▶ Acquired receptive aphasia
▶ Onset is between ages 3 and 6 years
▶ Electroechogram (EEG) abnormalities and seizures, spike waves in temporal loves
▶ Social interactivity and nonverbal communication is usually retained
▶ Also known as acquired epileptic aphasia

Learning disorders

▶ Reading disorder
▶ Mathematics disorder
▶ Disorder of written expression
▶ Learning disorder NOS

Mental retardation: function level

▶ Mild MR
  ▷ Sixth grade education
  ▷ Living independently as adults
  ▷ "Educable"
▶ Moderate MR
  ▷ Second grade education
  ▷ May live with supervision
  ▷ "Trainable"
▶ Severe MR
  ▷ Limited speech
  ▷ Close supervision
▶ Profound MR
  ▷ Minimal communication
  ▷ Constant supervision in highly structured setting

Phonological disorder

▶ Also known as developmental articulation disorder
▶ Impaired ability to produce proper sound as expected by age and other aspects of development
  ▷ Substituting some sounds
  ▷ Omitting some sounds
  ▷ Producing errors in sound
▶ If mental retardation, the symptoms are in excess of the expected difficulties given the developmental level

Pica

▶ Eating of inedible substances
▶ Symptom lasts for at least 1 month

Psychiatric conditions comorbid with ADHD

▶ Disruptive behavior disorders (most common)
▶ Depression
▶ Bipolar disorders
▶ Conduct disorder
▶ Learning disorders
▶ Substance related disorders

Psychostimulants: use in psychiatry

▶ ADHD
▶ Narcolepsy
▶ Depression in elderly and medically ill
▶ Exogenous obesity

Reactive attachment disorder of infancy or early childhood

▶ Inappropriate social interactions
▶ Lack of selective social attachments
▶ Reasonable clinical presumption that pathogenic pattern of care is responsible for the development of the symptoms
  ▷ Basic physical and emotional needs are neglected
  ▷ Frequent changes of primary caregiver prevent the formation of stable attachments
▶ No mental retardation or other pervasive developmental disorder

Reading disorder

▶ Reading ability is below the expected level given the age and intelligence as measured by standardized tests

Rett's disorder

Andreas Rett (1924–1997) was an Austrian pediatrician.

▶ Mutation on long arm of X chromosome
▶ X-linked dominant in girls or XXY boys; lethal in XY boys (one copy of normal allele is necessary)
▶ Onset 6–18 months
▶ Arrest or deterioration of mental and motor skills; purposeless stereotyped hand movements
▶ Progressive microcephaly
▶ Prenatal testing available

Rumination disorder

▶ Regurgitation and rechewing of food
▶ Symptoms last for at least 1 month

Selective mutism

▶ Also know as elective mutism
▶ Inability to speak in specific social situations
▶ Functional impairment
▶ Symptoms last for at least 1 month

Separation anxiety disorder

▶ Excessive distress with separation from major attachment figures
▶ Worry about losing major attachment figures
▶ Reluctance or refusal to leave home, to be alone or to go to sleep without the company of major attachment figures
▶ Complaints of nightmares or physical symptoms when separation occurs
▶ Symptoms last for at least 4 weeks

Stereotypic movement disorder

▶ Nonfunctional and repetitive movement
▶ Interferes with activities or causes self-inflicted injury
▶ Abnormal behavior persists for at least 4 weeks

Stuttering

▶ Repetitions
▶ Prolongations
▶ Interjections
▶ Broken words

Mental retardation: the most common causes

▶ Down's syndrome, fragile X syndrome and fetal alcohol syndrome are the three most common causes
  ▷ The most common genetic cause – Down's syndrome
  ▷ The most common inherited cause – Fragile X syndrome
  ▷ The most common preventable cause – Fetal alcohol syndrome

The Multimodal Treatment Study of Children with Attention Deficit Hyperactivity Disorder (MTA)

▶ An National Institute of Mental Health (NIMH) sponsored study started in 1998; the first stage of 14 month study was published in 1999; on-going follow-up is in process
▶ Patients were randomly assigned to four treatment modes
  ▷ Medication alone
  ▷ Psychosocial/behavioral treatment alone
  ▷ Combination of both
  ▷ Routine community care
▶ Preliminary conclusions
  ▷ In reducing ADHD symptoms – combination and medication alone are both significantly superior to intensive behavioral treatments and routine community care
  ▷ In multiple areas of functioning (academic performance, parent–child relations, and social skills, etc.) – combination was consistently superior to other modals of treatment
  ▷ Additional advantages of combination approach – required lower doses of medication compared to medication alone group

Tourette's syndrome

Georges de la Tourette (1857–1904) was a French neurologist.

▶ Inherited neurological disorder
▶ Onset before age 18 years, usually between 6 and 10 years
▶ Multiple motor tics and at least one vocal tic
▶ Wax and wane
▶ No tic-free period for more than 3 months

▶ Treatment
  ▷ Supportive psychobehavioral therapy, education, and reassurance may be sufficient for most cases
  ▷ Cognitive-behavioral therapy
  ▷ Typical or atypical antipsychotics, including pimozide
  ▷ Clonidine and guanfacine
  ▷ Antidepressants to treat comorbid symptoms

Transient tic disorder

▶ Motor and/or vocal tics
▶ At least 4 weeks, no longer than 12 months
▶ Onset before age 18 years

25 Psychosomatic Disorders and Consultation-Liaison Psychiatry

The interest in the interface between psychiatry and physical medicine, or the mind and the body, has been pursued since ancient time. The most intriguing case was hysteria, which for many centuries was believed to be a mental disorder caused by a wondering organ, the uterus. Though physical disorders have long been observed and proved to cause a wide spectrum of psychiatric conditions, the interest in psychosomatic medicine as a defined psychiatric specialty laid mostly in "psychological factors affecting medical condition," as described in DSM-IV-TR.

The causal relationship between psychological stresses and the physical disorders may sometimes be obvious, yet in other times vague. Consultation-liaison psychiatrists often face the challenge of the differentiation between physical and psychological etiologies. In most cases, however, combining both the psychiatric and general medical evaluation and treatment may be the most effective approach. Conditions frequently mentioned are reviewed in this chapter.

Acute intermittent porphyria

▶ Triad of symptoms
  ▷ Acute abdominal pain
  ▷ Polyneuropathy
  ▷ Psychosis and other mental symptoms
▶ Autosomal dominant disorder
▶ Inducers of porphyria – chemicals or situations that boost heme synthesis
  ▷ Fasting or strict diet
  ▷ Cytochrome P450 inducers – barbiturates, sulfonamides, and estrogens
  ▷ Alcohol
▶ Porphyria attacks may occur without any obvious provocation
▶ Barbiturates are absolutely contraindicated in persons with personal or family history of acute intermittent porphyria

Adrenal insufficiency: clinical features

Thomas Addison (1793–1860) was an English physician and scientist.

▶ Both primary (Addison's disease) and secondary adrenal failure
  ▷ Anorexia and weight loss
  ▷ Nausea and vomiting
  ▷ Weakness and fatigue
  ▷ Hypotension
  ▷ Hyponatremia

▶ Primary but not secondary adrenal failure
  ▷ Hyperpigmentation
  ▷ Hyperkalemia
  ▷ Volume depletion
▶ Psychiatric symptoms
  ▷ Mood disturbance – depression, apathy
  ▷ Social withdrawal
  ▷ Impaired sleep
  ▷ Cognitive impairments

Adrenal insufficiency: etiology

▶ Primary adrenal insufficiency, also known as Addison's disease
  ▷ Deficiency of both cortisol and aldosterone
  ▷ Elevated adrenocorticotropic hormone (ACTH)
  ▷ Infection – TB, fungal
  ▷ Hemorrhage
  ▷ Idiopathic atrophy – the most common, possible autoimmune in nature
  ▷ Congenital adrenal hyperplasia
  ▷ Cytotoxic agents (e.g., mitotane)
▶ Secondary adrenal insufficiency
  ▷ Deficiency of cortisol but not aldosterone
  ▷ ACTH deficiency
  ▷ Hypopituitarism
  ▷ Suppression of the hypothalamic-pituitary axis – exogenous steroids (the most common cause), or endogenous steroids such as from tumor
▶ Adrenal crisis
  ▷ Also known as acute adrenocortical insufficiency
  ▷ Acute exacerbation of chronic insufficiency – sepsis, surgical stress
  ▷ Adrenal hemorrhage
  ▷ Steroid withdrawal is the most common cause of acute adrenocortical insufficiency

Adrenal insufficiency: treatment

▶ Adrenal crisis
  ▷ Hydrocortisone intravenous (IV)
  ▷ Dexamethasone IV
▶ Maintenance therapy
  ▷ Prednisone
  ▷ Fludrocortisone

Agents causing QT/QTc prolongation

▶ LAAM (levo-α-acetylmethadol), a long acting opioid
▶ All new antipsychotics except aripiprazole
▶ Tricyclic antidepressants
▶ Trazodone

Autoimmune diseases: psychiatric presentations

▶ Giant cell arteritis – depression
▶ Systemic lupus erythematosus – affective lability, psychosis, delirium
▶ Anticardiolipin antibody syndrome – affective lability, cognitive decline
▶ Inflammatory bowel disease – disturbance in body image

Celiac disease and psychosis

▶ Celiac disease
  ▷ An autoimmune disease predisposed genetically
  ▷ Upon exposure to gliadin, a gluten protein in wheat, the immune system is triggered through cross reaction, which causes inflammatory response in small intestine
▶ Psychosis in celiac disease
  ▷ Elevated psychotic ratio among individuals with celiac disease
  ▷ Often not responsive to psychopharmacological therapy
  ▷ Withdrawal of gluten from the diet often resolves the psychosis

Central pontine myelinolysis (CPM): clinical presentation and diagnosis

▶ Disturbances of consciousness
▶ Affective and behavioral disturbances
▶ Signs of damage in the corticobulbar and corticospinal tracts in the basis pontis
▶ Paralysis of the lower cranial nerves (pseudobulbar palsy, dysarthria, dysphagia, tetraparesis)
▶ May also extend to extrapontine areas
▶ Diagnosis
  ▷ Computer tomography (CT) – hypodense areas within the central pons
  ▷ Magnetic resonance imaging (MRI) – hypointense on T1 and hyperintense on T2

Central pontine myelinolysis: etiology

▶ Also known as "osmotic demyelination syndrome"
▶ Etiology
  ▷ Multiple factors involved
  ▷ Hyponatremia and its inappropriate correction
  ▷ Chronic alcoholism

Central pontine myelinolysis: treatment

▶ Prevention and early diagnosis
▶ Correcting electrolytes at proper rate
▶ Multispecialty involvement, particularly neurology
▶ Possible advances in use of
  ▷ Thyrotropin releasing hormone (TRH)
  ▷ Plasmapheresis
  ▷ Corticosteroids
  ▷ Intravenous (IV) immunoglobulins

Creutzfeld–Jakob disease

Hans G. Creutzfeldt (1885–1964) and Alfons M. Jakob (1884–1931) were German neuropathologists.

▶ A spongiform encephalopathy transmitted by prion
  ▷ Also known as proteinaceous infective particle
▶ Psychiatric symptoms
  ▷ Fatigue
  ▷ Anxiety
  ▷ Depression
  ▷ Dementia (rapidly progressive)
▶ Neurological symptoms
  ▷ Incoordination
  ▷ Abnormal gait
  ▷ Myoclonus
▶ Electroencephalogram (EEG) – triphasic, sharp, synchronous discharges
▶ Prion is resistant to sterilization techniques, except autoclave or bleach
▶ Creutzfeld–Jakob (CJ) variant disease, also known as Mad Cow Disease, has similar clinical pictures

Folate deficiency: etiology

▶ Increased requirement
  ▷ Pregnancy and lactation
  ▷ Infection
  ▷ Anemia
▶ Decreased supply
  ▷ Alcoholism
  ▷ Malabsorption, e.g., celiac disease
▶ Impaired metabolism
  ▷ Medications – Phenytoin, primidone, metformin, methotrexate, etc.
  ▷ Hypothyroidism that may impair gastrointestinal (GI) absorption
▶ Increased loss
  ▷ Renal dialysis
  ▷ B12 deficiency (folate trap phenomenon)

Functional pituitary adenoma: classification and clinical features

▶ Growth hormone
  ▷ Deficiency – cardiovascular disease, obesity, reduced muscle strength and hyper-cholesterolemia; decreased height and growth rate in children; hypoglycemia in infants
  ▷ Overproduction – pituitary gigantism in children and adolescents; acromegaly in adults
▶ Gonadotrophin
  ▷ Deficiency – diminished libido, impotence in men and dyspareunia in women, testes shrink in size, breast atrophy, but spermatogenesis generally preserved; delayed or absence of puberty in children
  ▷ Overproduction – clinically not significant

- ▶ Thyrotropin
  - ▷ Deficiency – hypothyroidism
  - ▷ Overproduction – hyperthyroidism (rare)
- ▶ Corticotrophin
  - ▷ Deficiency – deficiency limited to glucocorticoids and adrenal androgens, but not mineralocorticoid function (which is dependent on the angiotensin-renin axis, and is affected significantly in primary adrenal insufficiency)
  - ▷ Overproduction – Cushing Disease; secondary arterial hypertension, diabetes, cataracts, glaucoma, and osteoporosis
- ▶ Prolactin
  - ▷ Deficiency – not clinically significant
  - ▷ Overproduction – hyperprolactinemia and hypogonadism; amenorrhea in women, impotence in men; galactorrhea (rare in men), decreased libido, and infertility in both genders

Hemodialysis: psychiatric conditions and treatment

- ▶ Reported increased suicide rate in patients receiving hemodialysis
- ▶ Stresses include dealing with preexisting depression and quality of life on hemodialysis
- ▶ Most psychotropics are metabolized by liver with secondary renal elimination, except lithium
- ▶ A generally accepted rule is to start with 50% dose with careful titration
- ▶ Lithium may be taken after dialysis only on dialysis days

HIV/AIDS-related psychiatric conditions

- ▶ Depression – prevalence 20%–25% in HIV/AIDS population
- ▶ Acute retroviral syndrome associated with depression and fatigue
- ▶ Psychiatric disorders are associated with higher rate of IV drug using, hence higher rate of HIV infection
- ▶ Depressive symptoms are an independent risk factor for HIV disease progression and mortality
- ▶ Reported markedly increased suicide rate among individuals with HIV infection; however, this was no longer true when appropriate control groups were compared with
- ▶ AIDS dementia complex
- ▶ End of life issues – five stages

HIV/AIDS: epidemiology

- ▶ Worldwide – 33 million infected population
- ▶ Sub-Saharan Africa – over 20 million infected population
- ▶ United States – 1 million infected, 0.4% of population
- ▶ Risk groups – IV drug users, history of multiple sexual partners, minority women
- ▶ Among psychiatric patients, schizophrenics may be at risk

Hyper-parathyroidism and depression

- ▶ Malignant hypercalcemia may be mistaken for depression
- ▶ Symptoms
  - ▷ Moans (depression)

▷ Bones (osteoporosis and bone pain)
▷ Groans (GI symptoms)
▷ Stones (kidney stones)

Hyperventilation syndrome

▶ Rapid and deep breathes last for several minutes
▶ Complaints of suffocation, lightheadedness, and anxiety
▶ Respiratory alkalosis symptoms
  ▷ Tetany
  ▷ Paresthesia
  ▷ Palpitations
▶ Treatment
  ▷ Breathing into a paper bag
  ▷ Education

Hypoglycemia: neuropsychiatric symptoms

▶ Delirium, confusion, amnesia
▶ Fatigue, weakness
▶ Mood
  ▷ Lability – irritability, belligerence, combativeness, rage
  ▷ Dysphoria, anxiety, and depression
  ▷ Apathy
▶ Neurologic
  ▷ Ataxia and incoordination
  ▷ Focal or general motor deficit, paralysis, or hemiparesis
  ▷ Paresthesias, headache
  ▷ Slurred speech
  ▷ Generalized or focal seizures
  ▷ Stupor and coma
  ▷ Permanent amnesia from hippocampal involvement

Interferon treatment and mental disorders

▶ Interferon treatment of hepatitis C may cause significant depression
▶ Serotonin-selective reuptake inhibitors (SSRIs) may be used for treatment or prevention
▶ Contraindications
  ▷ Active suicidal ideation
  ▷ Uncontrolled psychosis
  ▷ Significant psychiatric disease not under active treatment

Lyme disease: diagnosis

▶ Center for Disease Control (CDC) suggested two-step diagnosis
  ▷ Antibody titer
  ▷ Western blot

Lyme disease: mental symptoms

▶ Mania
▶ Panic symptoms
▶ Chronic fatigue
▶ Depression
▶ Dementia

Medical conditions associated with anxiety disorders

▶ Drugs and substances
  ▷ Caffeine
  ▷ Cocaine
  ▷ Corticosteroids
  ▷ Sympathomimetics
  ▷ Theophylline
  ▷ Thyroid hormones
  ▷ Withdrawal from alcohol, narcotics, benzodiazepines
▶ Endocrine
  ▷ Hyperthyroidism
  ▷ Hyperparathyroidism
  ▷ Pheochromocytoma
▶ Cardiovascular – arrhythmias, mitrovalve prolapse
▶ Pulmonary – pulmonary embolism, chronic obstructive pulmonary disease (COPD)

Multiple sclerosis: psychiatric symptoms

▶ Depression and irritability are most common
▶ Psychiatric symptoms may precede physical symptoms
▶ Psychiatric symptoms do not clear with remission of physical symptoms
▶ Psychiatric symptoms do not correlate with physical findings

Peptic ulcer disorder and psychiatric disorders

▶ Etiology
  ▷ Infection with *Helicobacter pylori* has been associated with 70%–95% of the cases
  ▷ Stress may reduce immune responses, and increase the vulnerability to infection with *H. pylori*
  ▷ Nonsteroidal antiinflammatory drugs (NSAID) use is another popular cause; NSAID blocks the cyclooxygenase-1, an enzyme essential for the production of prostaglandins; prostaglandins stimulate secretion of gastric-protective mucus
  ▷ Psychological stress increases the production of gastric acid excretion
▶ Treatment
  ▷ Antibiotic therapy is the treatment of choice
  ▷ Antacids
  ▷ H2-antagonists
  ▷ Avoid using NSAIDs, or combine with misoprostol (Cytotec), a prostaglandin analogue

Psoriasis

▶ Silvery scales with glossy, homogeneous erythema
▶ Chronic, relapsing condition
▶ Associated with stress, and produces more stress
▶ Comorbidity
  ▷ Anxiety and depression
  ▷ Personality disorders
  ▷ Alcohol-related conditions
▶ Treatment
  ▷ Stress management
  ▷ Relaxation therapy
  ▷ Dermatology therapy

Pulmonary condition and mental disorders

▶ Asthma and COPD
  ▷ May comorbid with panic disorder
▶ Corticosteroids treatment may cause
  ▷ Euphoria and mood lability
  ▷ Depression
  ▷ Psychosis
  ▷ Delirium
▶ SSRIs have been shown to improve COPD independent of improvement in mood and anxiety symptoms

Thyroid function tests

▶ Screening tests – thyroid stimulating hormone (TSH), T_4, T_3, and free thyroxine
▶ Hypothyroidism
  ▷ Elevated TSH – the most sensitive screening test
  ▷ Decreased T_4, T_3, free thyroxine index
▶ Hyperthyroidism
  ▷ Decreased TSH – the most sensitive screening test
  ▷ Elevated T_4, T_3, free thyroxine index
▶ Thyroxine binding globulin (TBG)
  ▷ T4 (RIA) – varies directly with TBG
  ▷ Resin uptake (T3RU) – varies inversely with TBG
  ▷ The product of FT_4 and T_3RU helps correct the abnormalities of thyroxine binding
▶ Advanced tests – immunology, radiology, pathology
▶ Immunology
  ▷ Antithyroglobulin
  ▷ Antithyroperoxidase antibodies
  ▷ Antimicrosomal antibodies
  ▷ TSH receptor antibody
▶ Radiology
  ▷ [123]I uptake and scan
  ▷ [99]mTc scan
  ▷ Ultrasonography
▶ Pathology
  ▷ Fine-needle aspiration

26 Psychosocial Therapies

In a broader sense of history, ancient complementary therapies using religious, magic, and other suggestive methods existed in many cultures over a millennium before the Common Era. Psychoanalysis is perhaps the first school of psychotherapy in a modern sense, which has a specifically defined theory and method, and targeted at altering the psychological process through mainly the conversation.

A wide variety of psychotherapies remain active in psychiatry, reflecting the complex of theoretical basis of mental illness. In general, psychotherapies seek for increasing the awareness, improving coping skills, and enhancing the resilience and functional level. Therapies usually base on certain psychological theories, and the practice of psychotherapies often provide test and feedback on the original theories.

The behavioral and emotional changes caused by psychotherapies were believed to be nonstructural and nonbiological. However, recent evidences suggested that through time, successful psychotherapies may cause neurobiological changes.

Commonly used psychotherapies include

▶ Biofeedback therapy
▶ Brief focal psychodynamic psychotherapy
▶ Cognitive behavior therapy (CBT)
▶ Dialectical behavioral therapy (DBT)
▶ Interpersonal psychotherapy
▶ Psychoanalytical psychotherapy
▶ Structural family therapy
▶ Supportive psychotherapy

Biofeedback therapy

▶ A form of alternative medicine purposed on conscious control of physiological activities
▶ Conditions with possible response to biofeedback
  ▷ Hypertension
  ▷ Tachycardia and bradycardia
  ▷ Raynaud's disease
  ▷ Anxiety and phobias
  ▷ Asthma
  ▷ Ulcers
  ▷ Stuttering
  ▷ Attention-deficit/hyperactivity disorder (ADHD)

Brief focal psychodynamic psychotherapy

▶ Also known as short-term dynamic psychotherapy
▶ Duration – usually 5–25 sessions
▶ Selection criteria
  ▷ High motivation
  ▷ Able to tolerate anxiety and guilt
  ▷ Flexible defenses, and lack of destructive defense such as projection, splitting, and denial
  ▷ Psychological mindedness
  ▷ Past meaningful relationship
  ▷ Good response to trial transference interpretation
▶ Goal – resolution of Oedipal conflict

Brief psychotherapy

▶ Duration – usually less than 20 sessions
▶ Focus not on the past, rather the present and future
▶ Focus on what clients want to achieve rather than on the problems that made them seek help
▶ Styles
  ▷ Brief focal or short-term dynamic psycotherapy
  ▷ Time-limited psychotherapy
  ▷ Short-term anxiety-provoking psychotherapy

Cognitive behavior therapy

▶ Assumption
  ▷ Negative thoughts promote pathological mood (mainly depression and anxiety)
  ▷ Disturbed emotions can be influenced through modifying cognitions, assumptions, beliefs and behaviors.
▶ Manual-driven
▶ Duration – usually 10–12 sessions
▶ Demonstrated efficacy in depression, obsessive-compulsive disorder (OCD), and other anxiety disorders

Confrontation

▶ An intervention strategy in psychotherapy
▶ To clarify the meaning of behavior that is not accepted, avoided, or minimized by the patient

Dialectical behavioral therapy

Marsha Linehan (1943–) is a contemporary U.S. psychologist.

▶ Designed by Marsha Linehan specifically to treat borderline personality disorder; it is, though, also used for other conditions
▶ Based largely on behaviorist theory and cognitive therapy
▶ A manual-driven therapy with a psychoeducational focus

► Essential elements
  ▷ Individual sessions – discussing issues that come up during the week, followed by therapy interfering behaviors
  ▷ Group sessions – learning to use specific skills
► Core skills
  ▷ Mindfulness skills
  ▷ Emotion regulation skills
  ▷ Interpersonal effectiveness skills
  ▷ Distress tolerance skills

Enmeshment vs. disengagement

Salvador Minuchin is an Argentina-born contemporary U.S. psychiatrist.

► Enmeshment is a concept from Minuchin's theory of structural family therapy
► Refers to overly closed relationship between family members that blur the ego boundaries
► It is considered ineffective and unhealthy, and widely viewed as a negative impact on child development
► Example
  ▷ In a doctor's office, a mother describes her child's disease as "our disease," and soothes the child "we will get well soon"
► Disengagement is a pattern opposite to enmeshment, refers to a relation with excessive distance

Focus of cognitive-behavioral therapy

► The goal is to identify and alter cognitive distortions that are believed to cause symptoms
► Common cognitive distortions and suggested intervention
  ▷ Overgeneralizing – intervention is to help patient expose faulty logic
  ▷ Selective abstraction – intervention is to identify successes patient ignored or forgot
  ▷ Assuming excessive responsibility – intervention is to help learn disattribution
  ▷ Predicting without sufficient evidence – intervention is to expose faulty logic
  ▷ Catastrophizing – intervention is to help calculate real probabilities

Free association

► A fundamental technique of psychoanalysis
► Patients are asked to say everything that comes to their minds
► The technique was designed as an alternative to hypnosis, to recover crucial memories while conscious, and to avoid false memories while hypnotized
► Resistance – in practice, patients often select and modify what they have to say, due to embarrassment or concerns about what the analyst may think
► Repression – some memories, even with the patient's genuine compliance, may still not be able to recover; these are usually repressed painful memories
► During free association, the therapist assumes not authoritarian role, but a supportive, encouraging, and understanding role

Functions of the psychiatric interview

▶ Assessing the nature of the problem
▶ Developing a therapeutic relationship
▶ Communicating information and treatment planning

Interpersonal psychotherapy

▶ A time-limited psychotherapy
▶ Used primarily in the treatment of depression
▶ Rooted in psychodynamic theory, but uses skills from cognitive-behavioral approaches
▶ Based on the belief that
  ▷ Psychological problems are due to inadequate communication
  ▷ Communication problems are formed due to attachment styles
▶ Common interpersonal issues
  ▷ Grief
  ▷ Role transition
  ▷ Role dispute
  ▷ Interpersonal deficits

Mindfulness

▶ A technique used in psychotherapy in which a person becomes intentionally aware of his or her thoughts and actions in the present moment, nonjudgmentally
▶ A fundamental skill of dialectical behavioral therapy

Psychoanalytical psychotherapy

▶ Also known as
  ▷ Psychodynamic psychotherapy
  ▷ Expressive psychotherapy
▶ Based on Sigmund Freud's theory on psychoanalysis
▶ Basic approach is focused on uncovering unconscious conflicts of the patient's mental life
▶ Difficulty in current life is believed to have a connection with childhood experience
▶ Basic technique is free association, with close attention paid to transference, counter-transference, and resistance
▶ Length of therapy varies from a few months to a few years
▶ Applied mostly to personality disorders, severe and chronic problems in coping with life events

Reaction to approaching death

Elisabeth Kubler-Ross (1926–2004) was a Swiss-born U.S. psychiatrist.

▶ Elisabeth Kubler-Ross described five stages of reaction a person typically encounter when facing approaching death
  1. Shock and denial
  2. Anger
  3. Bargaining
  4. Depression
  5. Acceptance

Reframing

▶ Also known as "positive connotation"
▶ Clarification and relabeling of negative thoughts and behavior in a positive meaning

Reparative therapy

▶ Also known as
  ▷ Conversion therapy
  ▷ Sexual reorientation therapy
▶ Psychotherapeutic approaches aimed at "repairing" homosexual people's sexual orientations
▶ Techniques include
  ▷ Behavior modification
  ▷ Aversion therapy
  ▷ Psychoanalysis
  ▷ Religious techniques
▶ The scientific consensus in the United States is that reparative therapy is not effective at changing sexual orientation and is potentially harmful
▶ Since 1970s, the American Psychiatric Association has held the position that homosexuality is a nonpathologic human behavior rather than a disorder

Resistance

▶ A psychoanalytic term coined by Sigmund Freud
▶ Unconscious repression of thoughts and impulses so to avoid conscious awareness

Structural family therapy

▶ Developed by Salvador Minuchin
▶ A family's ability to adapt to various stressors rests upon the clarity and appropriateness of its subsystem boundaries
▶ Family structure
  ▷ Hierarchy of power
  ▷ Subsystems
  ▷ Boundaries
▶ Dysfunctional families exhibit
  ▷ Mixed subsystems
  ▷ Improper power hierarchies
  ▷ Boundaries impairment – enmeshment, rigidity
  ▷ Example – an older child is brought in to the parental subsystem to replace an absent spouse
▶ The treatment
  ▷ The therapist enters the family system as a catalyst for positive change
  ▷ The goal is to restructure the family system

Supportive psychotherapy

▶ Brief
▶ Focus on assistance to deal with a life crisis

▶ Strategy
  ▷ Advice
  ▷ Sympathy
  ▷ Reinforcing the patient's strength
▶ Anecdotally especially effective for acute grief reactions

Systematic desensitization

▶ Based on the principle of counterconditioning
▶ Techniques
  ▷ Relaxation training
  ▷ A graded list of anxiety-provoking scenes, usually prepared by the therapist
  ▷ Exposing to the stimulus that elicits the anxiety response, while using relaxation techniques to inhibit the anxiety

Techniques used in psychiatric interviews

▶ Confrontation – helping the patient face what is missed or denied
▶ Continuation – encouraging the patient to continue
▶ Echoing – echoing part of the patient's words to emphasize or shift the emphasis
▶ Redirection – steering a patient to a more productive topic
▶ Silence – often providing accepting and supportive environment, but may be used in other ways
▶ Transition – encouraging the patient to continue on a different topic

Termination of psychodynamic psychotherapy

▶ Indicators for termination in psychodynamic psychotherapy are
  ▷ Presenting symptoms are eliminated
  ▷ Interpersonal relationships are improved
  ▷ Superego is modified
  ▷ Ability to examine conflicts is restored

Therapeutic neutrality

▶ A technique stance from psychoanalytical tradition, in which the therapist restrains him/herself from any directional response so to encourage free association to expose more unconscious contents
▶ It is no longer the rule in current trend of therapy, particularly in nondynamic schools

Transference and countertransference

▶ Both refer to the unconsciously retained feeling and desire in the childhood that is redirected to a new object
▶ Transference is the feeling from the patient toward the therapist
▶ Countertransference is the therapist's feeling to the patient; it is a distorted perception of the doctor–patient relationship

Triangle of insight

David Malan was a British psychologist.

▶ Concept brought up by David Malan in brief psychodynamic psychotherapy
▶ The model include
  ▷ Transference patterns
  ▷ Current relationships
  ▷ Past relationships

Triangulation

▶ A pathological family relationship that is usually noticed in family therapy
▶ Two parental authority figures have disagreements; rather than resolving the disagreements, they involve a third, less powerful party, usually a child, to diffuse the conflict; this involvement is called triangulation
▶ The triangulated child receives much of the frustration from parents, and develops behavior problems as a call for help

27 Antipsychotics

The term "antipsychotic" may well be an accepted misnomer, or at least not descriptive and inclusive enough to accommodate the current research and clinical trend. Many antipsychotics have effects as well as Food and Drug Administration (FDA) indication for nonpsychotic conditions. All the atypical antipsychotics have obtained indication for some part of treatment for bipolar disorders. Nonetheless, the most conventional and strict definition of the antipsychotic effect has to be the ability to reduce hallucinations, delusions and formal thought disorders. At this point in time, we have found no substance possesses such effect without dopamine D2 receptor blockade effect. The relationship between clinical efficacy and affinity to D2 receptors and other neuronal receptors have inspired much research interest and scientific insight to psychosis and other mental phenomena. However, with the single exception of clozapine, the difference between antipsychotics laying mainly not on their ability to control psychotic symptoms, but their side effect profiles, tolerability, effect on mood and cognitive symptoms. In large, the atypical antipsychotics possess advantage on most of these aspects. The following list summarizes antipsychotics currently available in the United States

- ▶ Typical antipsychotics
  - ▷ Aripiprazole (Abilify)
  - ▷ Clozapine (Clozaril, FazaClo ODT)
  - ▷ Olanzapine (Zyprexa)
  - ▷ Paliperidone (Invega)
  - ▷ Quetiapine (Seroquel)
  - ▷ Risperidone (Risperdal)
  - ▷ Ziprasidone (Geodon)
- ▶ Atypical antipsychotics
  - ▷ Chlorpromazine (Thorazine)
  - ▷ Fluphenazine (Prolixin)
  - ▷ Haloperidol (Haldol)
  - ▷ Loxapine (Loxitane)
  - ▷ Molindone (Moban)
  - ▷ Perphenazine (Trilafon)
  - ▷ Thioridazine (Mellaril)
  - ▷ Thiothixene (Navane)
  - ▷ Trifluoperazine (Stelazine)

Also described here are several dopamine blocking agents that are not used primarily as antipsychotics, but nonetheless believed to have antipsychotic effect, and certainly not immunized from adverse effects. These are Pimozide (Orap), indicated for Tourette's syndrome; prochlorperazine (Compazine) and droperidol (Inapsine), both used as antiemetics.

Antipsychotics for acute agitation: oral concentrate vs. injections

▶ Oral concentrate decreases feelings of traumatizing and helplessness
▶ Injections have more predictable absorption, and eliminate the need for hepatic metabolism

Aripiprazole

▶ Brand name
  ▷ Abilify (PO, IM)
  ▷ Abilify DiscMelt
▶ Dosage
  ▷ PO up to 30 mg/day
  ▷ IM 9.75 mg/2 h up to 30 mg/day
▶ Mechanism of action
  ▷ Partial agonist at D2 and 5-HT1A receptors
  ▷ Minimum affinity for cholinergic receptors
▶ Indicated for
  ▷ Schizophrenia – adults and adolescents (from 13 years of age)
  ▷ Bipolar – acute mania and maintenance
  ▷ Adjunct treatment of major depressive disorder
  ▷ Agitation
▶ Black box warning
  ▷ Increased mortality in elderly patients with dementia; risk of death is 1.6–1.7 times of that of placebo-treated patients; most of deaths are cardiovascular or infectious in nature
  ▷ Increased risk of suicidality in depressive patients under age 24 years, particularly during the first month of treatment
▶ Other safety caution and adverse effect
  ▷ Pregnancy – C
  ▷ Minimum weight gaining
▶ Metabolism
  ▷ CYP450: substrate of 2D6 and 3A4
  ▷ Half-life: approximately 75 hours

Atypical vs. typical antipsychotics

▶ All typical antipsychotics are mainly D2 blockers
▶ All atypicals are D2/5-HT2a blockers, and mostly have higher affinity to 5-HT2a than D2
▶ Advantages of atypical antipsychotics
  ▷ Efficacy for negative symptoms
  ▷ Less extrapyramidal symptoms (EPS)
  ▷ Efficacy for cognitive function impairment
  ▷ Evidence on mood stabilizing
▶ Advantages of typical antipsychotics
  ▷ Lower cost
  ▷ Relatively less weight gain and metabolic abnormalities

Chlorpromazine

The first antipsychotic approved (1954), hence the term "pre-" and "post-Thorazine era."

▶ Brand name
  ▷ Thorazine
▶ Dosage
  ▷ Up to 1,000 mg/day
▶ Mechanism
  ▷ Antagonizes dopamine D2 receptors
▶ Indicated for
  ▷ Psychosis
  ▷ Nausea and vomiting
  ▷ Preoperational sedation
  ▷ Intractable hiccups
  ▷ Adjunct treatment for tetanus
  ▷ Acute intermittent porphyria
▶ Black box warning
  ▷ Increased mortality in elderly patients with dementia; risk of death is 1.6–1.7 times of that of placebo-treated patients; most of deaths are cardiovascular or infectious in nature
▶ Other safety caution and adverse effect
  ▷ Pregnancy – C
  ▷ Sedation
  ▷ Hypotension
  ▷ Extrapyramidal syndrome
  ▷ Neuroleptic malignant syndrome
  ▷ Tardive dyskinesia
▶ Metabolism
  ▷ CYP450: substrate of 2D6
  ▷ Half-life: approximately 30 hours

Clozapine: clinical efficacy

▶ Effective for
  ▷ Both positive and negative symptoms
  ▷ Refractory psychosis
  ▷ Hostility and aggression
  ▷ The only antipsychotic that reduces suicidal behavior

Clozapine: adverse effects

▶ Black box warning
  ▷ Increased mortality in elderly patients with dementia; risk of death is 1.6–1.7 times of that of placebo-treated patients; most of deaths are cardiovascular or infectious in nature
  ▷ Agranulocytosis
  ▷ Seizures
  ▷ Myocarditis and congestive heart failure (CHF)
▶ Common adverse effects
  ▷ Sedation

▷ Orthostatic hypotension
▷ Anticholinergic effect
▷ Weight gain
▷ Metabolic abnormalities
▷ Sialorrhea
▶ Rare adverse effects
▷ Agranulocytosis (not dose related)
▷ Seizure (dose related)
▷ Myocarditis and fatal CHF
▶ Minimal or none
▷ EPS
▷ Prolactin elevation

Clozapine: white blood cell count and ANC monitoring (Figure 27–1)

▶ White blood cell (WBC) ≥ 3,500, ANC ≥ 2,000
▷ Weekly for 6 months, then every 2 weeks for 6 months, then monthly
▶ WBC: 3,500–3,000, or ANC: 2,000–1,500
▷ Continue drug, repeat to confirm, monitor twice per week
▶ WBC: 3,000–2,000, or ANC: 1,500–1,000
▷ Stop Clozapine, daily monitoring till WBC > 3,000 and ANC > 1,500; restart Clozapine, monitor twice weekly until WBC > 3,500, then weekly for 6 months
▶ WBC < 2,000 or ANC < 1,000 – stop clozapine permanently, daily WBC until normal, then repeat WBC weekly for 4 weeks; emergent medical care if fever or infection occurs

Droperidol

▶ Brand name
▷ Inapsine

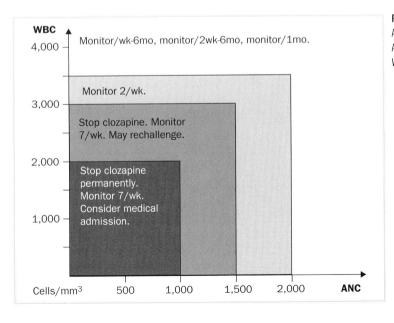

Figure 27-1 WBC count and ANC monitor frequency.
ANC, absolute neutrophil count; WBC, white blood cell.

▶ Dosage
 ▷ Intramuscular/intravenous (IM/IV) up to 2.5 mg/dose
▶ Mechanism
 ▷ Antagonizes dopamine D2 receptors
▶ Indication
 ▷ Nausea and vomiting
▶ Black box warning
 ▷ QT prolongation
▶ Other safety caution and adverse effect
 ▷ Pregnancy – C
 ▷ Extrapyramidal syndrome
 ▷ Neuroleptic malignant syndrome
 ▷ Tardive dyskinesia
▶ Metabolism
 ▷ CYP450 – substrate of 3A4
 ▷ Half-life – 1.5 hours

Fluphenazine

▶ Brand name
 ▷ Prolixin
▶ Dosage
 ▷ PO 0.5 mg tid up to 40 mg/day (tablets or oral concentrate)
 ▷ IM 1.25 mg/8 h up to 10 mg/day
 ▷ Decanoate IM 12.5 mg/3 wk up to 100 mg/dose/3–6 week
▶ Mechanism
 ▷ Antagonizes dopamine D2 receptors
▶ Indication
 ▷ Psychosis
▶ Black box warning
 ▷ Increased mortality in elderly patients with dementia; risk of death is 1.6–1.7 times of that of placebo-treated patients; most of deaths are cardiovascular or infectious in nature
▶ Other safety caution and adverse effect
 ▷ Pregnancy – C
 ▷ Extrapyramidal syndrome
 ▷ Neuroleptic malignant syndrome
 ▷ Tardive dyskinesia
 ▷ Pigmentary retinopathy, requires periodical ophthalmologic examination
 ▷ Seizure
 ▷ Blood dyscrasias
▶ Metabolism
 ▷ CYP450: substrate of 2D6
 ▷ Half-life: PO 15 hours; decanoate IM 6–10 days

Haloperidol

▶ Brand name
 ▷ Haldol

- ▶ Dosage
  - ▷ PO up to 100 mg/day
  - ▷ IM up to 100 mg/day
  - ▷ IV is not FDA approved
  - ▷ Decanoate IM – upto 450 mg/mo
- ▶ Mechanism
  - ▷ Antagonizes dopamine D2 receptors
- ▶ Indication
  - ▷ Psychosis
  - ▷ Tourette's syndrome
- ▶ Black box warning
  - ▷ Increased mortality in elderly patients with dementia; risk of death is 1.6–1.7 times of that of placebo-treated patients; most of deaths are cardiovascular or infectious in nature
- ▶ Other safety caution and adverse effect
  - ▷ Extrapyramidal syndrome
  - ▷ Neuroleptic malignant syndrome
  - ▷ Tardive dyskinesia
  - ▷ QT prolongation and Torsades de pointes; periodical electrocardiogram (ECG) monitoring is recommended
  - ▷ Pregnancy – C
- ▶ Metabolism
  - ▷ CYP450: 2D6 substrate and inhibitor
  - ▷ Half-life: PO/IM: 21 hours; decanoate: 21 days

Loxapine

- ▶ Brand name
  - ▷ Loxitane
- ▶ Dosage
  - ▷ PO 10 mg bid up to 250 mg/day
- ▶ Mechanism
  - ▷ Antagonizes dopamine D2 receptors
- ▶ Indication
  - ▷ Psychosis
- ▶ Black box warning
  - ▷ Increased mortality in elderly patients with dementia; risk of death is 1.6–1.7 times of that of placebo-treated patients; most of deaths are cardiovascular or infectious in nature
- ▶ Other safety caution and adverse effect
  - ▷ Pregnancy – C
  - ▷ Extrapyramidal syndrome
  - ▷ Neuroleptic malignant syndrome
  - ▷ Tardive dyskinesia
  - ▷ Anticholinergic effect
  - ▷ Orthostatic hypotension
  - ▷ Seizures
  - ▷ Agranulocytosis

▶ Metabolism
  ▷ CYP450: unknown
  ▷ Half-life: 3–4 hours

Molindone

▶ Brand name
  ▷ Moban
▶ Dosage
  ▷ Up to 225 mg/day, in divided doses
▶ Mechanism
  ▷ Antagonizes dopamine D2 receptors
▶ Indication
  ▷ Psychosis
▶ Black box warning
  ▷ Increased mortality in elderly patients with dementia; risk of death is 1.6–1.7 times of that of placebo-treated patients; most of deaths are cardiovascular or infectious in nature
▶ Other safety caution and adverse effect
  ▷ Pregnancy – C
  ▷ May cause leucopenia; periodical blood count follow-up is recommended
  ▷ Extrapyramidal syndrome
  ▷ Neuroleptic malignant syndrome
  ▷ Tardive dyskinesia
  ▷ Anticholinergic effect – moderate
  ▷ Orthostatic hypotension
  ▷ Weight gain – not expected
▶ Metabolism
  ▷ CYP450 – unknown
  ▷ Half-life – approximately 12 hours

Olanzapine

▶ Brand name and dosage
  ▷ Zyprexa – PO up to 20 mg/day, IM up to 30 mg/day
  ▷ Zyprexa Zydis – PO up to 20 mg/day
▶ Mechanism
  ▷ Antagonizes dopamine D2 and serotonin 5-HT2 receptors
▶ Indication
  ▷ Schizophrenia
  ▷ Bipolar mania
  ▷ Acute agitation
▶ Black box warning
  ▷ Increased mortality in elderly patients with dementia; risk of death is 1.6–1.7 times of that of placebo-treated patients; most of deaths are cardiovascular or infectious in nature
  ▷ Increased risk of suicidality in depressive patients under age 24 years, particularly during the first month of treatment
▶ Other safety caution and adverse effect
  ▷ Neuroleptic malignant syndrome

- ▷ EPS
- ▷ Tardive dyskinesia
- ▷ Hyperglycemia
- ▷ Diabetes mellitus
- ▷ Hyperlipidemia
- ▷ Weight gaining
- ▷ Pregnancy – C
- ▶ Absorption and metabolism
  - ▷ Absorption is not affected by food
  - ▷ Zyprexa tablet and Zydis are bioequivalents
  - ▷ Steady-state is achieved in 1 week
  - ▷ Protein binding – 93%
  - ▷ Direct glucoronidation
  - ▷ Flavin-containing monooxygenase pathway
  - ▷ CYP450: primarily 1A2
  - ▷ Half-life: approximately 30 hours

Paliperidone vs. Risperidone

- ▶ Brand name and dosage
  - ▷ Paliperidone – Invega, up to 12 mg/day
  - ▷ Risperidone – Risperdal, up to 16 mg/day
- ▶ Paliperidone is also known as 9-hydroxy-risperidone
- ▶ CYP 2D6 catalyzes the conversion from risperidone to paliperidone
- ▶ While paliperidone is an active metabolite of risperidone, it has no active metabolite from itself
- ▶ Besides the eliminated need for hepatic metabolism, paliperidone and risperidone are essentially the same medicine
- ▶ The marketed extended release version of paliperidone may have some advantage in smoother blood level
- ▶ Risperidone is approved as treatment of schizophrenia from age 13 year, and bipolar from age 10 year, and agitation in autism; while paliperidone is approved only as treatment of adult schizophrenia

Perphenazine

- ▶ Brand name
  - ▷ Trilafon
- ▶ Dosage
  - ▷ Up to 64 mg/day
- ▶ Mechanism
  - ▷ Antagonizes dopamine D2 receptors
- ▶ Indication
  - ▷ Schizophrenia
  - ▷ Nausea and vomiting
- ▶ Black box warning
  - ▷ Increased mortality in elderly patients with dementia; risk of death is 1.6–1.7 times of that of placebo-treated patients; most of deaths are cardiovascular or infectious in nature

▶ Other safety caution and adverse effect
  ▷ Pregnancy – C
  ▷ Neuroleptic malignant syndrome
  ▷ EPS
  ▷ Tardive dyskinesia
  ▷ Seizure
  ▷ Agranulocytosis
▶ Metabolism
  ▷ CYP450: 2D6 substrate/inhibitor
  ▷ Half-life: approximately 10 hours
▶ Used as a prototype of typical antipsychotic in CATIE and found to be equally as effective as most atypical antipsychotics, with a fraction of cost

Pimozide

▶ Brand name
  ▷ Orap
▶ Dosage
  ▷ Up to 10 mg/day
▶ Mechanism
  ▷ Antagonizes dopamine D2 receptors
▶ Indicated for Tourette's syndrome
▶ Black box warning
  ▷ Increased mortality in elderly patients with dementia; risk of death is 1.6–1.7 times of that of placebo-treated patients; most of deaths are cardiovascular or infectious in nature
▶ Other safety caution and adverse effect
  ▷ Contraindication – congenital QT prolongation, history of arrhythmia
  ▷ Pregnancy – C
  ▷ QT prolongation and Torsades de pointes; requires periodical ECG monitoring
  ▷ Neuroleptic malignant syndrome
  ▷ EPS
  ▷ Tardive dyskinesia
▶ Metabolism
  ▷ CYP450: 3A4 substrate
  ▷ Half-life: approximately 55 hours

Prochlorperazine

▶ Brand name
  ▷ Compazine
▶ Dosage
  ▷ PO/IM/IV 5 mg tid up to 150 mg/day
▶ Mechanism
  ▷ Antagonizes dopamine D2 receptors
▶ Indication
  ▷ Nausea and vomiting
  ▷ Anxiety
  ▷ Schizophrenia

- ▶ Black box warning
  - ▷ Increased mortality in elderly patients with dementia; risk of death is 1.6–1.7 times of that of placebo-treated patients; most of deaths are cardiovascular or infectious in nature
- ▶ Other safety caution and adverse effect
  - ▷ Pregnancy – C
  - ▷ Extrapyramidal syndrome
  - ▷ Neuroleptic malignant syndrome
  - ▷ Tardive dyskinesia
- ▶ Metabolism
  - ▷ CYP450: unknown
  - ▷ Half-life: 3–6 hours

Quetiapine

- ▶ Brand name
  - ▷ Seroquel, Seroquel XR
- ▶ Dosage
  - ▷ Up to PO 800 mg/day
- ▶ Mechanism
  - ▷ Antagonizes dopamine D2 and serotonin 5-HT2 receptors
- ▶ Indication
  - ▷ Schizophrenia
  - ▷ Bipolar mania
  - ▷ Bipolar maintenance
  - ▷ Bipolar depression
- ▶ Black box warning
  - ▷ Increased mortality in elderly patients with dementia; risk of death is 1.6–1.7 times of that of placebo-treated patients; most of deaths are cardiovascular or infectious in nature
  - ▷ Increased risk of suicidality in depressive patients under age 24 years, particularly during the first month of treatment
- ▶ Other safety caution and adverse effect
  - ▷ Pregnancy – C
  - ▷ Hyperglycemia
  - ▷ Diabetes mellitus
  - ▷ Hyperlipidemia
  - ▷ Weight gaining
  - ▷ Neuroleptic malignant syndrome (rare)
  - ▷ EPS (rare)
  - ▷ Tardive dyskinesia (rare)
- ▶ Metabolism
  - ▷ CYP450: 3A4 substrate
  - ▷ Half-life: approximately 6 hours

Risperidone

- ▶ Brand name and dosage
  - ▷ Risperdal and Risperdal M-Tab – up to PO 16 mg/daily
  - ▷ Risperdal Consta – up to IM 50 mg/2 weeks
- ▶ Mechanism
  - ▷ Antagonizes dopamine D2 and serotonin 5-HT2 receptors

  ▷ High affinity for D2, 5-HT2a, α-1, α-2
  ▷ Low affinity to M1
▶ Indication
  ▷ Schizophrenia
  ▷ Bipolar mania
▶ Black box warning
  ▷ Increased mortality in elderly patients with dementia; risk of death is 1.6–1.7 times of that of placebo-treated patients; most of deaths are cardiovascular or infectious in nature
▶ Other safety caution and adverse effect
  ▷ Contraindication
  ▷ Pregnancy – C
  ▷ Neuroleptic malignant syndrome
  ▷ EPS
  ▷ Tardive dyskinesia
  ▷ Hyperglycemia
  ▷ Diabetes mellitus
  ▷ Hyperlipidemia
  ▷ Weight gaining
▶ Metabolism
  ▷ CYP450: 2D6 substrate
  ▷ Active metabolite – Paliperidone (Invega)
  ▷ Half-life: 20 hours

Thioridazine

▶ Brand name
  ▷ Mellaril
▶ Dosage
▶ PO 50 mg tid up to 800 mg/day
▶ Mechanism
▶ Antagonizes dopamine D2 receptors
▶ Indication
  ▷ Schizophrenia
▶ Black box warning
  ▷ Most prominent among all the antipsychotics in causing QTc prolongation
  ▷ Increased mortality in elderly patients with dementia; risk of death is 1.6–1.7 times of that of placebo-treated patients; most of deaths are cardiovascular or infectious in nature
▶ Other safety caution and adverse effect
  ▷ May cause pigmentary retinopathy when dose is over 800 mg /day
  ▷ May cause photosensitivity and skin hyperpigmentation
  ▷ Rarely causes cholestatic jaundice
  ▷ Rarely causes agranulocytosis
  ▷ Neuroleptic malignant syndrome
  ▷ EPS
  ▷ Tardive dyskinesia
  ▷ Pregnancy – C
▶ Metabolism
  ▷ CYP450: 2D6 substrate/inhibitor
  ▷ Half-life: approximately 24 hours

Thiothixene

▶ Brand name
  ▷ Navane
▶ Dosage
  ▷ PO 2 mg tid up to 60 mg/day
▶ Mechanism
  ▷ Antagonizes dopamine D2 receptors
▶ Indication
  ▷ Psychosis
▶ Black box warning
  ▷ Increased mortality in elderly patients with dementia; risk of death is 1.6–1.7 times of that of placebo-treated patients; most of deaths are cardiovascular or infectious in nature
▶ Other safety caution and adverse effect
  ▷ Lowers seizure threshold
  ▷ May cause agranulocytosis; periodical WBC monitoring is recommended
  ▷ Neuroleptic malignant syndrome
  ▷ EPS
  ▷ Tardive dyskinesia
  ▷ Pregnancy – C
▶ Metabolism
  ▷ CYP450: unknown
  ▷ Half-life: approximately 34 hours

Trifluoperazine

▶ Brand name
  ▷ Stelazine
▶ Dosage
  ▷ PO 2 mg bid up to 40 mg/day
▶ Mechanism
  ▷ Antagonizes dopamine D2 receptors
▶ Indicated for psychosis and anxiety
▶ Black box warning
  ▷ Increased mortality in elderly dementia patients
▶ Other safety caution and adverse effect
  ▷ Pregnancy – C
  ▷ Neuroleptic malignant syndrome
  ▷ EPS
  ▷ Tardive dyskinesia
  ▷ Weight gain
  ▷ Moderate anticholinergic effect
▶ Half-life: 18 hours

Typical antipsychotics: side effects of high-potency vs. low-potency agents

▶ EPS
  ▷ High-potency agents have higher risk of EPS
  ▷ Low-potency agents have lower risk of EPS

▶ Side effects more common in low-potency agents
  ▷ Orthostatic hypotension
  ▷ Anticholinergic
  ▷ Antiadrenergic side effects
▶ Side effect more common in low-potency agents
  ▷ EPS
  ▷ Sedation

Ziprasidone

▶ Trade name
  ▷ Geodon (PO, IM)
▶ Dosage
  ▷ PO – up to 160 mg/day
  ▷ IM – up to 40 mg/day for up to 72 hours
▶ Black box warning
  ▷ Increased mortality in elderly patients with dementia; risk of death is 1.6–1.7 times of that of placebo-treated patients; most of deaths are cardiovascular or infectious in nature
▶ Other safety caution and adverse effect
  ▷ QT prolongation – avoid combination with medicines with potential of QT prolongation, including thioridazine, chlorpromazine, pimozide, and droperidol
  ▷ Neuroleptic malignant syndrome
  ▷ EPS
  ▷ Tardive dyskinesia
  ▷ Minimum weight gaining
  ▷ Low probability of sedation
  ▷ Pregnancy – C
▶ Metabolism
  ▷ CYP450: 3A4 substrate
  ▷ Half-life: approximately 7 hours

28 Lithium and Mood-Stabilizing Anticonvulsants

The term "mood stabilizer" is never officially defined, but is popularly used. It refers to a mixed collection of drugs used for the treatment of bipolar disorders; however, not all the medicines effective for bipolar disorders are termed mood stabilizer. Most mood stabilizers are primarily antimanic, but often also possess preventative effect for future mood episodes of either mania or depression, which is termed "maintenance" effect. Lamotrigine is the only one that is more effective in bipolar depression than mania. Clinical use of mood stabilizers is commonly extended to conditions characterized by volatile mood change, such as impulsive control disorders and cluster B personality disorders. The latter is sometimes called bipolar spectrum disorders.

Lithium is the oldest classic and the most tested member of mood stabilizers. Besides lithium, medicines of this group are all anticonvulsive agents with different mechanisms. Mood stabilizers are traditionally the first line treatment for bipolar disorders. In recent years, atypical antipsychotics emerged as new options for the treatment of bipolar disorders, with or without psychotic features. At present time, there is no practical reason to exclude atypical antipsychotics from the category of mood stabilizer, except the convenience of communication among clinicians who are too familiar with the traditional terminology.

Mood stabilizers in general refer to the following medicines

▶ Lithium (Eskalith, Lithobid)
▶ Valproic acid (Depakote, Depakene, Stavzor)
▶ Carbamazepine (Tegretol, Carbatrol, Epitol, Equetro)
▶ Lamotrigine (Lamictal)
▶ Oxcarbazepine (Trileptal)
▶ Topiramate (Topamax)

Carbamazepine

▶ Brand name
  ▷ Tegretol, Tegretol XR
  ▷ Carbatrol
  ▷ Epitol
  ▷ Equetro
▶ Dosage
  ▷ PO 200 mg bid up to 800 mg bid
▶ Mechanism
  ▷ Sodium channel blocker
  ▷ Reduces posttetanic potentiation
  ▷ Inhibits seizure spread

▶ Indication
  ▷ Partial seizure
  ▷ Grand mal seizure
  ▷ Mixed seizure
  ▷ Trigeminal neuralgia
  ▷ Acute mania
▶ Metabolism
  ▷ CYP450 – substrate and inducer of 3A4; induces its own metabolism (auto-induction)
  ▷ Half-life – initial doses 26–65 hours; repeated doses approximately 15 hours; variable half-life is associated with auto-induction

Carbamazepine: safety caution and adverse effects

Tip – has tricyclic structure similar to tricyclic antidepressants

▶ Black box warning
  ▷ HLA-B*1502 – may cause Stevens–Johnson syndrome and toxic epidermal necrolysis in patients with this allele; patients with ancestry from Asian areas should be screened for the HLA-B*1502 allele before starting treatment with carbamazepine
  ▷ Aplastic anemia and agranulocytosis – rare
▶ Contraindications
  ▷ Monoamine oxidase inhibitors (MAOI) use within 14 days (see tip)
  ▷ Narrow angle-closure glaucoma
  ▷ Hypersensitivity to tricyclic antidepressants
▶ Pregnancy
  ▷ Class D
  ▷ May cause spina bifida and developmental delay
▶ Weight change – possible in significant minority
▶ Hyponatremia
  ▷ Carbamazepine has antidiuretic effect, via activation of vasopressin type 2 receptors
▶ Bone marrow suppression
▶ Decrease in thyroid hormones
▶ Elevates cholesterol and high density lipopolysaccharides (HDL)
▶ Sedation, ataxia, dizziness
▶ Blurred vision
▶ Usually benign effects
  ▷ Elevations in liver function tests (LFTs)
  ▷ Decreases in white cell, red cell, and platelet counts
▶ Rare adverse effects
  ▷ Agranulocytosis
  ▷ Aplastic anemia
  ▷ Hepatitis
  ▷ Exfoliative dermatitis

Carbamazepine: laboratory

▶ Serum levels
  ▷ Therapeutic – 4–12 mcg/ml
  ▷ Toxic – >12 mcg/ml
  ▷ Time to steady state – >1 mo, due to induction of own metabolism

▶ Complete blood counts
▶ Platelet
▶ Reticulocytes
▶ Iron at baseline
▶ Blood urine nitrogen
▶ LFTs
▶ Urinalysis
▶ Lipid panel
▶ Creatinine in children

Lamotrigine

▶ Brand name
 ▷ Lamictal
 ▷ Lamictal CD
▶ Dosage
 ▷ PO from 25 mg/day to titrate up slowly
 ▷ Maximum 200 mg/day if monotherapy
 ▷ Maximum 100 mg/day if combined with valproate
 ▷ Maximum 400 mg/day if combined with enzyme-inducing antiepileptics (carbam-azepine, phenobarbital, phenytoin, primidone)
▶ Mechanisms
 ▷ Blocks Na^+ and Ca^{++} channels
▶ Indicated for
 ▷ Bipolar I disorder – maintenance
 ▷ Adjunctive therapy in partial or generalized epilepsy
 ▷ Generally believed more effective for bipolar depression and less effective for mania
▶ Black box warning
 ▷ Serious rash and Stevens–Johnson syndrome
▶ Other safety caution and adverse effect
 ▷ Pregnancy – C
 ▷ Weight change – not expected
 ▷ Headache
 ▷ Diplopia
 ▷ Ataxia
 ▷ Blurred vision
▶ Metabolism
 ▷ CYP450 – none; hepatic metabolism is through glucoronidation
 ▷ Half-life – approximately 25 hours

Lithium

▶ Brand name
 ▷ Eskalith, Eskalith CR
 ▷ Lithobid
▶ Dosage
 ▷ PO 300 mg bid up to 1,800 mg/day
▶ Mechanism
 ▷ Alters neuronal sodium transport

▷ Action through G-protein
▷ Not fully understood
▶ Indication
▷ Bipolar disorder
▶ Back box warning
▷ Lithium toxicity related to serum level
▶ Other safety caution and adverse effect
▷ Pregnancy – D
▷ Weight change – weight gain
▷ Tremor
▷ Confusion, syncope
▷ Hypothyroidism
▷ Hyperparathyroidism
▷ Arrhythmia
▷ Polydipsia and polyuria
▶ Metabolism
▷ CYP450 – none

Lithium: intoxication

▶ Serum concentration greater than 1.5 mEq/L
▶ Symptoms
▷ Lethargy
▷ Stuttering
▷ Muscle fasciculations
▷ Severe tremor
▷ Unsteadiness
▶ Treatment
▷ Medical support
▷ Stop lithium
▷ Maintenance of electrolyte balance
▷ Proximal segment-acting diuretics (aminophylline, acetazolamide)
▷ Hemodialysis if higher than 3.5 mEq/L or severe symptoms

Lithium: pharmacokinetics

▶ Filtered through the proximal tubules, competing with sodium
▶ A decrease in plasma sodium may increase lithium reabsorption and lead to an increase in plasma lithium levels
▶ Peak plasma levels – 1–4 hours
▶ Half-life – 24 hours

Lithium-induced polyuria and polydipsia

▶ Lithium suppresses the antidiuretic hormone (ADH)-induced resorption of free water from the distal tubules; this results in nephrogenic diabetes insipidus
▶ Treatment
▷ Use lowest possible dose of Lithium
▷ Use single daily dosing
▷ Use K^+ sparing diuretics, e.g., amiloride; or use thiazide diuretics

▶ Close monitoring on lithium level is essential
▶ If a diuretic is coadministered, also monitor K' level

Lithium: side effects in mental status

▶ Sedation
▶ Cognitive difficulties – poor concentration and memory
▶ Sense of mentally slowness and decreased creativity

Oxcarbazepine

Tip – has tricyclic structure similar to tricyclic antidepressants.

▶ Brand name
  ▷ Trileptal
▶ Dosage
  ▷ PO 300 mg bid to 1,200 mg bid
▶ Mechanism
  ▷ Sodium channel blocker
▶ Indication
  ▷ Partial seizures in adults and children aged 4–16 years
  ▷ May be useful as a second or third line mood stabilizer; limited data on bipolar disorder; believed by some to be a "non-toxic carbamazepine"
  ▷ May be effective for anxiety
▶ Safety caution and adverse effect
  ▷ Contraindication – MAOI use within 14 days; narrow angle-closure glaucoma; hypersensitivity to tricyclic antidepressants
  ▷ Pregnancy – C
  ▷ Weight change – possible in significant minority
  ▷ Hyponatremia – monitor sodium and creatine
  ▷ Sedation, dizziness, ataxia, nystagmus
  ▷ Nausea, vomiting
  ▷ Rash
  ▷ May reduce plasma levels of hormonal contraceptives
▶ Metabolism
  ▷ CYP450 – 2C19 inhibitor, 3A4 inducer
  ▷ Half-life – approximately 2 hours; active metabolite 9 hours

Pregnancy safety of mood stabilizers

▶ Lithium
  ▷ Ebstein's malformation – right ventricular hypoplasia and tricuspid insufficiency
  ▷ Risk category D
▶ Valproate
  ▷ Neural tube defects, e.g., spina bifida particularly if used in the first trimester
  ▷ Clotting abnormalities when used later in pregnancy
  ▷ Risk category D
▶ Lamotrigine
  ▷ Risk category C
▶ Carbamazepine
  ▷ Spina bifida and developmental delay
  ▷ Risk category D

▶ Oxcarbazepine
  ▷ Risk category C
▶ Atypical antipsychotics
  ▷ All are Risk category C

Topiramate

▶ Brand name
  ▷ Topamax
▶ Dosage
  ▷ PO 25 mg/day to 200 mg bid
▶ Mechanism
  ▷ Blocks voltage-sensitive sodium channel, and possible other mechanisms
▶ Indication
  ▷ Migraine prophylaxis
  ▷ Seizures – partial seizures, primary generalized tonic-clonic seizures, Lennox-Gastaut syndrome
  ▷ Possible off-label use for bipolar disorders
▶ Safety caution and adverse effect
  ▷ Pregnancy – C
  ▷ Weight change – possible weight loss
  ▷ Nausea and loss of appetite
  ▷ Sensation, asthenia
  ▷ Dizziness, ataxia
  ▷ Nystagmus, blurred vision
  ▷ Confusion
  ▷ Kidney stones
  ▷ Metabolic acidosis
▶ Metabolism
  ▷ Minimal liver metabolism
  ▷ Unchanged urinary excretion – 70%
  ▷ Half-life – approximately 21 hours

Valproate

▶ Brand names
  ▷ Depakote, Depakote ER (tablets)
  ▷ Depacon (IV)
  ▷ Depakene (syrup or capsules)
  ▷ Stavzor (soft gel capsules)
▶ Dosage
  ▷ PO 25 mg/kg/day to 60 mg/kg/day
  ▷ Intravenous (IV) 10 mg/kg/day to 60 mg/kg/day
▶ Mechanism
  ▷ Blocks voltage-sensitive sodium channel
  ▷ Increases gamma-aminobutyric acid (GABA) level
▶ Indication
  ▷ Bipolar disorder, acute mania
  ▷ Migraine prophylaxis
  ▷ Seizure disorders

▶ Monitoring
  ▷ Serum level – 50–100 mcg/ml for seizure, 50–125 mcg/ml for bipolar disorders
  ▷ Monitor baseline LFT, platelet, and coagulation
▶ Metabolism
  ▷ CYP450 – weak 2C9 inhibitor
  ▷ Half-life – approximately 12 hours

Valproate: safety caution and adverse effects

▶ Back box warning
  ▷ Hepatotoxicity
  ▷ Teratogenicity
  ▷ Pancreatitis
▶ Contraindication
  ▷ Hepatic function impairment
▶ Pregnancy – D
▶ Weight change – moderate weight gain
▶ Neurological
  ▷ Sedation, tremor, ataxia
▶ Gastrointestinal tract (GI)
  ▷ GI disturbance, benign increase in LFT, Hepatitis (rare), hemorrhagic pancreatitis (rare)
▶ Hematological
  ▷ Thrombocytopenia, bleeding abnormalities, agranulocytosis (rare)
▶ Dermatological
  ▷ Alopecia, erythema multiforme (rare)

29 Antidepressants

Antidepressants are medicines primarily designed and used for depression. Recent studies have found antidepressive effects from agents not traditionally categorized as antidepressants. Many antidepressants are proved to be effective in treating conditions other than depression. Nonetheless, at this point in time, when we talk about pharmacotherapy for depression, we are still in large talking about a consensually recognized group of agents.

The categorization of antidepressants is not as systematic, with a mixed emphasis on either chemical structure or mechanism of action. Four major groups of antidepressants are – tricyclic antidepressant (TCA), monoamine oxidase inhibitor (MAOI), serotonin specific reuptake inhibitor (SSRI), and serotonin-norepinephrine reuptake inhibitor (SNRI). The first two groups were invented before the birth of fluoxetine (1989), and the latter two after. They are therefore also called "old" and "new" antidepressants, respectively. The major advantage of the new vs. old antidepressants is the decreased toxic side effects and the lethality of overdose. Tetracyclics may be considered an extension from tricyclics. There are yet other antidepressants that cannot be easily included in any of the above four major groups.

TCAs have a characteristic molecular structure that contains a 3-ring component (Figure 29–1). Mechanism wise, TCAs are either norepinephrine reuptake inhibitors or SNRIs. However, we usually reserve the term of SNRI for those newer agents that do not have the characteristic tricyclic structure.

Maprotiline and amoxapine have the similar tricyclic structure and a fourth ring attached. They are called tetracyclics. Tetracyclics are structurally and chemically very close to the tricyclic group, and are sometimes referred to, together with TCAs, as "heterocyclic antidepressants."

There are other antidepressants with either three rings or four rings in their molecules, but are chemically irrelevant to TCAs due to lack of the characteristic tricyclic structure as in TCAs. Three SSRIs, sertraline, citalopram, and escitalopram, have three rings in molecular structure. Another SSRI, paroxetine, has four rings in its molecule. Mirtazapine, nefazodone, and trazodone also have four rings. But none of them are referred to as either tricyclic or tetracyclic antidepressants.

Nefazodone and trazodone are chemically and pharmacodynamically similar to each other and may be called 5-HT2a blockers.

Mirtazapine blocks presynaptic α-2 adrenergic receptors, a mechanism unique to any other antidepressant. It therefore forms its own one-member category. Similarly, bupropion also has a unique receptor profile. It has little impact on serotonergic system but mainly acts on adrenergic and dopaminergic systems.

The following is a list of antidepressants approved by Food and Drug Administration (FDA)

- ▶ TCA
    - ▷ Amitriptyline (Elavil)
    - ▷ Clomipramine (Anafranil)
    - ▷ Desipramine (Norpramin)
    - ▷ Doxepin (Sinequan)
    - ▷ Imipramine (Tofranil, Tofranil PM))
    - ▷ Nortriptyline (Aventyl, Pamelor)
    - ▷ Protriptyline (Vivactil)
    - ▷ Trimipramine (Surmontil)
- ▶ Tetracyclic antidepressant
    - ▷ Amoxapine (Asendin)
    - ▷ Maprotiline (Ludiomil)
- ▶ MAOI
    - ▷ Selegiline (Emsam)
    - ▷ Isocarboxazid (Marplan)
    - ▷ Phenelzine (Nardil)
    - ▷ Tranylcypromine (Parnate)
- ▶ SSRI
    - ▷ Citalopram (Celexa)
    - ▷ Fluvoxamine (Luvox, Luvox CR)
    - ▷ Escitalopram (Lexapro)
    - ▷ Fluoxetine (Prozac, Prozac Weekly, Sarafem)
    - ▷ Paroxetine (Paxil, Paxil CR, Paxeva))
    - ▷ Sertraline (Zoloft)
- ▶ SNRI
    - ▷ Desvenafaxine (Pristiq)
    - ▷ Duloxetine (Cymbalta)
    - ▷ Venlafaxine (Effexor, Effexor XR)
- ▶ Other
    - ▷ Bupropion (Wellbutrin, Wellbutrin SR, Wellbutrin XL, Budeprion SR, Budeprion XL)
    - ▷ Mirtazapine (Remeron, Remeron SolTab)
    - ▷ Nefazodone (Serzone)
    - ▷ Trazodone (Desyrel)

There have been suggestions of simplified, more systematic categorization. One alternative way is to simply call antidepressants "mono-action" or "dual-action" according to their major impact on either serotonergic system, or adrenergic system, or both. According to this categorization, SSRIs and bupropion are mono-action agents, and the rest of antidepressants are dual-action agents. Though possibly helpful in some clinical setting, this overly simplified categorization omits many important pharmacological characteristics of antidepressants. Most clinicians still prefer the current categorization, probably due to its descriptiveness, communicability, and a sense of historical evolvement.

Amitriptyline (See Figure 29–1 on page 218)

- ▶ Brand names
    - ▷ Elavil
- ▶ Dosage
    - ▷ PO 25 mg qhs up to 300 mg/day

Figure 29-1 Chemical structures of tricyclic antidepressants amitriptyline and nortriptyline, and tetracyclic antidepressant maprotiline. All have a similar core structure. Also notice the tertiary amine in amitriptyline (drawn with increased line weight) that is turned into secondary amine in nortriptyline through demethylation. This change eliminates the efficacy of serotonin reuptake inhibition. The same change happens when imipramine converts to desipramine.

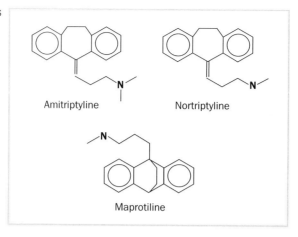

Amitriptyline   Nortriptyline

Maprotiline

- ▶ Mechanism
  - ▷ Inhibits norepinephrine (NE) and 5-HT reuptake
- ▶ Indication
  - ▷ Depression
  - ▷ Chronic pain
- ▶ Black box warning
  - ▷ Increased risk of suicidality in children, adolescents, and young adults ≤24-year-olds
  - ▷ Suicidal risk is not increased beyond 24-year-olds and decreased for patients above 64-year-olds
- ▶ Other safety caution and adverse effect
  - ▷ Contraindication – MAOI use within 14 days, recent myocardial infarction
  - ▷ Pregnancy – C
  - ▷ Orthostatic hypotension
  - ▷ QT prolongation
  - ▷ Anticholinergic effects
  - ▷ Sedation
  - ▷ Seizure
- ▶ Monitoring
  - ▷ Serum level – therapeutic level 120–250 ng/ml (amitriptyline + nortriptyline)
  - ▷ Electroencephalogram (ECG)
  - ▷ Blood pressure (BP)
- ▶ Metabolism
  - ▷ CYP450 – primarily 2D6
  - ▷ Active metabolite – nortriptyline
  - ▷ Half-life – approximately 18 hours

Amoxapine (Figure 29–2)

- ▶ Brand name
  - ▷ Asendin
- ▶ Dosage
  - ▷ PO 50 mg bid up to 600 mg/day

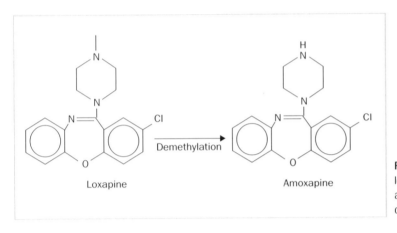

Figure 29–2 Antipsychotic loxapine converts to antidepressant amoxapine through demethylation.

▶ Mechanism
  ▷ Inhibits 5-HT and NE reuptake
  ▷ Also has postsynaptic dopamine blockade effect
▶ Indication
  ▷ Depression
▶ Black box warning
  ▷ Increased risk of suicidality in children, adolescents, and young adults ≤24-year-olds
  ▷ Suicidal risk is not increased beyond 24-year-olds and decreased for patients 65-year-olds
▶ Adverse effect and safety caution
  ▷ Contraindication – MAOI use within 14 days, recent myocardial infarction
  ▷ Pregnancy – C
  ▷ May cause extrapyramidal syndrome and tardive dyskinesia
  ▷ Sedation
▶ Metabolism
  ▷ Amoxapine is the metabolite of loxapine (Loxitane), an antipsychotic
  ▷ CYP450 – unknown
  ▷ Half-life – approximately 8 hours
▶ Note
  ▷ Due to its dopamine blockade effect, amoxapine was used to treat depression with psychotic features

Bupropion

▶ Brand names
  ▷ Wellbutrin, Wellbutrin SR, Wellbutrin XL
  ▷ Zyban
  ▷ Buproban
  ▷ Budeprion SR, Budeprion XL
▶ Dosage
  ▷ PO 100 mg/day up to 450 mg/day
▶ Mechanism
  ▷ Reuptake blockage to dopamine and norepinephrine

▶ Indication
▷ Major depressive disorder
▷ Seasonal affective disorder
▷ Smoke cessation
▶ Black box warning
▷ Increased risk of suicidality in children, adolescents, and young adults ≤24-year-olds
▷ Suicidal risk is not increased beyond 24-year-olds and decreased for patients above 64-year-olds
▶ Adverse effect and safety caution
▷ Contraindication – seizure disorders, eating disorders, MAOI use with in 14 days
▷ Pregnancy – C
▷ Adverse effects – agitation, insomnia, anxiety, gastrointestinal tract (GI) distress
▷ Not associated with sexual dysfunction, weight gain, and anticholinergic activity
▶ Metabolism
▷ CYP450 – 2D6 inhibitor
▷ Half-life – approximately 21 hours

Cardiac monitoring for tricyclic antidepressants

▶ All patients with cardiac conditions – ECG follow-up
▶ Age over 40 years – ECG follow-up
▶ Bundle branch block – relative contraindication

Citalopram

▶ Brand name
▷ Celexa
▶ Dosage
▷ PO 20 mg/day up to 60 mg/day
▶ Mechanism
▷ SSRI
▶ Indication
▷ Major depressive disorder
▶ Black box warning
▷ Increased risk of suicidality in children, adolescents, and young adults ≤24-year-olds
▷ Suicidal risk is not increased beyond 24-year-olds and decreased for patients above 65-year-olds
▶ Adverse effect and safety caution
▷ Contraindication – MAOI use within 14 days
▷ Pregnancy – C; caution if pregnancy over 20 weeks
▷ Abrupt withdrawal may cause discontinuation symptoms
▶ Metabolism
▷ CYP450 – weak 2D6 interaction
▷ Half-life – approximately 35 hours

Clomipramine

▶ Brand name
▷ Anafranil

▶ Dosage
  ▷ PO 25 mg qd up to 100 mg/day in the first 2 weeks, up to 250 mg/day maintenance
▶ Mechanism
  ▷ Inhibits 5-HT and NE reuptake
▶ Indication
  ▷ Obsessive-compulsive disorder (OCD)
▶ Black box warning
  ▷ Increased risk of suicidality in children, adolescents, and young adults ≤24-year-olds
  ▷ Suicidal risk is not increased beyond 24-year-olds and decreased for patients above 65-year-olds
▶ Adverse effect and safety caution
  ▷ Contraindication – MAOI use within 14 days, recent myocardial infarction
  ▷ Pregnancy – C
  ▷ Orthostatic hypotension
  ▷ QT prolongation
  ▷ Anticholinergic effects
  ▷ Sedation
  ▷ Seizure (rare)
▶ Metabolism
  ▷ CYP450 – extensive hepatic metabolism; substrate of primarily 2D6
  ▷ Half-life – approximately 32 hours or longer

Desipramine

▶ Brand name
  ▷ Norpramin
▶ Dosage
  ▷ PO 25 mg qd up to 300 mg/day
▶ Mechanism
  ▷ Inhibits 5-HT and NE reuptake
▶ Indication
  ▷ Depression
▶ Black box warning
  ▷ Increased risk of suicidality in children, adolescents, and young adults ≤24-year-olds
  ▷ Suicidal risk is not increased beyond 24-year-olds and decreased for patients above 65-year-olds
▶ Safety caution and adverse effect
  ▷ Contraindication – MAOI use within 14 days, recent myocardial infarction
  ▷ Pregnancy – D
  ▷ Therapeutic level 180–350 ng/ml
  ▷ Orthostatic hypotension
  ▷ QT prolongation
  ▷ Anticholinergic effects
  ▷ Sedation
  ▷ Seizure
▶ Metabolism
  ▷ A metabolite of imipramine
  ▷ CYP450 – substrate of 2D6 and 2C19
  ▷ Half-life – approximately 18 hours

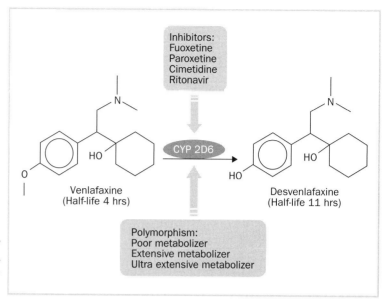

Figure 29-3 Metabolic pathway from venlafaxine to desvenlafaxine. The efficacy of CYP 2D6 is influenced by multiple factors.

Desvenlafaxine (Figure 29-3)

▶ Brand name
  ▷ Pristiq
▶ Dosage
  ▷ PO 50 mg qd up to 100 mg/day
▶ Mechanism
  ▷ Inhibits 5-HT, NE and dopamine (DA) reuptake
▶ Indication
  ▷ Major depressive disorder
▶ Black box warning
  ▷ Increased risk of suicidality in children, adolescents, and young adults ≤24-year-olds
  ▷ Suicidal risk is not increased beyond 24-year-olds and decreased for patients above 65-year-olds
▶ Safety caution and adverse effect
  ▷ Contraindication – MAOI use within 14 days
  ▷ Pregnancy – C
  ▷ Abrupt withdrawal may cause discontinuation symptoms
  ▷ Generally well tolerated
▶ Metabolism
  ▷ A metabolite of venlafaxine
  ▷ CYP450 – 3A4; no active metabolite
  ▷ Half-life – approximately 11 hours

Doxepin

▶ Brand name
  ▷ Sinequan

▶ Dosage
  ▷ PO 25 mg qhs up to 300 mg/day
▶ Mechanism
  ▷ Inhibits 5-HT and NE reuptake
▶ Indication
  ▷ Depression
  ▷ Anxiety
▶ Black box warning
  ▷ Increased risk of suicidality in children, adolescents, and young adults ≤24-year-olds
  ▷ Suicidal risk is not increased beyond 24-year-olds and decreased for patients above 65-year-olds
▶ Safety caution and adverse effect
  ▷ Contraindication – MAOI use within 14 days, recent myocardial infarction, glaucoma
  ▷ Pregnancy – C
  ▷ Orthostatic hypotension
  ▷ QT prolongation; need to monitor ECG
  ▷ Anticholinergic effects
  ▷ Sedation
  ▷ Seizure
▶ Metabolism
  ▷ CYP450 – primarily 2D6
  ▷ Half-life – approximately 7 hours

Duloxetine

▶ Brand name
  ▷ Cymbalta
▶ Dosage
  ▷ PO 30 mg qd up to 120 mg/day
▶ Mechanism
  ▷ 5-HT and NE reuptake inhibitor
▶ Indication
  ▷ Major depressive disorder
  ▷ Diabetic neuropathic pain
  ▷ Generalized anxiety disorder
  ▷ Fibromyalgia
▶ Black box warning
  ▷ Increased risk of suicidality in children, adolescents, and young adults ≤24-year-olds
  ▷ Suicidal risk is not increased beyond 24-year-olds and decreased for patients above 65-year-olds
▶ Safety caution and adverse effect
  ▷ Contraindication – MAOI use within 14 days
  ▷ Pregnancy – C
  ▷ Nausea
  ▷ Dry mouth
▶ Metabolism
  ▷ CYP450 – 1A2 and 2D6 substrate and inhibitor
  ▷ Half-life – Approximately 12 hours

Escitalopram

▶ Brand name
  ▷ Lexapro
▶ Dosage
  ▷ PO 10 mg qd up to 20 mg/day
▶ Mechanism
  ▷ 5-HT reuptake inhibitor
▶ Indication
  ▷ Major depressive disorder
  ▷ Generalized anxiety disorder
▶ Black box warning
  ▷ Increased risk of suicidality in children, adolescents, and young adults ≤24-year-olds
  ▷ Suicidal risk is not increased beyond 24-year-olds and decreased for patients above 65-year-olds
▶ Safety caution and adverse effect
  ▷ Contraindication – MAOI use within 14 days
  ▷ Pregnancy – C
  ▷ Nausea
  ▷ Insomnia
▶ Metabolism
  ▷ CYP450 – 2D6
  ▷ Half-life – approximately 30 hours

Fluoxetine

▶ Brand name
  ▷ Prozac, Prozac Weekly, Sarafem
▶ Dosage
  ▷ PO 20 mg qd up to 80 mg/day
  ▷ Prozac weekly – PO 90 mg qwk
▶ Mechanism
  ▷ 5-HT reuptake inhibitor
▶ Indication
  ▷ Major depressive disorder
  ▷ OCD
  ▷ Bulimia nervosa
  ▷ Panic disorder
  ▷ Premenstrual dysphoric disorder
▶ Black box warning
  ▷ Increased risk of suicidality in children, adolescents, and young adults ≤24-year-olds
  ▷ Suicidal risk is not increased beyond 24-year-olds and decreased for patients above 65-year-olds
▶ Safety caution and adverse effect
  ▷ Contraindication – MAOI use with 5 weeks
  ▷ Pregnancy – C
  ▷ Nausea
  ▷ Headache

▶ Metabolism
  ▷ CYP450 – 2D6, 2C19 substrate and inhibitor
  ▷ Half-life – approximately 5 days

Fluvoxamine

▶ Brand name
  ▷ Luvox, Luvox CR
▶ Dosage
  ▷ PO 50 mg qhs up to 300 mg/day
▶ Mechanism
  ▷ 5-HT reuptake inhibitor
▶ Indication
  ▷ OCD
▶ Black box warning
  ▷ Increased risk of suicidality in children, adolescents, and young adults ≤24-year-olds
  ▷ Suicidal risk is not increased beyond 24-year-olds and decreased for patients above 65-year-olds
▶ Safety caution and adverse effect
  ▷ Contraindication – MAOI use within 14 days
  ▷ Pregnancy – C
  ▷ Nausea
  ▷ Headache
▶ Metabolism
  ▷ CYP450 – 1A2, 2D6
  ▷ Half-life – approximately 16 hour

Heterocyclic antidepressants: mechanism profile

▶ All are norepinephrine reuptake inhibitors, with desipramine the strongest
▶ Clomipramine and amitriptyline are strong serotonin reuptake inhibitors; Imipramine and doxepin are moderate ones
▶ Amoxapine is a moderate D2 blocker, and is believed to have antipsychotic effect
▶ Amitriptyline has the strongest α-1 blockade, antihistaminergic, and anticholinergic effects

Imipramine

▶ Brand name
  ▷ Tofranil, Tofranil PM
▶ Dosage
  ▷ PO 25 mg qhs up to 300 mg/day
▶ Mechanism
  ▷ Inhibits 5-HT and NE reuptake
▶ Indication
  ▷ Depression
▶ Black box warning
  ▷ Increased risk of suicidality in children, adolescents, and young adults ≤24-year-olds
  ▷ Suicidal risk is not increased beyond 24-year-olds and decreased for patients above 65-year-olds

▶ Safety caution and adverse effect
  ▷ Contraindication – MAOI use within 14 days, recent myocardial infarction
  ▷ Pregnancy – D
  ▷ Therapeutic level 180–350 ng/ml
  ▷ Orthostatic hypotension
  ▷ QT prolongation
  ▷ Anticholinergic effects
  ▷ Sedation
  ▷ Seizure
▶ Metabolism
  ▷ Active metabolite – Desipramine
  ▷ CYP450 – substrate of 2D6 and 2C19
  ▷ Half-life – approximately 18 hours

Isocarboxazid

▶ Brand name
  ▷ Marplan
▶ Dosage
  ▷ PO 10 mg bid up to 60 mg/day
▶ Mechanism
  ▷ Nonselective monoamine oxidase inhibitor
▶ Indication
  ▷ Depression
▶ Black box warning
  ▷ Increased risk of suicidality in children, adolescents, and young adults ≤24-year-olds
  ▷ Suicidal risk is not increased beyond 24-year-olds and decreased for patients above 65-year-olds
▶ Safety caution and adverse effect
  ▷ Contraindication – general anesthesia within 10 days; elective surgery within 10 days; pheochromocytoma; hypertension
  ▷ Pregnancy – C
  ▷ Monitoring – blood pressure (BP) and liver function tests (LFTs)
  ▷ Orthostatic hypotension
  ▷ Hypertensive crisis
  ▷ Dizziness
  ▷ Nausea
▶ Metabolism
  ▷ CYP450 – unknown
  ▷ Half-life – unknown

Maprotiline

▶ Brand name
  ▷ Ludiomil
▶ Dosage
  ▷ PO 25 mg qhs up to 225 mg/day
▶ Mechanism
  ▷ Inhibits NE reuptake

▶ Indication
  ▷ Depression
▶ Black box warning
  ▷ Increased risk of suicidality in children, adolescents, and young adults ≤24-year-olds
  ▷ Suicidal risk is not increased beyond 24-year-olds and decreased for patients above 65-year-olds
▶ Safety caution and adverse effect
  ▷ Contraindication – MAOI use within 14 days, recent myocardial infarction
  ▷ Pregnancy – B
  ▷ Orthostatic hypotension
  ▷ Cardiac arrhythmia
  ▷ Sedation
  ▷ Anticholinergic effects
  ▷ Rare extrapyramidal syndrome
  ▷ Rare seizure
▶ Metabolism
  ▷ CYP450 – 2D6 substrate
  ▷ Half-life – approximately 43 hour

Mirtazapine

▶ Brand name
  ▷ Remeron, Remeron SolTab
▶ Dosage
  ▷ PO 15 mg qhs up to 45 mg/day
▶ Mechanism
  ▷ Presynaptic effect – antagonism at α-2 NE autoreceptors causes reduced negative feedback, resulting in increased 5-HT and NE activity
  ▷ Postsynaptic effect – antagonism at 5-HT2a and 5-HT2c receptors results in net activation of 5-HT1a receptors
  ▷ Also blocks 5-HT3 and histamine receptors
▶ Indication – major depressive disorder
▶ Black box warning
  ▷ Increased risk of suicidality in children, adolescents, and young adults ≤24-year-olds
  ▷ Suicidal risk is not increased beyond 24-year-olds and decreased for patients above 65-year-olds
▶ Safety caution and adverse effect
  ▷ Contraindication – MAOI use within 14 days
  ▷ Pregnancy – C
  ▷ Sedation
  ▷ Increased appetite and weight gain
  ▷ Not associated with sexual dysfunction
  ▷ Minimal anticholinergic effects
▶ Metabolism
  ▷ CYP450 – 1A2, 2D6, 3A4
  ▷ Half-life – approximately 30 hours

Nefazodone

▶ Brand name
  ▷ Serzone
▶ Dosage
  ▷ PO 100 mg bid up to 600 mg/day
▶ Mechanism
  ▷ Blocks postsynaptic 5-HT2 receptors
  ▷ Weakly inhibits reuptake of 5-HT and NE
  ▷ The combination of neurotransmitter interaction results in selective activation of 5-HT1 receptors (comparable to trazodone)
  ▷ Antagonism of α-1 adrenergic receptors
▶ Indication – depression
▶ Black box warning
  ▷ May cause hepatotoxicity and hepatic failure
  ▷ Increased risk of suicidality in children, adolescents, and young adults ≤24-year-olds
  ▷ Suicidal risk is not increased beyond 24-year-olds and decreased for patients above 65-year-olds
▶ Adverse effect and safety caution
  ▷ Contraindication – liver diseases, MAOI use within 14 days
  ▷ Pregnancy – C
  ▷ Orthostatic hypotension
  ▷ Not associated with sexual dysfunction or weight gain
▶ Metabolism
  ▷ CYP450 – 3A4 substrate and inhibitor
  ▷ Half-life – approximately 3 hours

Norepinephrine in the treatment of depression

▶ TCA, venlafaxine, desvenlafaxine, bupropion, and nefazodone block NE and 5-HT reuptake
▶ MAOIs block the catabolism of NE and 5-HT
▶ Mirtazapine blocks presynaptic α-2 receptors, therefore reduces the negative feedback, and enhances the release of NE to synaptic cleft
▶ Down regulation of postsynaptic β-adrenergic receptors is found correlated with clinical improvement

Nortriptyline

▶ Brand name
  ▷ Aventyl, Pamelor
▶ Dosage
  ▷ PO 25 mg qhs up to 150 mg/day
▶ Mechanism
  ▷ Inhibits NE and 5-HT reuptake
▶ Indication – depression
▶ Black box warning
  ▷ Increased risk of suicidality in children, adolescents, and young adults ≤24-year-olds
  ▷ Suicidal risk is not increased beyond 24-year-olds and decreased for patients above 65-year-olds

▶ Safety caution and adverse effect
  ▷ Contraindication – MAOI use within 14 days, recent myocardial infarction
  ▷ Pregnancy – C
  ▷ Plasma concentration between 50 ng/ml and 150 ng/ml is most effective; higher level not only increases risk of toxicity, it also decreases therapeutic response; toxic level – ≥500 ng/ml
  ▷ It is the TCA least likely to cause orthostatic hypotension
▶ Metabolism
  ▷ CYP450 – 2D6
  ▷ It is a metabolite of amitriptyline
  ▷ Half-life – 31 hours

Paroxetine

▶ Brand name
  ▷ Paxil, Paxil CR, Paxeva
▶ Dosage
  ▷ PO 10 mg qd up to 50 mg/day
  ▷ CR – PO 12.5 mg qd up to 62.5 mg/day
▶ Mechanism – inhibits 5-HT reuptake
▶ Indication
  ▷ Major depression
  ▷ OCD
  ▷ Social anxiety disorder
  ▷ Panic disorder
  ▷ Generalized anxiety disorder
▶ Black box warning
  ▷ Increased risk of suicidality in children, adolescents, and young adults ≤24-year-olds
  ▷ Suicidal risk is not increased beyond 24-year-olds and decreased for patients above 65-year-olds
▶ Safety caution and adverse effect
  ▷ Contraindication – MAOI us in 14 days
  ▷ Pregnancy – D
  ▷ Significant discontinuation symptoms
▶ Metabolism
  ▷ CYP450 – substrate and inhibitor of 2D6
  ▷ Half-life – approximately 21 hours

Phenelzine

▶ Brand name
  ▷ Nardil
▶ Dosage
  ▷ PO 15 mg tid up to 90 mg/day
▶ Mechanism
  ▷ Nonselective monoamine oxidase inhibitor
▶ Black box warning
  ▷ Increased risk of suicidality in children, adolescents, and young adults ≤24-year-olds
  ▷ Suicidal risk is not increased beyond 24-year-olds and decreased for patients above 65-year-olds

- ▶ Safety caution and adverse effect
  - ▷ Contraindication – pheochromocytoma
  - ▷ Pregnancy – C
  - ▷ Hypertensive crisis
  - ▷ Orthostatic hypotension
  - ▷ Serotonin syndrome
  - ▷ Seizures
  - ▷ Sedation
  - ▷ Avoid high tyramine-content food
- ▶ Monitoring – BP, LFTs
- ▶ Metabolism
  - ▷ CYP450 – unknown
  - ▷ Half-life – approximately 12 hours

Protriptyline

- ▶ Trade name
  - ▷ Vivactil
- ▶ Dosage
  - ▷ PO 5–10 mg tid up to 60 mg/day
- ▶ Mechanism
  - ▷ Inhibits NE and 5-HT reuptake
- ▶ Indication
  - ▷ Depression
- ▶ Black box warning
  - ▷ Increased risk of suicidality in children, adolescents, and young adults ≤24-year-olds
  - ▷ Suicidal risk is not increased beyond 24-year-olds and decreased for patients above 65-year-olds
- ▶ Safety caution and adverse effect
  - ▷ Contraindication – MAOI use within 14 days, recent myocardial infarction
  - ▷ Pregnancy – C
  - ▷ Orthostatic hypotension
  - ▷ QT prolongation
  - ▷ Sedation
  - ▷ Anticholinergic effects
- ▶ Metabolism
  - ▷ CYP450 – unknown
  - ▷ Half-life – approximately 70 hours

Selegiline (transdermal)

- ▶ Brand name
  - ▷ EMSAM
- ▶ Dosage
  - ▷ 6 mg/24h up to 12 mg/24 h
- ▶ Mechanism
  - ▷ Selective inhibitor of monoamine oxidase
- ▶ Indication
  - ▷ Major depressive disorder

- ▶ Black box warning
  - ▷ Increased risk of suicidality in children, adolescents, and young adults ≤24-year-olds
  - ▷ Suicidal risk is not increased beyond 24-year-olds and decreased for patients above 65-year-olds
- ▶ Safety caution and adverse effect
  - ▷ Contraindication – pheochromocytoma, elective surgery in 10 days
  - ▷ Pregnancy – C
  - ▷ Headache
  - ▷ Insomnia
  - ▷ Hypertensive crisis
  - ▷ Avoid high tyramine foods if dose above 6 mg/24h
- ▶ Metabolism
  - ▷ CYP450 – primarily 3A4
  - ▷ Half-life – approximately 21 hours
- ▶ Note
  - ▷ Wash in – 1 week after discontinue of most other antidepressants, 5 weeks for fluoxetine
  - ▷ Wash out – discontinue selegiline transdermal 2 week before initiating another antidepressant

Sertraline

- ▶ Trade name
  - ▷ Zoloft
- ▶ Dosage
  - ▷ PO 50 mg qd up to 200 mg/day
- ▶ Mechanism
  - ▷ 5-HT reuptake inhibitor
- ▶ Indications
  - ▷ Major depression
  - ▷ OCD
  - ▷ Panic disorder
  - ▷ Posttraumatic stress disorder (PTSD)
  - ▷ Premenstrual dysphoric disorder
- ▶ Age – approved down to 6-year-olds
- ▶ Black box warning
  - ▷ Increased risk of suicidality in children, adolescents, and young adults ≤24-year-olds
  - ▷ Suicidal risk is not increased beyond 24-year-olds and decreased for patients above 65-year-olds
- ▶ Safety caution and adverse effect
  - ▷ Contraindication – MAOI use within 14 days, use with pimozide
  - ▷ Pregnancy – C
  - ▷ Nausea
  - ▷ Headache
- ▶ Metabolism
  - ▷ CYP450 – weak 2D6 and 3A4 inhibitor
  - ▷ Half-life – 26 hours

Tranylcypromine

▶ Brand name
  ▷ Parnate
▶ Dosage
  ▷ PO 10 mg tid up to 60 mg/day
▶ Mechanism
  ▷ Nonselective monoamine oxidase inhibitor
▶ Indication
  ▷ Depression
▶ Black box warning
  ▷ Increased risk of suicidality in children, adolescents, and young adults ≤24-year-olds
  ▷ Suicidal risk is not increased beyond 24-year-olds and decreased for patients above 65-year-olds
▶ Adverse effects
  ▷ Contraindication – pheochromocytoma
  ▷ Pregnancy – C
  ▷ Hypertensive crisis
  ▷ Orthostatic hypotension
  ▷ Serotonin syndrome
  ▷ Seizures
  ▷ Sedation
  ▷ Avoid high tyramine-content food
  ▷ Monitoring: BP, LFTs
▶ Metabolism
  ▷ CYP450 – unknown
  ▷ Half-life – 2.5 hours

Trazodone

▶ Brand name
  ▷ Desyrel
▶ Dosage
  ▷ PO 50 mg qhs up to 400 mg/day outpatient, 600 mg/day inpatient
▶ Mechanism
  ▷ Blocks postsynaptic 5-HT2 receptors
  ▷ Weakly inhibits reuptake of 5-HT and NE
  ▷ The combination of neurotransmitter interaction results in selective activation of 5-HT1 receptors (comparable to nefazodone)
▶ Indication
  ▷ Depression
▶ Black box warning
  ▷ Increased risk of suicidality in children, adolescents, and young adults ≤24-year-olds
  ▷ Suicidal risk is not increased beyond 24-year-olds and decreased for patients above 65-year-olds
▶ Adverse effect and safety caution
  ▷ Contraindication – myocardial infarction
  ▷ Pregnancy – C
  ▷ Rare incident of priapism

▷ Sedation
▷ Anticholinergic effects
▶ Metabolism
▷ CYP450 – 3A4 substrate
▷ Half-life – 6 hours

Tricyclic antidepressants: Secondary amine vs. Tertiary amine (Figure 29–1)

▶ Secondary amine TCAs
▷ Desipramine
▷ Nortriptyline
▷ Protriptyline
▶ Tertiary amine TCAs
▷ Amitriptyline
▷ Clomipramine
▷ Doxepin
▷ Imipramine
▶ Secondary amine TCAs have more potent NE reuptake blockade; tertiary amine TCAs have more 5-HT reuptake blockade
▶ Tertiary TCAs tend to have more side effects than the secondary TCAs

Trimipramine

▶ Brand name
▷ Surmontil
▶ Dosage
▷ Up to 300 mg/day
▶ Mechanism
▷ Inhibits reuptake of norepinephrine and serotonin
▶ Indication
▷ Depression
▶ Adverse effect and safety caution
▷ Contraindication – MAOI use within 14 days, recent myocardial infarction
▷ Pregnancy – C
▷ Monitor ECG
▷ QT prolongation
▷ Anticholinergic effects
▶ Metabolism
▷ CYP450 – 2C19, 2D6, 3A4
▷ Half-life – approximately 10 hours

Venlafaxine (Figure 29–3)

▶ Brand name
▷ Effexor, Effexor XR
▶ Dosage
▷ PO 37.5 mg qd up to 375 mg/day for immediate release, 225 mg/day for XR version
▶ Mechanism
▷ At low dose, inhibits reuptake of 5-HT
▷ At mediate to high dose, inhibits reuptake of 5-HT, NE, and DA

▶ Indication
  ▷ Major depressive disorder
  ▷ Generalized anxiety disorder
  ▷ Panic disorder
  ▷ Social anxiety disorder
▶ Black box warning
  ▷ Increased risk of suicidality in children, adolescents, and young adults ≤24-year-olds
  ▷ Suicidal risk is not increased beyond 24-year-olds and decreased for patients above 65-year-olds
▶ Safety caution and adverse effect
  ▷ Contraindication – MAOI use within 14 days; uncontrolled narrow angle-closure glaucoma
  ▷ Pregnancy – C
  ▷ Abrupt withdrawal may cause discontinuation symptoms
  ▷ Elevation of blood pressure (dose-dependent)
  ▷ Reduces (i.e., worsens) heart rate variability
  ▷ No anticholinergic, antihistaminic, or adrenergic blocking effects
▶ Metabolism
  ▷ Active metabolite – desvenlafaxine
  ▷ CYP450 – substrate of 2D6, no significant CYP inhibition
  ▷ Half-life – 5 hours, 12 hours for desvenlafaxine

30   Anxielytics and Hypnotics

Psychotropics are no longer easy to be sorted in single-functioning slots. Most anti-depressants, some anticonvulsants, and even antipsychotics, have been used for the treatment of anxiety. This chapter focuses chiefly on the large family of benzodiazepines, which serves as the most frequently used anxielytics and hypnotics. Nonbenzodiazepine gamma-aminobutyric acid (GABA) receptor binding agents are also reviewed here, along with a few other relevant anxielytics and hypnotics.

Benzodiazepines were first developed by Roche Laboratories in 1950s. The first ben-zodiazepine introduced was chlordiazepoxide (Librium), followed by diazepam (Valium) in a few years. Continued laboratory study developed a large group of agents, which share the same core structure (Figure 30–1) and broad spectrum of clinical effects as hypnotics, muscle relaxants, sedatives, anxielytics, and anticonvulsants. All the ben-zodiazepines have the same mechanism of action, and all bear risk of addiction. The difference between one benzodiazepine and another lays mainly on the half-life. The rate of absorption and lipophilicity also play important roles in these agents' individual personality. Benzodiazepines have their naturally occurring receptors in human brain. Some fungi may be able to synthesize benzodiazepine. However, at this point, no endog-enous ligands for benzodiazepine receptors have been found. Commonly used benzo-diazepines include

- ▶ Alprazolam (Xanax, Xanax XR, Niravam)
- ▶ Midazolam (Versed)
- ▶ Oxazepam (Serax)
- ▶ Triazolam (Halcion)
- ▶ Lorazepam (Ativan)
- ▶ Estazolam (ProSom)
- ▶ Temazepam (Restoril)
- ▶ Chlordiazepoxide (Librium)
- ▶ Clonazepam (Klonopin, Klonopin Wafers)
- ▶ Clorazepate (Tranxene SD, Tranxene T-Tab)
- ▶ Diazepam (Valium)
- ▶ Flurazepam (Dalmane)

A new group of nonbenzodiazepine, selective GABA-binding hypnotics has been gain-ing popularity with relative safety and probable less tendency of abuse. These include

- ▶ Zolpidem (Ambien, Ambien CR)
- ▶ Eszopiclone (Lunesta)
- ▶ Ramelteon (Rozerem)
- ▶ Zaleplon (Sonata)

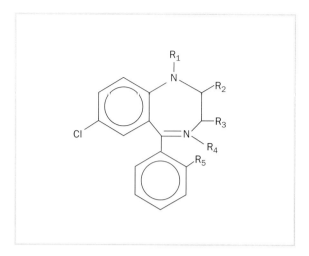

Figure 30–1 Core structure of benzodiazepines.

A few other frequently mentioned anxielytics and hypnotics are also discussed here

▶ Gamma-hydroxybutyrate (Xyrem)
▶ Hydroxyzine (Atarax, Vistaril)
▶ Buspirone (BuSpar)
▶ Chloral Hydrate (Aquachloral Supprettes)

Alprazolam

▶ Brand name
  ▷ Xanax, Xanax XR, Niravam
▶ Dosage
  ▷ PO 0.25 mg TID up to 4 mg/day
▶ Mechanism
  ▷ Binds to benzodiazepine binding site on GABA-A receptor complex
  ▷ Enhances GABA effect in opening ligand-regulated chloride channel
▶ Indication
  ▷ Anxiety
  ▷ Panic disorder
▶ Safety caution and adverse effect
  ▷ Contraindication – angel-closed glaucoma, pregnancy
  ▷ Pregnancy risk category – D
  ▷ Drug Enforcement Administration (DEA) schedule – IV
  ▷ Significant withdrawal upon abrupt cessation
▶ Metabolism
  ▷ CYP450 – substrate of p450 3A4
  ▷ Half-life – approximately 10–15 hours

Benzodiazepines: general consideration (See Figure 2–4 on page 14)

▶ Binds to benzodiazepine binding site on GABA-A receptor complex
▶ Enhances GABA effect in opening ligand-regulated chloride channel
▶ All are category D in pregnancy risk

▶ All are DEA schedule IV
▶ Major differences lay in absorption, hepatic metabolism, half-life, and onset of action

Benzodiazepines with long half life

▶ Usually 30–100 hours; up to 200 hours in slow metabolizer
  ▷ Chlordiazepoxide (Librium)
  ▷ Clonazepam (Klonopin)
  ▷ Clorazepate (Tranxene)
  ▷ Diazepam (Valium)
  ▷ Flurazepam (Dalmane)
  ▷ Halazepam (Paxipam)
  ▷ Prazepam (Centrax)
  ▷ Quazepam (Doral)

Benzodiazepines with medium– to short–half-life

▶ Triazolam (Halcion): 2–3 hours
▶ Alprazolam (Xanax): 10–15 hours
▶ Half-life: 8–30 hours
  ▷ Lorazepam (Ativan)
  ▷ Oxazepam (Serax)
  ▷ Temazepam (Restoril)
  ▷ Estazolam (ProSom)

Buspirone

▶ Brand name
  ▷ BuSpar
▶ Dosage
  ▷ 7.5 mg bid to 30 mg bid
  ▷ Mechanism5-HT1a partial agonist
▶ Indication
  ▷ Anxiety
▶ Safety caution and adverse effect
  ▷ Pregnancy – B
  ▷ Dizziness
  ▷ Nausea
  ▷ Serotonin syndrome (rare)
▶ Metabolism
  ▷ CYP450 – 3A4 substrate
  ▷ Half-life – approximately 2.5 hours

Chloral hydrate

▶ Brand names and dosage
  ▷ Generic – PO 500 mg QHS up to 1,000 mg Q6h
  ▷ Aquachloral Supprettes (rectal), PR, up to 1,950 mg/day

▶ Mechanism
  ▷ Exact mechanism unknown; it is assumed its active metabolite trichloroethanol has central nervous system (CNS) suppressive effect
▶ Indicated for insomnia and alcohol withdrawal
▶ Safety caution and adverse effect
  ▷ Pregnancy risk category – C
  ▷ DEA schedule – IV
  ▷ Nausea, vomiting
  ▷ Confusion, delirium
  ▷ Respiratory depression
▶ Metabolism
  ▷ CYP450: unknown
  ▷ Half-life: 8–11 hours

Chlordiazepoxide

The first benzodiazepine to be introduced in 1960

▶ Brand name
  ▷ Librium
▶ Dosage
  ▷ PO 5 mg tid to maximum 300 mg/day
▶ Mechanism
  ▷ Binds to benzodiazepine binding site on GABA-A receptor complex
  ▷ Enhances GABA effect in opening ligand-regulated chloride channel
▶ Indication
  ▷ Anxiety
  ▷ Alcohol withdrawal
▶ Safety caution and adverse effect
  ▷ Pregnancy risk category – D
  ▷ Sedation
  ▷ Rarely reported agranulocytosis
▶ Metabolism
  ▷ CYP450: 3A4 substrate
  ▷ Half-life: 5–30 hours; active metabolite up to 200 hours

Clonazepam

▶ Trade name
  ▷ Klonopin
  ▷ Klonopin Wafers
▶ Dosage
  ▷ PO 0.5 mg BID up to 4 mg/day for anxiety disorders
  ▷ Up to 20 mg/day for seizure disorders
▶ Mechanism
  ▷ Binds to benzodiazepine binding site on GABA-A receptor complex
  ▷ Enhances GABA effect in opening ligand-regulated chloride channel
▶ Indication
  ▷ Seizure disorder
  ▷ Panic disorder
  ▷ Anxiety

▶ Safety caution and adverse effect
  ▷ Contraindication
  ▷ Pregnancy risk category – D
  ▷ Weight change
  ▷ Considered less potential in developing addiction and abusive pattern than alprazolam
▶ Metabolism
  ▷ CYP450: 3A4 substrate
  ▷ Half-life: 20–50 hours
▶ Note – the only benzodiazepine can be used in solo maintenance for seizure disorders

Clorazepate

▶ Brand name
  ▷ Tranxene SD, Tranxene T-Tab
▶ Dosage
▶ PO 15–30 mg/day QHS or divided, up to 90 mg/day
▶ Mechanism
  ▷ Binds to benzodiazepine binding site on GABA-A receptor complex
  ▷ Enhances GABA effect in opening ligand-regulated chloride channel
▶ Indication
  ▷ Anxiety
  ▷ Alcohol withdrawal
  ▷ Adjunct therapy for partial seizures
▶ Safety caution and adverse effect
  ▷ Contraindication – acute angle-close glaucoma
  ▷ Pregnancy risk category – D
  ▷ Drowsiness
  ▷ Hepatotoxicity
▶ Metabolism
  ▷ CYP450: unknown
  ▷ Half-life: 40–50 hours

Diazepam

▶ Brand name
  ▷ Valium, Diastat
▶ Dosage
  ▷ PO 2 mg BID up to 40 mg/day
▶ Mechanism
  ▷ Binds to benzodiazepine binding site on GABA-A receptor complex
  ▷ Enhances GABA effect in opening ligand-regulated chloride channel
▶ Indication
  ▷ Anxiety
  ▷ Alcohol withdrawal
  ▷ Muscle spasm
  ▷ Seizure disorders
▶ Safety caution and adverse effect
  ▷ Pregnancy risk category – D
  ▷ Respiratory depression

▷ Depression
▷ Sedation, confusion
▶ Metabolism
▷ CYP450: substrate of 2C19 and 3A4
▷ Half-life: 30–60 hours; active metabolite (desmethyldiazepam) up to 100 hours

Estazolam

▶ Brand name
▷ ProSom
▶ Dosage
▷ PO 1–2 mg QHS
▶ Mechanism
▷ Binds to benzodiazepine binding site on GABA-A receptor complex
▷ Enhances GABA effect in opening ligand-regulated chloride channel
▶ Indication
▷ Short-term treatment for insomnia
▶ Safety caution and adverse effect
▷ Pregnancy risk category – D
▷ Respiratory depression
▶ Metabolism
▷ CYP450: substrate of 3A4
▷ Half-life: 10–24 hours

Eszopiclone

▶ Brand name
▷ Lunesta
▶ Dosage
▷ PO 2–3 mg QHS
▶ Mechanism
▷ Acts on α-1 isoform of GABA-A receptor
▶ Indication
▷ Insomnia
▶ Safety caution and adverse effect
▷ Contraindication
▷ Pregnancy risk category – C
▷ Minimal tolerance, discontinuation reaction or sleep rebound
▷ Depression, suicidal ideas
▷ Agitation
▷ Unpleasant taste is one of the notable side effects
▶ Metabolism
▷ CYP450: substrate of 2E1, 3A4
▷ Half-life: 6 hours

Flurazepam

▶ Brand name
▷ Dalmane

▶ Dosage
  ▷ PO 15–30 mg QHS
▶ Mechanism
  ▷ Binds to benzodiazepine binding site on GABA-A receptor complex
  ▷ Enhances GABA effect in opening ligand-regulated chloride channel
▶ Indication
  ▷ Insomnia
▶ Safety caution and adverse effect
  ▷ Pregnancy risk category – D
  ▷ Sedation
  ▷ Headache
▶ Metabolism
  ▷ CYP450: substrate of 3A4
  ▷ Half-life: 2–3 hours; active metabolite: 40–100 QHS

Gamma-hydroxybutyrate (Figure 30–2)

Also known as oxybate

▶ Brand name
  ▷ Xyrem
▶ Dosage
  ▷ PO 2.25 g QHS and second dose 2–4 hours later, up to 9 g/day
▶ Mechanisms
  ▷ Gamma-hydroxybutyrate (GHB) receptors – excitatory, require low concentration
  ▷ GABA-B receptors – inhibitory, require high concentration
▶ Indicated for excessive daytime sleepiness and narcolepsy
▶ Back box warning
  ▷ Restricted distribution through Xyrem Success Program
  ▷ CNS depressant with abuse potential

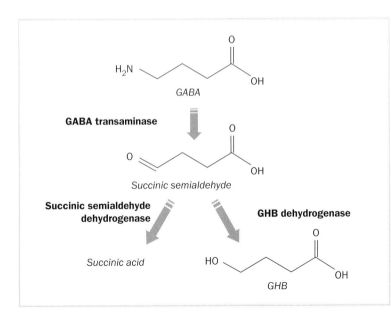

Figure 30–2 The degradation of GABA and the production of GHB. Normally, GABA is converted to succinic semialdehyde and then to succinic acid, which is utilized in Krebs cycle. In the case of genetic deficiency in succinic semialdehyde dehydrogenase, succinic semialdehyde accumulates and is reduced to GHB. Patients with genetic succinic semialdehyde dehydrogenase deficiency should not take GHB. GABA, gamma aminobutyric acid; GHB, gamma-hydroxybutyric acid.

- ▶ Other safety caution and adverse effect
  - ▷ Contraindication – CNS depressant use, succinic semialdehyde dehydrogenase deficiency
  - ▷ Pregnancy risk category – D
  - ▷ Respiratory depression
  - ▷ Seizure
- ▶ Metabolism
  - ▷ CYP450: unknown
  - ▷ Half-life: 14 hours
- ▶ Note
  - ▷ Rapid acting hypnotic
  - ▷ Reduces cataplexy
  - ▷ Increases slow wave sleep while has not effect on rapid eye movement (REM)
- ▶ The only drug receives two schedules
  - ▷ Schedule I – GHB (generic)
  - ▷ Schedule III – when marketed and prescribed as Xyrem

Hydroxyzine

- ▶ Trade name
  - ▷ Atarax, Vistaril
- ▶ Dosage
  - ▷ PO 25 mg q6h prn up to 600 mg/day
- ▶ Mechanism
  - ▷ Antagonist to H1 receptors
- ▶ Indicated for anxiety and pruritus
- ▶ Safety caution and adverse effect
  - ▷ Pregnancy risk category – C
  - ▷ Monitoring – Creatinine at baseline
  - ▷ Dry mouth
  - ▷ Dyspnea
- ▶ Metabolism
  - ▷ CYP450: unknown
  - ▷ Half-life: 20–25 hours

Lorazepam

Tip – one of the three benzodiazepines that have no active metabolite and that are relatively safe for impaired livers; the other two are oxazepam and temazepam

- ▶ Brand name
  - ▷ Ativan
- ▶ Dosage
  - ▷ IV/IM/PO 0.5 mg q6–8h up to 10 mg/day
- ▶ Mechanism
  - ▷ Binds to benzodiazepine binding site on GABA receptor complex, enhances GAGAergic effect
- ▶ Indication
  - ▷ Anxiety
  - ▷ Insomnia
  - ▷ Status epilepticus

▶ Safety caution and adverse effect
  ▷ Contraindication – acute angle-closure glaucoma
  ▷ Pregnancy – D
  ▷ Sedation
  ▷ Respiratory suppression
  ▷ Addiction
▶ Metabolism
  ▷ CYP450: none
  ▷ Half-life: 14 hours

Oxazepam

▶ Brand name
  ▷ Serax
▶ Dosage
  ▷ PO 10 mg tid to 30 mg qid
▶ Mechanism
  ▷ Binds to benzodiazepine binding site on GABA-A receptor complex
  ▷ Enhances GABA effect in opening ligand-regulated chloride channel
▶ Indication
  ▷ Anxiety
  ▷ Alcohol withdrawal
▶ Safety caution and adverse effect
  ▷ Pregnancy risk category – D
  ▷ Sedation, confusion
  ▷ Withdrawal
▶ Metabolism
  ▷ No active metabolite
  ▷ CYP450: unknown
  ▷ Half-life: 8 hours

Quick onset of action in benzodiazepines

▶ Quick onset of action is often desired for symptom relief; however, the quick onset of euphoria may raise the risk of abuse
▶ Usually implies lipophilic character of the molecule, which facilitates crossing of the blood-brain barrier
▶ Quick onset does not always mean short half-life
  ▷ Alprazolam (Xanax) – short half-life
  ▷ Diazepam (Valium) – long half-life
  ▷ Estazolam (ProSom) – medium half-life
  ▷ Lorazepam (Ativan) – medium half life
  ▷ Triazolam (Halcion) – very short half-life

Ramelteon

▶ Brand name
  ▷ Rozerem
▶ Dosage
  ▷ 8 mg/day

▶ Mechanism
  ▷ A melatonin receptor agonist, with much higher affinity than melatonin
▶ Indicated for insomnia
▶ Safety caution and adverse effect
  ▷ Pregnancy risk category – C
  ▷ Depression, suicidal ideation
  ▷ Headache
  ▷ Fatigue
▶ Metabolism
  ▷ CYP450: 1A2 substrate
  ▷ Half-life: 1–2.6 hours, 2–5 hours for active metabolite

Temazepam

▶ Brand name
  ▷ Restoril
▶ Dosage
  ▷ PO 7.5–30 mg qhs
▶ Mechanism
  ▷ Binds to benzodiazepine binding site on GABA-A receptor complex
  ▷ Enhances GABA effect in opening ligand-regulated chloride channel
▶ Indication
  ▷ Insomnia
▶ Safety caution and adverse effect
  ▷ Pregnancy – D
  ▷ Respiratory depression
▶ Metabolism
  ▷ CYP450: none
  ▷ Half-life: 9 hours

Triazolam

▶ Brand name
  ▷ Halcion
▶ Dosage
  ▷ PO 0.125 up to 0.5 mg qhs
▶ Mechanism
  ▷ Binds to benzodiazepine binding site on GABA-A receptor complex
  ▷ Enhances GABA effect in opening ligand-regulated chloride channel
▶ Indication
  ▷ Insomnia
▶ Safety caution and adverse effect
  ▷ Pregnancy risk category – D
  ▷ Respiratory depression
  ▷ Movement impairment
▶ Metabolism
  ▷ CYP450: 3A4 substrate
  ▷ Half-life: 1.5–5.5 hours

Use of benzodiazepines with impaired liver

▶ Any benzodiazepines that require oxidation in metabolism should be limited in use in patients with compromised hepatic function
▶ Benzodiazepines metabolized via glucoronidation and require no oxidation are relatively safe for impaired livers
  ▷ Temazepam (Restoril)
  ▷ Oxazepam (Serax)
  ▷ Lorazepam (Ativan)

Withdrawal of benzodiazepine

▶ Common benzodiazepine withdrawal symptoms
  ▷ Anxiety
  ▷ Diaphoresis
  ▷ Fatigue
  ▷ Insomnia
  ▷ Irritability
  ▷ Light-headedness
  ▷ Restlessness
  ▷ Tremor
▶ Abrupt discontinuation of benzodiazepines, particularly those with short half-lives, or use of flumazenil, are associated with severe withdrawal symptoms
  ▷ Delirium
  ▷ Depression
  ▷ Paranoia
  ▷ Seizures
▶ Management
  ▷ Tapering slowly (25% a week)
  ▷ Psychological support
  ▷ Concurrent use of carbamazepine (Tegretol) during benzodiazepine discontinuation
  ▷ Reported particular difficulty in discontinuing alprazolam may be resolved by switching to clonazepam, which is then tapered

Zaleplon

▶ Brand name
  ▷ Sonata
▶ Dosage
  ▷ PO 5–20 mg qhs
▶ Mechanism
  ▷ Nonbenzodiazepine GABA antagonist
▶ Indication
  ▷ Insomnia
▶ Safety caution and adverse effect
  ▷ Pregnancy risk category – C
  ▷ Headache
  ▷ Depression, suicidal ideation

▶ Metabolism
  ▷ CYP450: substrate of 3A4
  ▷ Half-life: 1 hour

Zolpidem

▶ Brand names and dosage
  ▷ Ambien – up to 10 mg/day
  ▷ Ambien CR – up to 12.5 mg/day
▶ Mechanism
  ▷ Nonbenzodiazepine GABA antagonist
▶ Indication
  ▷ Insomnia
▶ Safety caution and adverse effect
  ▷ Pregnancy risk category C
  ▷ Depression, suicidal ideation
  ▷ Headache
▶ Metabolism
  ▷ CYP450: substrate of 3A4
  ▷ Half-life: 2.5 hours

31 Pharmacotherapy for Substance-Related Conditions

Until recently, there were not enough medicines to form a category designated to the treatment of substance abuse and dependence. Traditional treatment relies on a combination of symptomatic pharmacotherapy, psychosocial therapy, and behavioral rehabilitation. Institutionalization and incarceration may sometimes play a therapeutic role in the recovery. Symptomatic treatment for the comorbid psychiatric conditions is another important area; however the medicines used are not substance specific. Opioid receptor blocker and replacement treatment have probably the longest history since the 1970s. Recent years have witnessed new development of several substance-specific agents targeting the conditions related to alcohol, nicotine, and opioid. In large, we still have not enough effective remedies and aggressive new development should be desired. The medicines included in this chapter are

▶ Treatment for opioid-related conditions (See Figure 31–1 on page 248)
  ▷ Buprenorphine
  ▷ Methadone
  ▷ Naloxone
  ▷ Naltrexone (ReVia, Vivitrol, also for alcohol treatment)
▶ Treatment for alcohol-related conditions
  ▷ Acamprosate (Campral)
  ▷ Disulfiram (Antabuse)
  ▷ Naltrexone (ReVia, Vivitrol)
▶ Treatment for nicotine-related conditions
  ▷ Varenicline (Chantix)
▶ Other agents
  ▷ Flumazenil
  ▷ Clonidine

Acamprosate

▶ Brand name
  ▷ Campral
▶ Dosage
  ▷ PO 333 mg tid to 666 mg tid
▶ Mechanism
  ▷ Reduces alcohol intake without aversive reaction
  ▷ Interacts with glutamate and gamma aminobutyric acid (GABA) system
▶ Indication
  ▷ Alcohol dependence

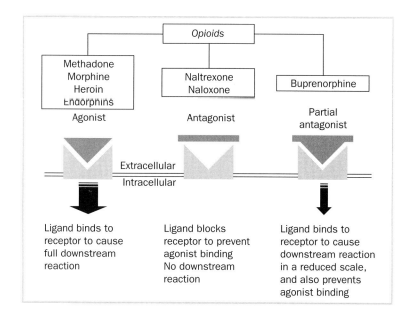

Figure 31–1 Summary of receptor mechanisms of opioid agents.

▷ Adverse effect and safety caution
    ▷ Contraindication – creatinine clearance lower than 30 ml/min
    ▷ Pregnancy risk category – C
    ▷ Diarrhea
    ▷ Insomnia
    ▷ Possible induction of depression and psychosis
▷ Metabolism
    ▷ No hepatic metabolism; excreted from kidney
    ▷ Half-life: 20–33 hours

Buprenorphine

▷ Brand name
    ▷ Buprenex
    ▷ Subutex, SL
    ▷ Suboxone (Buprenorphine/naloxone)
▷ Dosage
    ▷ IM or IV, 300 mcg q8h. Up to 600 mcg per dose, IV only
    ▷ up to 16 mg per day
    ▷ SL 2 mg/0.5 mg to 24 mg/6 mg daily
▷ Mechanism
    ▷ Partial antagonist of opioid receptors
▷ Safety caution and adverse effect
    ▷ Pregnancy – C
    ▷ Respiratory depression
    ▷ Withdrawal symptoms
    ▷ Pain
    ▷ Constipation

▶ Metabolism
  ▷ CYP450: 3A4 substrate
  ▷ Half-life: 22–44 hours
▶ Ceiling effect equivalent to 40 mg methadone, therefore individuals taking more than 40 mg methadone equivalent should first be tapered to near 40 mg/day
▶ Long acting – single dose acts for 3 days; the advantage of this is the enforced commitment
▶ Sublingual formula available for prescribing in office-based setting

Clonidine

▶ Brand name
  ▷ Catapres, Catapres TTS (transdermal)
▶ Dosage
  ▷ PO up to 2.4 mg/day
  ▷ Transdermal up to 0.6 mg/day
▶ Mechanism
  ▷ Agonizes on presynaptic α-2 adrenergic receptor
▶ Indication
  ▷ Approved for hypertension
  ▷ Has been used off-label for attention deficit hyperactivity disorder (ADHD), Tourette's syndrome, alcohol and opioid withdrawal, anxiety disorders, and clozapine-induced hypersalivation
▶ Safety caution and adverse effect
  ▷ Contraindication
  ▷ Pregnancy – C
  ▷ Monitor blood pressure
  ▷ Monitor creatinine (Cr) at baseline
  ▷ Avoid abrupt cessation to prevent rebound hypertension
  ▷ Dry mouth
  ▷ Dizziness
▶ Metabolism
  ▷ CYP450: unknown
  ▷ Half-life: 12 hours
▶ Note – effective in suppressing autonomic symptoms during opioid withdrawal, but not subjective craving

Disulfiram (See Figure 12–1 on page 87)

▶ Brand name
  ▷ Antabuse
▶ Dosage
  ▷ PO 125–500 mg/day
▶ Mechanism
  ▷ Disulfiram inhibits acetaldehyde dehydrogenase (an enzyme degrades alcohol) and therefore raises acetaldehyde level in the blood and tissues
  ▷ Acetaldehyde causes severe intoxicating symptoms, and may cause autonomous destabilization
▶ Indication
  ▷ Alcohol dependence

▶ Back box warning
  ▷ Alcohol contraindicated
▶ Other safety caution and adverse effect
  ▷ Contraindication – alcohol use within 12 hour
  ▷ Pregnancy – C
  ▷ Respiratory depression
  ▷ Cardiovascular collapse
  ▷ Seizures
▶ Metabolism
  ▷ CYP450: 2A9 inhibitor
  ▷ Half-life: known
▶ Note –the clinical effects last for up to 2 weeks after the last dose
  ▷ Disulfiram also inhibits dopamine-β-hydroxylase, an enzyme converts dopamine to norepinephrine; it may be useful in reducing cocaine use

Flumazenil

▶ Brand name
  ▷ Romazicon
▶ Dosage
  ▷ Intravenous (IV) 0.2 mg/min up to 1 mg/dose, 1 dose per 20 minute up to 3 mg/h
▶ Mechanism
  ▷ Antagonizes benzodiazepine receptors
▶ Indication
  ▷ Benzodiazepine overdose
▶ Back box warning
  ▷ Seizure risk
▶ Other safety caution and adverse effect
  ▷ Contraindication – tricyclic antidepressant overdose
  ▷ Pregnancy risk category – C
  ▷ Seizure and withdrawal symptoms
  ▷ Nauseas
  ▷ Headache
▶ Metabolism
  ▷ CYP450: unknown
  ▷ Half-life: 54 minutes

Methadone

▶ Brand name
  ▷ Dolophine, Methadose
▶ Dosage
  ▷ Up to 40 mg/day on day 1
  ▷ Above 100 mg/day requires proper documentation
  ▷ No mandated maximum dosage
▶ Mechanism Opioid agonist
▶ Indication
  ▷ Opioid dependence
  ▷ Severe pain

▶ Back box warning
  ▷ Cross-tolerance with other opioids
  ▷ Respiratory depression
  ▷ Cardiac conduction blockade – QT prolongation, arrhythmias including Torsades de pointes
  ▷ Certification requirement for addiction treatment
▶ Pregnancy – C
▶ Metabolism
  ▷ CYP450: multiple p450 metabolisms, primarily 3A4; may induce own metabolism in chronic use
▶ Half-life: 8–59 hours

Naloxone

▶ Trade name
  ▷ Narcan
▶ Dosage
  ▷ SC, IM, IV, 0.4–2 mg/2–3 minutes
▶ Mechanism
  ▷ Opioid antagonist used for opioid overdose and postoperational opioid reversal
▶ Indication
▶ Back box warning
▶ Other safety caution and adverse effect
  ▷ Contraindication
  ▷ Pregnancy
▶ Metabolism
  ▷ CYP450
  ▷ Half-life: 1 hour

Naltrexone

▶ Trade name
  ▷ ReVia (PO), Vivitrol (IM)
▶ Dosage
  ▷ PO 50 mg/day
  ▷ IM 380 mg every 4 weeks
▶ Mechanism
  ▷ Opioid receptor antagonist
▶ Indication
  ▷ Opioid addiction
  ▷ Alcohol dependence
▶ Black box warning
  ▷ Hepatotoxicity
▶ Other safety caution and adverse effect
  ▷ Pregnancy risk category – C
  ▷ Depression, suicidality
  ▷ Nausea
  ▷ Abdominal pain
  ▷ Withdrawal symptoms

▶ Metabolism
  ▷ CYP450: none
  ▷ Half-life: 4 hours, active metabolite: 13 hours

Varenicline

▶ Brand name
  ▷ Chantix
▶ Dosage: up to 2 mg/day
▶ Mechanism
  ▷ Agonizes and blocks nicotinic acetylcholine receptors
▶ Indicated for smoke cessation
▶ Safety caution and adverse effect
  ▷ Pregnancy – C
  ▷ Possible induction of depression and suicidality
  ▷ Rare case of renal failure
  ▷ Depression
  ▷ Nausea, vomiting
▶ Metabolism
  ▷ Minimum hepatic metabolism; largely excreted from urine
  ▷ CYP450: none
  ▷ Half-life: 24 hours

32 Cognitive Enhancers

Research on cognitive enhancement has been fostered in large by the temptation of hope in reaching a cure for Alzheimer's disease. Consistent findings of central cholinergic depletion in patients with Alzheimer's disease led to many studies rushing to the track of cholinergic replenishment. Through the past decade, cholinesterase inhibitor has been the primary group of cognitive enhancers. Palliative treatment focusing on other neurotransmitters has also been explored. At this point in time, the N-Methyl-D-aspartate (NMDA) partial agonist memantine is the only one received official approval.

Cognitive enhancers and stimulants reviewed in this chapter include

▶ Tacrine (Cognex)
▶ Memantine (Namenda)
▶ Donepezil (Aricept)
▶ Galantamine (Razadyne)
▶ Rivastigmine (Exelon)

Cholinesterase inhibitors: class effects

▶ May provide 6–9 month of delay in dementia progression
▶ In addition to cognitive protection, may also be effective in behavioral stabilization
▶ Class side effects
  ▷ Nausea
  ▷ Diarrhea
  ▷ Vomiting

Donepezil

▶ Brand name
  ▷ Aricept
▶ Dosage
  ▷ PO 5–10 mg/day
▶ Mechanism
  ▷ Cholinesterase inhibitor
▶ Indication
  ▷ Alzheimer's dementia, mild to severe
▶ Safety caution and adverse effect
  ▷ Pregnancy risk category – C
  ▷ Not hepatotoxic
  ▷ Gastrointestinal tract (GI) symptoms including bleeding
  ▷ Headache

▶ Metabolism
  ▷ CYP450: primarily 3A4 substrate
  ▷ Half-life: 70 hours

Galantamine

▶ Brand name
  ▷ Razadyne, Razadyne ER
▶ Dosage
  ▷ PO 4 mg BID up to 12 mg BID
  ▷ Razadyne ER – PO 8 mg qam up to 24 mg/day
▶ Mechanism
  ▷ Cholinesterase inhibitor
  ▷ Also a nicotinic acetylcholine receptor modulator
  ▷ The only cholinesterase inhibitor that acts also on postsynaptic neurons
▶ Indication
  ▷ Dementia of Alzheimer's type, mild to moderate
▶ Safety caution and adverse effect
  ▷ Pregnancy risk category – B
  ▷ Urinary obstruction, monitor creatinine
  ▷ Nausea, vomiting, GI bleeding
  ▷ Syncope, fatigue
▶ Metabolism
  ▷ CYP450: 2D6 and 3A4 substrate
  ▷ Half-life: 7 hours

Memantine

▶ Brand name
  ▷ Namenda
▶ Dosage
  ▷ PO 5 mg/day up to 20 mg/day
▶ Indication
  ▷ Alzheimer's dementia, moderate to severe
▶ Safety caution and adverse effect
  ▷ Pregnancy risk category – B
  ▷ Stevens–Johnson syndrome
  ▷ Dizziness
  ▷ Headache
  ▷ In general well tolerated
  ▷ Needs creatinine (Cr) monitoring
▶ Metabolism
  ▷ CYP450: none
  ▷ Active tubular secretion
  ▷ Half-life: 60–80 hours

Memantine: mechanisms

▶ A noncompetitive NMDA receptor antagonist
▶ Moderate affinity to NMDA receptor to enhance the physiological function of Mg^{++}, which is to reduce calcium influx

▶ By reducing, but not complete blocking, the calcium influx, memantine blocks neural toxicity yet allows normal function necessary for memory and other cognition

Rivastigmine

▶ Brand name
  ▷ Exelon, Exelon Patch
▶ Dosage
  ▷ PO 1.5 mg BID up to 12 mg/day
▶ Mechanism
  ▷ Inhibits cholinesterase
  ▷ Inhibits butyrylcholinesterase, a theoretic advantage
▶ Indication
  ▷ Alzheimer's dementia, mild to moderate
  ▷ Parkinson's dementia, mild to moderate
▶ Safety caution and adverse effect
  ▷ Pregnancy risk category – B
  ▷ GI symptoms including GI bleeding
  ▷ Dizziness
▶ Metabolism
  ▷ CYP450: none
  ▷ Half-life: 1.5 hours

Tacrine

▶ Brand name
  ▷ Cognex
▶ Dosage
  ▷ PO 10 mg QID up to 40 mg QID
▶ Mechanism
  ▷ Cholinesterase inhibitor
▶ Indication
  ▷ Alzheimer's dementia, mild to moderate
▶ Safety caution and adverse effect
  ▷ Pregnancy risk category – C
  ▷ Severe hepatic toxicity; need close liver function test (LFT) monitoring.
  ▷ GI symptoms
▶ Metabolism
  ▷ CYP450: 1A2 substrate and inhibitor, has active metabolite
  ▷ Half-life: 2–4 hours
▶ Note – Tacrine use has significantly decreased in recent years due to its hepatic toxicity and inconvenience in dosing

33 Stimulants

Stimulants, as prototyped by amphetamine, may be considered in an aspect as cognitive enhancing agents. Stimulants do not work on primary memory loss, but are potent in improving wakefulness, concentration, and learning abilities. In spite of controversy due to the potential of addiction, stimulants have been the mainstay therapeutics for attention-deficit/hyperactivity disorder (ADHD), narcolepsy, and obesity. Stimulants were also proposed to be optional augmenting agents in treating severe depression, and lethargy induced by brain injury or opioid medications.

Stimulants reviewed in this chapter include

▶ Amphetamine or dextroamphetamine (Adderall, Dexadrine)
▶ Benzphetamine (Didrex)
▶ Lisdexamfetamine (Vyvanse)
▶ Methamphetamine (Desoxyn)
▶ Methylphenidate or dexmethylphenidate (Ritalin, Concerta, Daytrana, Metadate, Focalin)
▶ Phentermine (Adipex-P)
▶ Sibutramine (Meridia)

Atomoxetine (Strattera) is the only Food and Drug Administration (FDA)-approved medicine for ADHD that is not Drug Enforcement Administration (DEA) scheduled. It is not a stimulant but nonetheless discussed here due to its therapeutic association with stimulants.

Amphetamine/dextroamphetamine

▶ Brand name
  ▷ Adderall, Adderall XR
▶ Dosage
  ▷ Adderall – PO 5 mg BID up to 60 mg/day
  ▷ Adderall XR – 6–12-year-olds, PO 10 mg/day up to 30 mg/day; 13-year-olds and beyond, PO 10 mg/day up to 40 mg/day
▶ Mechanism
  ▷ Blocks norepinephrine and dopamine reuptake
  ▷ Enhances presynaptic release of norepinephrine and dopamine
▶ Indication
  ▷ ADHD
  ▷ Narcolepsy
▶ Back box warning
  ▷ High addiction potential

▶ Other safety caution and adverse effect
  ▷ Contraindication – MAOI use in 14 days
  ▷ Pregnancy risk category – C
  ▷ Weight change – weight loss or growth suppression, need to monitor height and weight
  ▷ Baseline cardiac evaluation
  ▷ Caution with cardiovascular diseases
  ▷ Blood pressure (BP) and heart rate (HR) elevation
  ▷ Dependence, abuse, withdrawal
  ▷ Psychosis
  ▷ Anorexia
  ▷ Aggression
  ▷ Worsening of tics, Tourette's syndrome
  ▷ Seizure risk – low
▶ Metabolism
  ▷ CYP450: 2D6 substrate with active metabolites
  ▷ Half-life: 9–14 hours

Atomoxetine

▶ Trade name
  ▷ Strattera
▶ Dosage
  ▷ Children above 6 years and less than 70 kg – PO 0.5 mg/kg/day up to 1.4 mg/kg/day
  ▷ Adults or children above 6 years and more then 70 kg – PO 40 mg/day up to 100 mg/day
▶ The only medicine indicated for ADHD that is not scheduled
  ▷ Mechanism
▶ Selectively inhibits norepinephrine reuptake
▶ Indication
  ▷ ADHD
▶ Back box warning
  ▷ Increased suicidality in children and adolescents, particularly in the first month of treatment
▶ Other safety caution and adverse effect
  ▷ Contraindication – MAOI use in 14 days; angle-closure glaucoma
  ▷ Pregnancy risk category – C
  ▷ Baseline cardiac evaluation
  ▷ Psychosis
  ▷ BP elevation
  ▷ Tachycardia
  ▷ Aggressive behavior
  ▷ Nausea/vomiting
▶ Metabolism
  ▷ CYP450: 2C19 and 2D6 substrate
  ▷ Half-life: 5.2 hours, 21 hours in poor 2D6 metabolizers

Benzphetamine

▶ Brand name
  ▷ Didrex

▶ Dosage
  ▷ PO 25 mg qd up to 50 mg tid
▶ Mechanism
  ▷ Sympathomimetic stimulant
  ▷ Suppresses appetite
▶ Indicated for obesity
▶ Safety caution and adverse effect
  ▷ Contraindication – MAOI use in 14 days
  ▷ Pregnancy – X
  ▷ Consider cardiovascular evaluation before start treatment
  ▷ Addiction tendency – schedule III
  ▷ Palpitation
  ▷ Escalated BP
  ▷ Insomnia
▶ Metabolism
  ▷ CYP450: unknown
  ▷ Half-life: unknown

Dextroamphetamine

▶ Brand name
  ▷ Dexedrine
▶ Dosage
  ▷ PO 10 mg/day up to 60 mg/day
  ▷ Children above 6 years – PO 5 mg/day up to 60 mg/day
▶ Mechanism
  ▷ Blocks dopamine and norepinephrine reuptake
  ▷ Enhances presynaptic release of norepinephrine and dopamine
▶ Indication
  ▷ ADHD, narcolepsy, obesity
▶ Other safety caution and adverse effect
  ▷ Contraindication – MAOI use in 14 days
  ▷ Pregnancy risk category – C
  ▷ Weight change – weight loss or growth suppression, need to monitor height and weight
  ▷ Baseline cardiac evaluation
  ▷ Caution with cardiovascular diseases
  ▷ BP and HR elevation
  ▷ Dependence, abuse, withdrawal
  ▷ Psychosis
  ▷ Anorexia
  ▷ Aggression
  ▷ Worsening of tics, Tourette's syndrome
  ▷ Seizure risk – low
▶ Metabolism
  ▷ CYP450: minimal
  ▷ Half-life: 12 hours

Lisdexamfetamine

▶ Brand name
  ▷ Vyvanse
▶ Dosage
  ▷ Up to 70 mg/day
▶ Mechanism
  ▷ It is a prodrug to be hydrolysed to dextroamphetamine
  ▷ Blockade of dopamine and norepinephrine reuptake
  ▷ Enhances presynaptic release of norepinephrine and dopamine
▶ Indication
  ▷ ADHD
▶ Back box warning
  ▷ High addiction potential
▶ Other safety caution and adverse effect
  ▷ Contraindication – MAOI use in 14 days
  ▷ Pregnancy risk category – C
  ▷ Weight change – weight loss or growth suppression, need to monitor height and weight
  ▷ Baseline cardiac evaluation
  ▷ Caution with cardiovascular diseases
  ▷ BP and HR elevation
  ▷ Dependence, abuse, withdrawal
  ▷ Psychosis
  ▷ Anorexia
  ▷ Aggression
  ▷ Worsening of tics, Tourette's syndrome
  ▷ Seizure risk – low
▶ Metabolism
  ▷ CYP450: minor
  ▷ Half-life: 1 hour for lisdexamfetamine, 12 hours for dextroamphetamine

Methamphetamine

▶ Brand name
  ▷ Desoxyn
▶ Dosage
  ▷ PO 5 mg BID up to 20 mg/day
▶ Mechanism
  ▷ Increases cleft level of 5-HT, DA, and NE (relative ratio 60/2/1) probably through reversing the reuptake transporter and other mechanisms
▶ Indication
  ▷ ADHD for children age 6 years or older
  ▷ Obesity, short-term treatment from age 12 years
▶ Back box warning
  ▷ High potential for abuse
▶ Other safety caution and adverse effect
  ▷ Contraindication – MAOI in 14 days, glaucoma, advanced arteriosclerosis, symptomatic cardiovascular disease, moderate to severe hypertension, hyperthyroidism
  ▷ Pregnancy risk category – C

▷ Hypertension
▷ Headache
▷ Gastrointestinal tract (GI) symptoms
▷ Change of libido
▶ Metabolism
▷ CYP450: unknown
▷ Half-life: 4–5 hours
▶ Note – more addictive than the rest of the stimulants; methamphetamine is rarely used in psychiatry; under strict supervision, it may be useful for treatment resistant cases

Methylphenidate

▶ Brand name
▷ Concerta
▷ Metadate CD, Metadate ER
▷ Methylin, Methylin ER
▷ Ritalin, Ritalin LA, Ritalin SR
▷ Daytrana (transdermal)
▶ Dosage
▷ PO 5 mg/day or BID up to 40–70 mg/day
▷ Transdermal 10–30 mg/day
▶ Mechanism
▷ Blocks NE and DA reuptake
▷ Enhances presynaptic release of norepinephrine and dopamine
▶ Indication
▷ ADHD
▷ Narcolepsy
▶ Back box warning
▷ High addiction potential
▶ Other safety caution and adverse effect
▷ Contraindication – MAOI use in 14 days
▷ Pregnancy risk category – C
▷ Weight change – weight loss or growth suppression, need to monitor height and weight
▷ Baseline cardiac evaluation
▷ Caution with cardiovascular diseases
▷ BP and HR elevation
▷ Dependence, abuse, withdrawal
▷ Psychosis
▷ Anorexia
▷ Aggression
▷ Worsening of tics, Tourette's syndrome
▷ Seizure risk – low
▶ Metabolism
▷ CYP450: none
▷ Half-life: 3–4 hours

Phentermine

▶ Brand name
▷ Adipex-P

▶ Dosage
　▷ PO 18.75–37.5mg/day
▶ Mechanism
　▷ Sympathomimetic stimulant
　▷ Suppresses appetite
▶ Indicated for short-term treatment of obesity
▶ Safety caution and adverse effect
　▷ Contraindication – MAOI use in 14 days
　▷ Pregnancy risk category – C
　▷ Consider cardiovascular evaluation before starting treatment
　▷ Hypertension
　▷ Tachycardia
　▷ Cardiomyopathy
　▷ Insomnia
　▷ Addiction risk – schedule IV
▶ Metabolism
　▷ CYP450: unknown
　▷ Half-life: 19–24 hours

Sibutramine

▶ Brand name
　▷ Meridia
▶ Dosage
　▷ PO 5–15 mg/day
▶ Mechanism
　▷ Stimulant; inhibits norepinephrine, serotonin, and dopamine reuptake
▶ Indicated for obesity
▶ Safety caution and adverse effect
　▷ Contraindication – MAOI use in 14 days
　▷ Pregnancy risk category – C
　▷ Tachycardia
　▷ Hypertension
　▷ Insomnia
　▷ Seizures
▶ Metabolism
　▷ CYP450: substrate of 3A4; has active metabolite
　▷ Half-life: 1 hour; 14–16 hours for active metabolites

34 Drug Interactions

Drug interactions change the pharmacokinetics or pharmacodynamics of concurrently administered agents. Some drug interactions may be used to improve clinical efficacy. There have been reports on combination of enzyme-suppressing antifungal agents with expensive antibiotics that reached the cost-saving goals. However, in most cases, drug interactions complicate the treatment, reduce the effectiveness, and often result in unwanted side effects. Drug interactions may be categorized as

▶ Idiosyncratic interaction
▶ Pharmacodynamic interaction – alteration at the action mechanism level
▶ Pharmacokinetic interaction – alteration of absorption, distribution, metabolism, and elimination

Pharmacokinetic interaction is the most common and arguably the most important drug interaction. Of the growing understanding and clinical importance is the cytochrome P450 (CYP450) system. CYP450 is a large family of oxidases that is involved in drug metabolism, primarily deactivation and detoxification. Approximately 40–50 CYP450 enzymes have been identified in humans. Only six of these enzymes are responsible for the majority of drug oxidation. These are – CYP 1A2, CYP 3A4, CYP 2C9, CYP 2C19, CYP 2D6, and CYP 2E1. CYP 3A4 is the most commonly seen among the CYP450 interactions.

Antiretroviral agents

▶ Inhibition of CYP 3A4 by protease inhibitors "-navirs"
  ▷ Indinavir
  ▷ Nelfinavir
  ▷ Ritonavir
  ▷ Saquinavir
  ▷ Amprenavir
▶ Inhibition of CYP 2D6 by ritonavir
  ▷ Increases tricyclic antidepressants (TCAs) levels
  ▷ Prevents the metabolism of codeine to morphine, and reduces effect
▶ Induction of CYP 3A4 by efavirenz and nevirapine
  ▷ Methadone and most benzodiazepines are substrates of CYP 3A4; coadministration may cause methadone and/or benzodiazepines withdrawl

Carbamazepine

▶ Carbamazepine induces metabolic enzymes and causes decreased serum levels of
  ▷ Bupropion
  ▷ Clozapine

    ▷ Haloperidol
    ▷ Lamotrigine
    ▷ Oral contraceptive pills
    ▷ Valproate
    ▷ Warfarin
▶ Avoid coadministration with clozapine due to risk of agranulocytosis
▶ Contraindicated for coadministration with monoamine oxidase inhibitors (MAOIs)

Clozapine and carbamazepine: combination

▶ This combination should be avoided because
    ▷ May lower clozapine blood level; carbamazepine is a CYP 1A2 and 3A4 inducer, while clozapine is a 1A2, and 3A4 substrate
    ▷ May have additive bone marrow toxicity

Codeine

▶ Codeine is a substrate for CYP 2D6, which converts it to morphine
▶ Analgesic effect is diminished by CYP 2D6 inhibitors
    ▷ TCAs
    ▷ Serotonin selective reuptake inhibitors (SSRIs) – paroxetine, fluoxetine, sertraline
    ▷ Other antidepressants – bupropion, duloxetine
    ▷ Protease inhibitor – ritonavir
    ▷ Quinidine

CYP450 substrates: atypical antipsychotics

▶ CYP 1A2 – clozapine, olanzapine
▶ CYP 3A4 – quetiapine, ziprasidone, aripiprazole
▶ CYP 2D6 – risperidone, paliperidone

Hepatic metabolism: common inducers

▶ Anticonvulsants
    ▷ Carbamazepine
    ▷ Phenobarbital
    ▷ Phenytoin
▶ Rifampin
▶ St. John's wort

Hepatic metabolism: common inhibitors

▶ Antibiotics
    ▷ Erythromycin
    ▷ Ciprofloxacin
▶ Anticonvulsants
    ▷ Valproate
▶ Antidepressants
    ▷ Fluoxetine
    ▷ Paroxetine
    ▷ TCAs

- ▶ Antifungals
  - ▷ Ketoconazole
  - ▷ Miconazole
- ▶ β-blockers
  - ▷ Propranolol
  - ▷ Labetalol
- ▶ Calcium blockers
  - ▷ Diltiazem
  - ▷ Verapamil
- ▶ Grapefruit juice
- ▶ Histamine blockers – cimetidine

Lamotrigine

- ▶ Lamotrigine dose not have significant impact on CYP450 enzymes
- ▶ Level increased by – valproate (enzyme inducer)
- ▶ Level decreased by – carbamazepine and phenytoin (enzyme suppressors)

Lithium

- ▶ Drugs that increase lithium level
  - ▷ Angiotensin converting enzyme inhibitors – captopril, enalapril, lisinopril, etc.
  - ▷ Fluoxetine
  - ▷ Ibuprofen
  - ▷ Indomethacin
  - ▷ Spironolactone
  - ▷ Thiazide diuretics
- ▶ Drugs that decrease lithium level
  - ▷ Theophylline
  - ▷ Caffeine
  - ▷ Laxatives
- ▶ Idiosyncratic neurotoxicity when combination with
  - ▷ Verapamil and other calcium channel blockers
  - ▷ Antipsychotics
  - ▷ Carbamazepine

MAOIs and over the counter medications

- ▶ Safe over-the-counter (OTC) medications
  - ▷ Guaifenesin (Robitussin)
- ▶ Unsafe OTC medications
  - ▷ Oxymetazoline (Afrin)
  - ▷ Pseudoephedrine (Sudafed)
  - ▷ Phenylephrine (Sudafed PE, Neo-Synephrine)
  - ▷ Dextromethorphan (Delsym, Silphen DM, Robitussin DM)

MAOIs and serotonin elevating agents

- ▶ Serotonin syndrome may occur when combined with
  - ▷ SSRIs
  - ▷ Venlafaxine

▷ Clomipramine
▷ Linezolid (brand name Zyvox, an antibiotic with serotonin reuptake inhibiting effect)
▶ Wash-out interval
  ▷ Following discontinuation of another serotonin elevating agent – 2 weeks
  ▷ Following discontinuation of fluoxetine – 5 weeks

Phosphodiesterase type 5 inhibitors

▶ Agents
  ▷ Sildenafil (Viagra, Revatio)
  ▷ Tadalafil (Cialis)
  ▷ Vardenafil (Levitra)
▶ Potentiate the hypotensive effects of nitrates, therefore coadministration is absolutely contraindicated

Pimozide and sertraline (Figure 34–1)

▶ Pimozide may prolong QTc and cause Torsades de pointes
▶ Contraindicated for combination with sertraline due to increase QTc prolongation, probably associated with metabolism inhibition (CYP 3A4 interaction)
▶ Pimozide is also contraindicated for coadministration with ziprasidone due to the additive QTc prolongation

Protein-binding characters of psychotropic drugs

▶ Most psychotropic drugs are moderate to high protein-bound
▶ For most drugs, only the unbound state is available for pharmacological activity

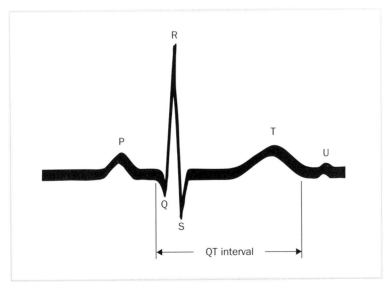

Figure 34–1 QT and QTc intervals. The QT interval is measured from the beginning of the QRS complex to the terminal of the T wave. It is markedly affected by heart rate. The QTc, or corrected QT interval, is calculated from formulas in correspondence to heart rate. The QTc interval with heart rates of 60–100/minute is usually between 310–440 milliseconds. When QTc interval approaches 500 milliseconds, the risk of cardiac arrhythmia and developing Torsade de pointes is significantly increased.

▶ Protein-binding drugs may displace other protein bound drugs, and potentially vital to the dosing and monitoring
▶ Warfarin deserves particular close monitoring, as it has low therapeutic index
▶ Psychiatric drugs with minimal protein binding
  ▷ Gabapentin
  ▷ Lithium
  ▷ Oxcarbazine
  ▷ Topiramate
  ▷ Venlafaxine

Valproic acid involved drug interactions

▶ Valproic acid is an inhibitor of hepatic metabolism, and a moderate protein binder
▶ Increases serum level of coadministered agents through metabolic inhibition
  ▷ Benzodiazepines
  ▷ Lamotrigine
  ▷ Carbamazepine
  ▷ Phenobarbital
  ▷ Warfarin
  ▷ Zidovudine
▶ Increases serum level of coadministered agents through displacement of protein-binding
  ▷ Phenytoin
  ▷ Tolbutamide
  ▷ Warfarin
  ▷ Carbamazepine
  ▷ Aspirin
▶ Level decreased by coadministered agents through induction of metabolism
  ▷ Carbamazepine
  ▷ Cimetidine
  ▷ Ibuprofen
▶ Level decreased by coadministered agents through displacement of protein-binding
  ▷ Aspirin
▶ Note – carbamazepine decreases valproic acid level through metabolic induction, while valproic acid increases carbamazepine level through both metabolic inhibition and protein-binding competition

Ziprasidone: additive QT prolongation with other antipsychotics

▶ Coadministration of ziprasidone and other antipsychotics with QT-prolongation effect may induce cardiac arrhythmia; frequently mentioned antipsychotics include
  ▷ Chlorpromazine (Thorazine)
  ▷ Droperidol (Inapsine)
  ▷ Pimozide (Orap); also contraindicated for combination with sertraline
  ▷ Thioridazine (Mellaril)

35 Evaluation and Treatment for Adverse Effects

As in any medical treatment, the clinical decision of psychopharmacotherapy relies on the weighing benefits and risks. Important clinical presentation, medical evaluation, and management of common adverse effects from psychiatric drugs are reviewed here. Included are also several nonpsychotropic medicines that are used primarily for the management of psychotropic side effects. Those include

▶ Amantadine (Symmetrel)
▶ Benztropine (Cogentin)
▶ Diphenhydramine (Benadryl)
▶ Dantrolene (Dantrium)
▶ Propranolol (Inderal)
▶ Trihexyphenidyl (Artane)

Amantadine

▶ Trade name
  ▷ Symmetrel
▶ Dosage
  ▷ PO 100 mg bid up to 400 mg/day
▶ Mechanisms
  ▷ Potentiates central nervous system (CNS) dopaminergic responses
  ▷ Blocks viral particle uncoating and nucleic acid release into host cell, inhibiting viral replication
▶ Indicated for
  ▷ Parkinsonism, essential or drug-induced
  ▷ Influenza A infection
▶ Safety caution and adverse effect
  ▷ Pregnancy risk category – C
  ▷ Congestive heart failure
  ▷ Arrhythmia
  ▷ Psychosis
  ▷ Nausea, vomiting
  ▷ Irritability
  ▷ Monitor serum creatinine
▶ Metabolism
  ▷ CYP450: unknown
  ▷ Half-life: 17 hours

Anticholinergic intoxication

▶ Symptoms
  ▷ Fever
  ▷ Tachycardia
  ▷ Dry mouth
  ▷ Urinary retention
  ▷ Dilated and unresponsive pupils
▶ Treatment – physostigmine

Anticholinergic symptoms in antipsychotics

▶ High probability
  ▷ Clozapine
▶ Moderate probability
  ▷ Olanzapine
▶ Low probability
  ▷ Risperidone, quetiapine, ziprasidone, aripiprazole, and paliperidone

Benztropine

▶ Trade name
  ▷ Cogentin
▶ Dosage
  ▷ PO/IM/IV 1–6 mg/day
▶ Mechanism
  ▷ Anticholinergic and antihistaminergic agent
▶ Indicated for
  ▷ Parkinsonism and acute dystonic reaction
▶ Safety caution and adverse effect
  ▷ Contraindication – angle-closure glaucoma, tardive dyskinesia, ileus, obstructive uropathy, benign prostate hypertrophy
  ▷ Pregnancy risk category – C
  ▷ Tachycardia
  ▷ Anticholinergic symptoms
▶ Metabolism
  ▷ CYP450: unknown
  ▷ Half-life: unknown

Dantrolene

▶ Brand name
  ▷ Dantrium
▶ Dosage
  ▷ PO 25 mg/day up to 400 mg/day
  ▷ Intravenous (IV) 2.5 mg/kg prn; follow the guidelines of the Malignant Hyperthermia Association of the United States (MHAUS)
▶ Mechanism
  ▷ Direct muscle relaxant

- ▶ Indication
  - ▷ Acute malignant hyperthermia
  - ▷ Chronic spasticity
- ▶ Back box warning
  - ▷ Hepatotoxicity
- ▶ Other safety caution and adverse effect
  - ▷ Contraindication
  - ▷ Pregnancy risk category – C
  - ▷ Incoordination, dizziness
  - ▷ Diarrhea
  - ▷ Fatigue
  - ▷ Nausea, vomiting, abdominal pain
- ▶ Metabolism
  - ▷ CYP450: unknown
  - ▷ Half-life: 4–8 hours

Diphenhydramine

- ▶ Trade name
  - ▷ Benadryl
- ▶ Dosage
  - ▷ PO/IM/IV up to 400 mg/day
- ▶ Indicated for
  - ▷ Extrapyramidal symptoms
  - ▷ Upper respiratory symptoms
  - ▷ Allergic reactions
  - ▷ Insomnia
  - ▷ Motion sickness prevention
- ▶ Mechanisms
  - ▷ Antagonizes central and peripheral H1 receptors (nonselective antihistamine)
  - ▷ Suppresses the medulla cough center (antitussive)
- ▶ Safety caution and adverse effect
  - ▷ Pregnancy risk category – B
  - ▷ Hypotension
  - ▷ Sedation
  - ▷ Blurred vision
  - ▷ Wheezing, thickening of bronchial secretions
- ▶ Metabolism
  - ▷ CYP450: inhibitor of 2D6
  - ▷ Half-life: 2–8 hours

Discontinuation syndromes

- ▶ Usually occurs with abrupt discontinuation of antidepressants
- ▶ Most common with paroxetine and venlafaxine, least likely with fluoxetine
- ▶ Self-limited, usually resolves within 2 weeks
- ▶ Symptoms
  - ▷ Malaise
  - ▷ Headache
  - ▷ Dizziness

▷ Nausea
▷ Paresthesias
▷ Mood symptoms

Glaucoma, uncontrolled narrow-angle: precaution for use of antidepressants

▶ The antidepressants, which have precaution for use in uncontrolled narrow-angle glaucoma are
  ▷ Duloxetine
  ▷ Venlafaxine
  ▷ Paroxetine
  ▷ All tricyclic antidepressants (TCAs)
▶ Antidepressants have no package insert warning for glaucoma
  ▷ serotonin-selective reuptake inhibitors (SSRIs) except paroxetine
  ▷ Monoamine oxidase inhibitors (MAOIs)
  ▷ Mirtazapine (Remeron)
  ▷ Bupropion (Wellbutrin)
  ▷ Nefazodone (Serzone)

Hypertensive crisis related to MAOIs

▶ MAOIs block tyramine metabolism in gastrointestinal (GI) tract
▶ Increased tyramine absorption
▶ High level of tyramine can result in hypertension, potentially hypertensive crisis
▶ Dietary restrictions on tyramine-rich food significantly reduce risk of hypertensive crisis
▶ Treatment
  ▷ Phentolamine (central α-blocker)
  ▷ Nifedipine

Leukopenia, neutropenia, and agranulocytosis related to atypical antipsychotics

▶ Clozapine
  ▷ Prevalence of agranulocytosis – 1.2%
  ▷ Not dose related
  ▷ Strict monitoring required – white blood cell (WBC) and absolute neutrophil count (ANC) weekly for 6 months, then biweekly for 6 months, then every 4 weeks; continue blood monitoring for 4 weeks after discontinuation of clozapine
▶ Other atypical antipsychotics
  ▷ Leukopenia, neutropenia, and fatal agranulocytosis have also been reported to be related to quetiapine
  ▷ Complete blood count (CBC) periodical monitoring is recommended for individuals with history of low white cell count

MAOIs: common side effects

▶ Most common – orthostatic hypotension
▶ Insomnia
▶ Sedation

▶ Weight gain
▶ Sexual dysfunction (anorgasmia or impotence)
▶ Headache
▶ Dry mouth

Neuroleptic malignant syndrome

▶ Epidemiology
  ▷ Prevalence ranged from 0.02% to 2%
  ▷ Untreated neuroleptic malignant syndrome (NMS) carries a mortality rate of 21%
  ▷ The majority of cases occur within 2 weeks of the initiation of dosing or after a rapid increase in the dose
▶ Risk factors include
  ▷ Female
  ▷ Older age
  ▷ Mood disorder
  ▷ Dementia
  ▷ Delirium
  ▷ Dehydration
  ▷ Rapid dose titration
▶ Symptoms and signs
  ▷ Fever
  ▷ Severe muscle "lead pipe" rigidity
  ▷ Increased creatine phosphokinase
  ▷ May cause acute renal failure
▶ Treatment
  ▷ Supportive treatment
  ▷ Discontinue offending medicine
  ▷ Electroconvulsive therapy (ECT) (controversial)
▶ Recurrence prevention
  ▷ Avoid the offending agent during resumption of psychiatric treatment

Orthostatic hypotension: probability among atypical antipsychotics

▶ High
  ▷ Clozapine
▶ Moderate
  ▷ Risperidone
  ▷ Quetiapine
  ▷ Paliperidone
▶ Low
  ▷ Olanzapine
  ▷ Ziprasidone
  ▷ Aripiprazole

Propranolol

▶ Brand name
  ▷ Inderal, Inderal LA, InnoPran XL

▶ Dosage
  ▷ PO 40 mg bid up to 640 mg/day
▶ Mechanism
  ▷ Nonselective β-1 and β-2 adrenergic antagonist
▶ Indication
  ▷ Hypertension
  ▷ Angina
  ▷ Myocardial infarction
  ▷ Cardiac arrhythmia
  ▷ Migraine headache
  ▷ Essential tremor
  ▷ Pheochromocytoma
  ▷ Idiopathic hypertrophic subaotic stenosis (IHSS)
▶ Off-label use
  ▷ Effective for akathisia and tremor induced by antipsychotics and lithium
  ▷ Have been used to treat posttraumatic stress disorder (PTSD), especially nightmares and exaggerated startle response
  ▷ Have been used for restless leg syndrome
▶ Back box warning
  ▷ Avoid abrupt discontinuation
▶ Other safety caution and adverse effect
  ▷ Contraindication – sinus bradycardia, atrioventricular (AV) block, sick sinus syndrome
  ▷ Pregnancy risk category – C
  ▷ Fatigue
  ▷ Dizziness
  ▷ Constipation
▶ Metabolism
  ▷ CYP450: primarily 2D6 substrate
  ▷ Half-life: 3–5 hours
▶ Note
  ▷ The antihypertensive effects can be blocked by TCAs

Rabbit syndrome

▶ A variant of extrapyramidal symptoms (EPS)
▶ Fine, rapid, vermiform movements of the lips

Sedation in atypical antipsychotics

▶ High probability
  ▷ Clozapine
  ▷ Quetiapine
▶ Moderate probability
  ▷ Olanzapine
  ▷ Aripiprazole
▶ Low probability
  ▷ Risperidone
  ▷ Ziprasidone
  ▷ Paliperidone

Seizure threshold influenced by antipsychotics

▶ Low potency first generation antipsychotics may lower seizure threshold
▶ This is a dose-related effect

Serotonin Syndrome

▶ Significant increase of extracellular serotonin level is proposed as mechanism
▶ Onset – with hours to days after start or increase in dose
▶ Neuromuscular symptoms – myoclonus, tremor, hyperreflexia, hypertonicity, rigidity, gait unsteadiness
▶ Autonomic instability – fever, hypo-/hypertension, tachycardia, diaphoresis
▶ Mental status changes – delirium, excitement, coma, and death
▶ Lab findings – leukocytosis, elevated creatine phosphokinase (CPK)
▶ Precautions
   ▷ MAOIs coadministered with meperidine (Demerol)
   ▷ Switches between MAOIs and any other antidepressants without proper washout
   ▷ Combination of two antidepressants
   ▷ Other serotonergic agents, e.g., Dihydroergotamine (DHE), buspirone (BuSpar), sumatriptan (Imitrex), etc.

Syndrome of inappropriate secretion of antidiuretic hormone (SIADH)

▶ May be associated with antipsychotics, carbamazepine, SSRIs, and other psychotropics
▶ More common in alcoholics and older patients
▶ Laboratory
   ▷ Serum Na^+ <122 mEq/L
   ▷ Increased K^+
   ▷ Decreased serum osmolality
   ▷ Increased urine osmolality
▶ Symptoms
   ▷ Polyuria, polydipsia
   ▷ Fatigue
   ▷ Muscle cramps
   ▷ Nausea, vomiting
   ▷ Headache
   ▷ Confusion
   ▷ Seizures
   ▷ Coma
▶ Treatment
   ▷ Stop offensive agent, if known
   ▷ Fluid restriction
   ▷ Demeclocycline (Declomycin)
   ▷ IV NaCl

Tardive dyskinesia: anatomy

▶ Anatomic localization
   ▷ Basal ganglia, particularly striatal nuclears, are hypothesized to be the pathological location
   ▷ Also involved is the thalamocortical pathway

▶ Receptors
  ▷ Dopamine D2 receptor is traditionally been implicated in the pathogenesis
  ▷ However, there are evidence implied the involvement of D4 and D5 receptors

Tardive dyskinesia: epidemiology

▶ Patients on long-term treatment with typical antipsychotics: 20%–30%
▶ There is a slightly lower risk of tardive dyskinesia with atypical antipsychotics
▶ Young patients: 3%–5%
▶ Elderly patients: generally much higher
▶ Other at risk populations
  ▷ Individuals who are more sensitive to acute extrapyramidal side effects
  ▷ Patients with comorbid cognitive or mood disorders

Tardive dyskinesia: hypothesized pathology

▶ Dopamine receptor supersensitivity
  ▷ Up-regulation (or disinhibition) of dopamine receptor responsiveness following chronic dopamine blockade
▶ Imbalance of D1 and D2 receptors
  ▷ Chronic D2 blockade may cause the imbalance in the thalamocortical pathway
▶ Neurodegeneration
  ▷ Secondary to lipid peroxidation or excitotoxic mechanisms
▶ Genetic traits may produce vulnerability
▶ Brain-derived neurotrophic factor (BDNF) may have a protective effect

Tardive dyskinesia: management

▶ Prevention
  ▷ Try atypical neuroleptics first
  ▷ Using the lowest effective dose of antipsychotic
  ▷ Prescribing cautiously with children, elderly patients, and patients with mood disorders
  ▷ Examining patients on a regular basis
  ▷ Avoid abrupt cessation of antipsychotic treatment
  ▷ Avoid ignoring tardive dyskinesia (TD)-like diseases – syphilis, thyroid diseases, seizure disorders, Wilson disease
▶ Management
  ▷ Reducing dosage
  ▷ Discontinuing the antipsychotic
  ▷ Switching to a different drug, such as clozapine
▶ Record keeping
  ▷ Written informed consent before start of antipsychotic treatment
  ▷ If typical antipsychotics have to be used, document the reason

Tardive dyskinesia: onset

▶ Usual onset
  ▷ While the patient is receiving an antipsychotic
  ▷ Within 4 weeks of discontinuing an oral antipsychotic
  ▷ Within 8 weeks after the withdrawal of a depot antipsychotic

Tardive dyskinesia: risk factors

▶ Typical antipsychotics
▶ Greater duration of treatment
▶ Female gender
▶ Advanced age
▶ Presence of mood or cognitive disorders

Trihexyphenidyl

▶ Brand name
  ▷ Artane
▶ Dosage
  ▷ PO 1–15 mg/day
▶ Mechanism
  ▷ Antagonist to acetylcholine receptors
▶ Indicated for
  ▷ Parkinson's diseases and extrapyramidal reactions
▶ Safety caution and adverse effect
  ▷ Contraindication – angle-closure glaucoma
  ▷ Pregnancy risk category – C
  ▷ Anticholinergic symptoms
▶ Metabolism
  ▷ CYP450: unknown
  ▷ Half-life: 5–10 hours

Weight gain and metabolic abnormalities associated with atypical antipsychotics

▶ High probability
  ▷ Clozapine
  ▷ Olanzapine
▶ Moderate probability
  ▷ Risperidone
  ▷ Quetiapine
  ▷ Paliperidone
▶ Low probability
  ▷ Ziprasidone
  ▷ Aripiprazole

36 Electroconvulsive Therapy, Brain Stimulation Therapies, and Other Novel Treatments

Treating mental illness with physical technologies provides effective alternatives to psychopharmacology. Physical technologies were used before and around the birth of psychopharmacology to bring impact on impaired brain function. Though considered by some to be antiquated, several of these treatments have gone through continuous technical refinement and remain active in mainstay psychiatry. New technologies have been developed in recent years and offered hope for more powerful and safer treatment.

Among the old treatments, the most prominent and publicized one is the electroconvulsive therapy (ECT). ECT is also probably the most controversial treatment in psychiatry. The negative perception of ECT may be traced to its historical stages of crude technology, and further, largely influenced by motion pictures that rarely depicted ECT in reasonable resemblance to modern practice. The use of anesthesia, muscle relaxant, and brief pulse are among the technical advancements that have made ECT a much safer procedure. Research has proved ECT the most effective treatment for major depression, a rapidly effective treatment for a spectrum of life-threatening psychiatric conditions, and under many circumstances a safer option of treatment.

Psychosurgery, though not a brain stimulation therapy, bore similar scrutiny as ECT did, and remains active because of its efficacy in a small group of severe cases.

New developments described here include vagus nerve stimulation and transcranial magnetic stimulation, both are Food and Drug Administration (FDA) approved treatments for depression, and deep brain stimulation, which is FDA approved for treatment-resistant, obsessive-compulsive disorder, and Parkinson's disease.

Cognitive impairment in ECT

▶ Postictal/postanesthetic confusion
  ▷ 30 minutes–hours
  ▷ Severe agitation may occur
  ▷ Treatment – benzodiazepines and/or antipsychotics combined with intensive nursing care
▶ Memory loss
  ▷ A major adverse effect of ECT
  ▷ Retrograde and anterograde
  ▷ Usually improve within 6 weeks, but may last for months
  ▷ Bilateral treatment is associated with greater verbal memory impairment
▶ Memory loss is not correlated with the treatment efficacy

Conditions considered appropriate for ECT

▶ Depression, unipolar or bipolar; treatment of choice for psychotic and catatonic depression
▶ Mania
▶ Psychotic agitation
▶ Treatment-resistant positive symptoms
▶ Parkinson's disease
▶ Organic affective disorders
▶ Intractable seizures
▶ Chronic pain

Contraindications for ECT

▶ No absolute contraindications
▶ Relative contraindications are related to risks from anesthesia and increases in intracranial pressure (intracranial space occupying lesions, increased cerebrospinal fluid [CSF])
▶ Cerebral vascular
   ▷ Recent cerebral vascular accidents
   ▷ Vascular aneurysms or malformations
▶ Cardiovascular
   ▷ Recent myocardial infarction (MI)
   ▷ Unstable angina
   ▷ Uncompensated congestive heart failure
▶ Hemorrhages
▶ Retinal detachment
▶ Pheochromocytoma

Deep brain stimulation (DBS): indications

▶ FDA approved indications
   ▷ Essential tremor
   ▷ Parkinson's disease
   ▷ Dystonia
   ▷ Obsessive-compulsive disorder
▶ Potential applications
   ▷ Chronic pain
   ▷ Depression

Deep brain stimulation: potential complications and adverse effects

▶ Altered executive function
   ▷ Word generation
   ▷ Attention
   ▷ Learning
▶ Infection
▶ Seizures and paralysis

ECT indications

▶ Lack of adequate response to less-intrusive treatment (medicines and psychotherapy)
▶ Rapid response is desired (severe and endangering symptoms, e.g., high suicide risk)
▶ Intolerable side effects or higher risk from less intrusive treatment (e.g., pregnancy and other physical conditions)
▶ History of good response to ECT
▶ Patient preference

Electrical factors in ECT

▶ The highest static impedance in the ECT circuit is in the bony skull
▶ The combination of impedance in the skin and the brain tissue is only 1%–2% of the skull
▶ Only less than 20% of the stimulus enters the brain
▶ Brief-pulse stimuli drive neuronal firing more efficiently than either constant-step pulse or sine wave stimuli
▶ The preferred duration of a brief pulse is 0.5–2 milliseconds

Electrode placement in ECT (Figure 36–1)

▶ Bilateral (Bitemporal)
  ▷ Using minimal suprathreshold electrical dose
  ▷ Indicated for poor prior response to unilateral treatment, or favorable prior response to bilateral ECT
  ▷ Severe symptoms require aggressive treatment
▶ Unilateral at nondominant side (also known as d'Elia placement)
  ▷ Preferred initial mode due to its reduced chance of memory impairment
  ▷ Electrical charges 2.5–5.0 times the seizure threshold

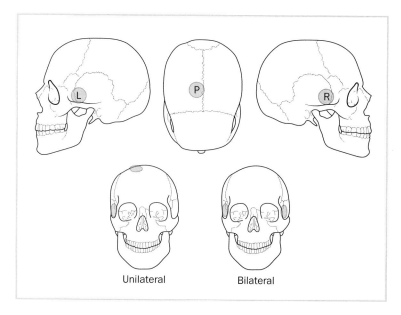

Figure 36–1 Electrode placement for ECT. Left temporal (L), right temporal (R), and nondominant parietal (P) placements are shown. ECT, electroconvulsive therapy.

Unilateral   Bilateral

Interaction of psychotropic medication with ECT

▶ Lack of strong evidence, but with clinical concern
▶ Lithium
  ▷ Increased cerebral toxicity and prolonged confusion
  ▷ Prolonged duration of succinylcholine through interference with pseudo-cholinesterase
▶ Clozapine, bupropion, maprotiline, and low-potency antipsychotics
  ▷ Potentially lower seizure threshold and prolong seizure
▶ Benzodiazepines
  ▷ Elevated seizure threshold
▶ MAOIs
  ▷ Difficulty with blood pressure management

Mechanism of ECT

▶ Not completely understood
▶ Full brain seizure is required as a curative agent
▶ Proposed potential mechanisms
  ▷ Alteration in the concentration of serotonin and norepinephrine, and upregulation of their receptors
  ▷ Enhanced gamma-aminobutyric acid (GABA)ergic transmission, which causes the rise in seizure threshold
  ▷ Hippocampal neurogenesis
  ▷ Increased release of brain derived neurotrophic factor (BDNF)
  ▷ Upregulated opioid receptors
▶ Scientifically dismissed historical hypotheses
  ▷ Fear
  ▷ Ego regression
  ▷ Memory loss

Mortality of ECT

▶ Similar to general anesthesia – 1/25,000
▶ Common causes of death
  ▷ Cardiovascular complication (most common)
  ▷ Brain herniation
  ▷ Respiratory complications
  ▷ Ruptured aneurysms (rare)

Potential adverse effects of succinylcholine during ECT

▶ Headache
  ▷ Associated with muscle soreness caused by fasciculation
▶ Cardiac arrhythmia
  ▷ Depolarization of the neuromuscular junction is associated with elevated extracellular potassium, which may suppress cardiac conductivity
▶ Prolonged apnea
  ▷ Particularly in patients with pseudocholinesterase deficiency

Pregnancy and ECT

▶ ECT is often preferred due to the limit of medication use during pregnancy
▶ Risk of aspiration due to mass effect in third trimester

Pseudocholinesterase deficiency

▶ Pseudocholinesterase is an enzyme hydrolyzes exogenous choline esters, such as succinylcholine; it has no known physiological function
▶ Pseudocholinesterase deficiency is a rare genetic deficiency, most common in people of European descent
▶ Clinical significance
  ▷ Prolongs the recovery of muscle strength hence the ability of autonomic respiration
▶ Tests
  ▷ Quick screening test – acholest paper test
  ▷ Confirmation – serum pseudocholinesterase activity
  ▷ Genotype – allele specific polymerase chain reaction (PCR), available only in advanced research laboratories
▶ Management
  ▷ Supportive measures including mechanical ventilation

Psychosurgery: efficacy and adverse effect

▶ Efficacy
  ▷ Between 50% and 70% have significant improvement
  ▷ Fewer than 3% become worse
  ▷ Continued improvement from 1 to 2 years after surgery
  ▷ Improved response to pharmacological and behavioral treatment
  ▷ Improved cognitive ability
▶ Adverse effects
  ▷ Postoperative seizures <1%
  ▷ No undesired changes in personality have been noted with modern techniques

Psychosurgery: indications

▶ Major depressive disorder and obsessive-compulsive disorder (OCD)
▶ Chronic and debilitating symptoms
▶ Failure of a wide variety of noninvasive treatments
▶ At least 5 years of history
▶ Treatment for intractable aggression is controversial

Psychosurgery: history and new trend

Egas Moniz (1874–1955) was a Portuguese psychiatrist and neurosurgeon, Nobel Prize laureate in 1949 for his work in developing psychosurgical techniques.

▶ Pioneers
  ▷ Jacobsen and Fulton – demonstrated in 1935 that frontal lobe ablation in a monkey had a calming effect
  ▷ Antonio Moniz – reported a decrease in tension and psychotic symptoms by severing frontal lobe white matter in 20 cases

  ▷ Walter Freeman and James Watts – introduced prefrontal lobotomy in 1936
  ▷ Freeman later developed the technique of transorbital leukotomy
► The decline
  ▷ The introduction of antipsychotics
  ▷ Public concern about the ethics of psychosurgery
► The renewed interest in recent years is based on
  ▷ Modern techniques to make stereotactically defined lesions
  ▷ Improved preoperative diagnoses including comprehensive psychological assessments
► Modern technique of making the precise lesions
  ▷ Radioactive implants
  ▷ Cryoprobes
  ▷ Electrical coagulation
  ▷ Proton beams
  ▷ Ultrasonic waves

Psychosurgery: techniques

► Common procedures
  ▷ Subcaudate tractotomy
  ▷ Anterior cingulotomy
  ▷ Limbic leucotomy
  ▷ Anterior capsulotomy

Quality of seizure in ECT (See Figure 36–2 on page 282)

► The quality of seizure refers to the clinical efficacy in treating target symptoms
► Though lack of data, consensus of expert opinion agreed that a seizure of good quality is
  ▷ Symmetrical
  ▷ Synchronous
  ▷ High-amplitude
  ▷ With high interhemispheric coherence
  ▷ With marked postictal suppression
  ▷ Accompanied by a prominent tachycardia response
► The minimum required duration of seizure is controversial
  ▷ No objective criteria are established
  ▷ Many agreed on the range 25–30 seconds
  ▷ APA Task Force Report on ECT (2001) defined a seizure lower than 15 seconds as "abortive"

Risks and adverse effects of ECT

► Mortality is equivalent to brief anesthesia, approximately 1/25,000
► Neurological
  ▷ Headache – the most common
  ▷ Status epilepticus
  ▷ Brain herniation
► Cardiovascular
  ▷ MI
  ▷ Arrhythmia

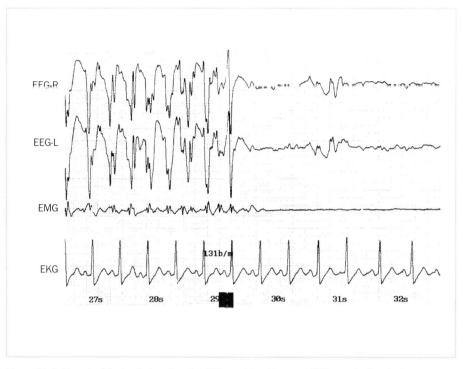

Figure 36-2 Example of the terminal portion of an EEG record from Thymatron IV. The termination of seizure occurs at around 30 seconds. The recorded seizure shows the consensus signs of a good-quality seizure – symmetrical, synchronous, high-amplitude, with high interhemispheric coherence, with marked postictal suppression, and accompanied by a prominent tachycardia response.
EEG, electroencephalogram; ECG, electrocardiogram; EMG, electromyogram.

▶ Respiratory
  ▷ Prolonged apnea
▶ Musculoskeletal
  ▷ Musculoskeletal pain
  ▷ Fractures (rare with modern techniques)
▶ Mental/cognitive
  ▷ Postictal confusion and delirium
  ▷ Memory impairment
  ▷ Treatment emergent mania – approximately 7%

Seizure threshold in ECT

▶ Seizure threshold is the minimum charge required to generate a grand mal seizure
▶ Seizure threshold is
  ▷ Higher in men than in women
  ▷ Higher in older individuals
  ▷ Higher with bilateral electrode placement
▶ Threshold-raising agents
  ▷ Anticonvulsants
  ▷ Benzodiazepines
  ▷ Barbiturates
  ▷ Antiarrhythmic drugs

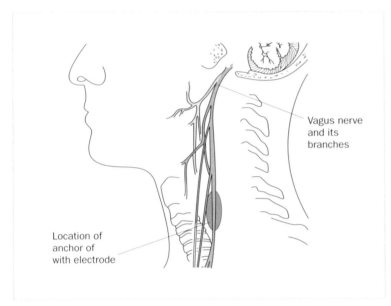

Figure 36–3 Vagus nerve stimulation.

Labels in figure: Vagus nerve and its branches; Location of anchor of with electrode

- ▶ Threshold-lowering agents
  - ▷ Theophylline
  - ▷ Lithium
  - ▷ Clozapine
  - ▷ Bupropion
  - ▷ Maprotiline
  - ▷ Low-potency antipsychotics
- ▶ Shorter pulse duration and lower frequency produce lower threshold

Structural brain damage and ECT

- ▶ No evidence indicates ECT produces structural damage to the brain
- ▶ Prolonged seizure, such as status epilepticus, may cause hypoxic brain damage; however, ECT seizures are brief and under aggressive oxygenation

Transcranial magnetic stimulation and repetitive transcranial magnetic stimulation

- ▶ A noninvasive method to excite neurons by weak electric currents induced in the tissue by rapidly changing magnetic fields
- ▶ Risks and advers effects of transcranial magnetic stimulation (TMS) and repetitive transcranial magnetic stimulation (rTMS)
  - ▷ Seizure; the risk is significantly higher in rTMS
  - ▷ Discomfort or pain from the stimulation of the scalp
- ▶ Potential treatment for
  - ▷ Neurological conditions – movement disorders, seizures, chronic headache
  - ▷ Depression, as an alternative for ECT

Vagus nerve stimulation (VNS): indications

▶ Adjunctive treatment for partial-onset epilepsy
▶ Treatment-resistant (refractory) depression

Vagus nerve stimulation: mechanisms (See Figure 36–3 on page 283)

▶ Not completely understood
▶ Affect blood flow to different parts of the brain, including limbic system
▶ Affect neurotransmitters including serotonin and norepinephrine which are implicated in depression

Vagus nerve stimulation: side effects

▶ Generally mild and temporal; mostly associated with disturbance of vagus nerve
  ▷ Alteration of voice quality, hoarseness
  ▷ Throat pain
  ▷ Cough
  ▷ Dyspnea
  ▷ Paresthesia in neck area

37 Congenital Neuropsychiatric Disorders

Congenital disorders refer to pathological processes initiated before the time of birth. Genetic abnormalities and less than protective intrauterine environment are often attributed to. Etiologies of many congenital disorders are still not fully understood. Psychiatric treatment is targeted on management of behavior disturbance and secondary, often stress-related, mood disturbance, as well as functional preservation. Patients with congenital disorders are certainly not immune from other mental disorders. Selected congenital disorders with neuropsychiatric symptoms are reviewed in this chapter, including

▶ Disorders associated with chromosomal abnormality (See Figure 37–1 on page 286)
  ▷ Angelman's syndrome
  ▷ Cri-du-Chat
  ▷ Fragile X syndrome
  ▷ Huntington's disease
  ▷ Klinefelter's syndrome
  ▷ Machado-Joseph disease (Spinocerebellar ataxia type 3)
  ▷ Myotonic dystrophy (type 1 and 2)
  ▷ Phenylketonuria
  ▷ Prader-Willi syndrome
  ▷ Seckel syndrome
  ▷ Spinobulbar muscular atrophy (Kennedy disease)
  ▷ Spinocerebellar ataxia type 1
  ▷ Turner's syndrome
  ▷ William's Syndrome
▶ Disorders with no known chromosomal abnormality
  ▷ Arnold-Chiari malformation
  ▷ Cerebral palsy
  ▷ Dandy-Walker syndrome
  ▷ Sturge-Weber syndrome

Angelman's syndrome

Harry Angelman (1915–1996) was an English pediatrician.

▶ Characteristics
  ▷ Intellectual and developmental delay
  ▷ Speech impediment
  ▷ Sleep disturbance
  ▷ Unstable jerky gait
  ▷ Seizures

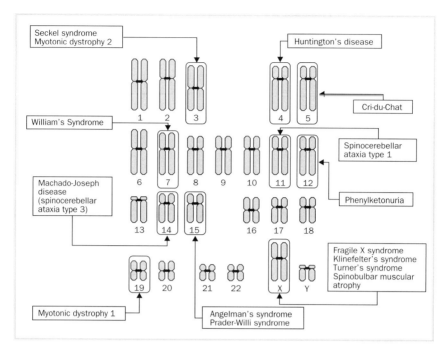

Figure 37-1 Chromosomal abnormality of congenital neuropsychiatric disorders. Diseases associated with trinucleotide expansion are shaded.

> ▷ Hand flapping movements
> ▷ Frequent laughter/smiling and usually a happy demeanor
▶ Deletion or inactivation of critical genes on the maternally inherited chromosome 15
▶ The sister syndrome is called Prader-Willi syndrome, and is caused by loss of paternal genes

Arnold-Chiari malformation (Figure 37–2)

Julius Arnold, (1835–1915) and Hans Chiari (1851–1916) were German pathologists.

▶ A congenital anomaly of brain
▶ The cerebellar tonsils are elongated and pushed down through foramen magnum
▶ The brainstem, cranial nerves, and the lower portion of the cerebellum may be stretched or compressed
▶ The blockage of cerebrospinal fluid (CSF) flow may also cause a syrinx to form
▶ Symptoms
> ▷ May be asymptomatic
> ▷ Swallowing and breathing difficulties
> ▷ Headaches and neck pain
> ▷ Dizziness and vertigo
> ▷ Neuropathic pain
> ▷ Fatigue and muscle weakness
> ▷ Impaired fine motor skills
▶ Treatment – decompression surgery

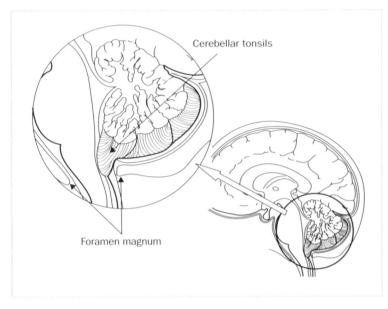

Figure 37–2 Arnold-Chiari malformation. The cerebellar tonsils are elongated and pushed down through foramen magnum and compress structures around.

Cerebral palsy: spastic

▶ Neurologic motor system impairments due to brain injuries in early stage of life
▶ The injuries occur in uterus, around delivery, or in early childhood
▶ Irreversible and nonprogressive
▶ Subtypes
  ▷ Spastic – diplegia, hemiplegia, or quadriplegia
  ▷ Extrapyramidal – athetosis, chorea, ataxia
  ▷ Mixed – high incidence of mental retardation and epilepsy
▶ Possible associated conditions
  ▷ Mental retardation
  ▷ Epilepsy
  ▷ Impairment of visual and auditory sensations

Cri-du-Chat

▶ Also known as 5p minus
▶ Abnormality on short arm of chromosome 5 (5p)
▶ Moderate to severe mental retardation
▶ Cat-like cry

Dandy-Walker syndrome

Walter Dandy (1886–1946) and Arthur Walker (1907–1995) were American neuro-surgeons.

▶ Failure in development of the posterior portion of the upper neural tube
▶ Abnormalities
  ▷ Enlarged fourth ventricle
  ▷ Absence of cerebellar vermis
  ▷ Cyst formation near the internal base of the skull

▶ Symptoms
  ▷ Increased intracranial pressure – vomiting, convulsion, irritability
  ▷ Cerebellar dysfunction – ataxia, poor motor coordination
  ▷ Hydrocephalus
  ▷ Mental retardation

Fragile X syndrome

▶ X-linked mental retardation
▶ Triplet expansion of FMR1 gene in the Long arm of x chromosome
▶ Prevalence – 1/4,000–6,000, slightly higher incidence in boys
▶ 80% comorbid with attention deficit/hyperactivity disorder (ADHD)
▶ Clinical features
  ▷ Facial features – prognathism (jaw projects markedly); large ears; long face; high-arched palate; malocclusion (faulty contact between the upper and lower teeth when the jaw is closed)
  ▷ Secondary sexual signs –macroorchidism (large testicles); gynecomastia
  ▷ Mental features – mental retardation; ADHD (the most common comorbid); autism
  ▷ Other physical features – hypotonia; flat feet; lordosis (abnormally forwarded curvature of the lumbar spine)

Klinefelter's syndrome

Harry Klinefelter (born 1912) was an American endocrinologist.

▶ Chromosome – 47, XXY
▶ Patients usually have a normal intelligence quotient (IQ)
▶ Weakened male habits
▶ Behavior and mood symptoms
  ▷ Impulsivity
  ▷ Anxiety
  ▷ Aggression
  ▷ Difficulty in socialization

Mental retardation associated with autosomal-recessive inheritance pattern

▶ Adrenogenital syndrome
▶ Hurler's syndrome
▶ Tay-sachs disease
▶ Phenylketonuria

Phenylketonuria

▶ An autosomal-recessive inherited disease located on chromosome 12
▶ Deficiency in hepatic phenylalanine hydroxylase, which catalyzes the conversion from phenylalanine to tyrosine
▶ Accumulated phenylalanine saturates the large neutral amino acid (LNAA) transporters and decreases LNAA levels in the brain; the latter disrupts brain development, and causes mental retardation
▶ Treatment
  ▷ Low phenylalanine diet to be started early and continued for the rest of life

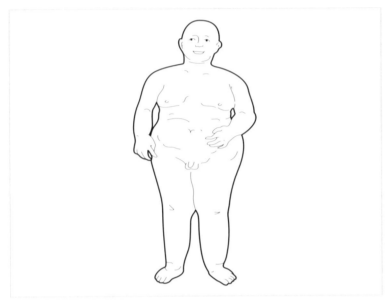

Figure 37–3 Prader-Willi syndrome.

Prader-Willi syndrome (Figure 37–3)

Andrea Prader (1919–2001) and Heinrich Willi (1900–1971) were Swiss pediatricians.

▶ Deletions in chromosome 15
▶ Clinical features
  ▷ Mental retardation
  ▷ Obesity
  ▷ Short stature
  ▷ Small hands and feet
  ▷ Hypotonia
  ▷ Hypogonadotropic hypogonadism
  ▷ Strabismus (one eye cannot focus with the other on an object because of imbalance of the eye muscles)
▶ Prevalence – approximately 1/20,000

Seckel syndrome

Helmut Seckel (1900–1960) was a Germany-born U.S. pediatrician.

▶ Also known as "bird-headed dwarfism"
▶ Inherited in autosomal-recessive manner
▶ Probable genes on chromosomes 3 and 18
▶ Clinical features
  ▷ Low birth weight
  ▷ Short stature
  ▷ Microcephaly
  ▷ Receding forehead, large eyes, low ears, prominent beaklike protrusion of the nose, and smallish chin
  ▷ Defects of bones in the arms and legs, dislocations of the elbow and hip, and inability to straighten the knees

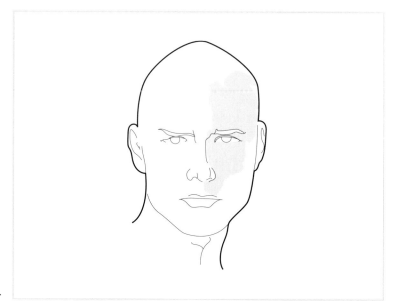

Figure 37–4 Sturge-Weber syndrome – facial cutaneous angioma in trigeminal distribution.

▷ Cryptorchidism (failure of the testes to descend into the scrotum).
▷ Mental retardation
▷ Behavior – usually friendly and pleasant, often hyperactive

Sturge-Weber syndrome (Figure 37–4)

William Sturge (1850–1919) and Frederick Weber (1863–1962) were English physicians.

▶ Cutaneous angioma – port wine stain in trigeminal distribution
▶ Physical features are limited to central nervous system
  ▷ Seizure
  ▷ Glaucoma, and buphthalmos (the eyeball enlarges and bulges out of its socket) because of higher intraocular pressure
  ▷ Possible developmental delay and mental retardation
▶ Characteristic pattern of clacifications on skull X-ray – railroad track calcifications

Triplet (trinucleotide) repeat expansion

▶ DNA sequences that contain repeated trinucleotide, e.g., CAGCAGCAG…, may expand from the original repeating number, usually 8–15, up to hundreds
▶ This expansion may cause change in cellular structure and function, and is important mechanism of a number of neurological conditions, that include
  ▷ Huntington's disease
  ▷ Fragile X syndrome
  ▷ Myotonic dystrophy
  ▷ Spinobulbar muscular atrophy
  ▷ Spinocerebellar ataxia type 1
  ▷ Machado-Joseph disease

Turner's syndrome

Henry Turner (1892–1970) was a U.S. endocrinologist.

▶ Monosomy X, or labeled as 45 X
▶ Physical features
  ▷ Short stature
  ▷ Obesity
  ▷ Low hairline
  ▷ Low-set ears
  ▷ Simian crease – single transverse crease same as seen in Down's syndrome and fetal alcohol syndrome
  ▷ Drooping eyelids
  ▷ Webbed neck
  ▷ Broad chest (shield chest) and widely-spaced nipples
▶ Physiological impairment
  ▷ Lymphoedema (swelling) of the hands and feet
  ▷ Reproductive sterility
  ▷ Amenorrhea

William's Syndrome

J. William is a New Zealand cardiologist.

▶ Chromosome 7 deletion
▶ Mental features
  ▷ Mild to moderate mental retardation
  ▷ Learning difficulties
  ▷ Unique personality that combines overfriendliness and high levels of empathy with anxiety
▶ Physical features
  ▷ Distinctive facial appearance
  ▷ Broad range of vascular stenosis, including supravalvular aortic stenos and pulmonary artery stenosis

38 Infections of the Nervous System

A wide variety of infectious agents, including viruses, bacteria, fungi, and other organisms may cause central nervous system (CNS) infection. Diffusely distributed infections are the most common, such as meningitis and encephalitis. Localized infections, such as abscess, are less common. Human immunodeficiency virus (HIV) has drawn particular attention in recent years due to not only the infection, but also the suppression of immunological system that makes the individual vulnerable to secondary infections. CNS infections are medical emergencies. Prompt diagnosis and treatment, at times trial treatment based on preliminary diagnosis, are often life-saving.

Selected infections frequently encountered in psychiatric practice are reviewed here.

Acquired immunodeficiency syndrome: CNS lymphoma

▶ The most common neoplasm in acquired immunodeficiency syndrome (AIDS)
▶ Highly malignant B-cell tumors
▶ Associated with Epstein-Barr virus infection
▶ Slowly progressing multifocal deficits
▶ Multiple enhancing lesions with diffuse or ring pattern, similar to toxoplasmosis
▶ Single photon emission computed tomography (SPECT)
  ▷ Lymphoma is hot
  ▷ Toxoplasmosis is cold

AIDS: cryptococcus infection

▶ The most common CNS fungal infection in AIDS
▶ Symptoms
  ▷ Headache
  ▷ Fever
  ▷ Meningeal signs
  ▷ Mental status changes
▶ No focal abnormalities
▶ Diagnosis
  ▷ Cerebrospinal fluid (CSF) cultures
  ▷ Cryptococcal antigens
▶ Treatment – amphotericin
▶ Mortality – 10%–20%

AIDS: cytomegalovirus infections

▶ Cyomegalovirus (CMV) encephalitis

▶ CMV retinitis – the most common cause of blindness in HIV
▶ CMV lumbo-sacral radiculoplexopathy

AIDS: presentation of CNS complications

▶ Toxoplasmosis
  ▷ Fever
  ▷ Headache
  ▷ Prominent focal signs
▶ Lymphoma or progressive multifocal leukoencephalopathy (PML)
  ▷ No fever
  ▷ No headache
  ▷ Mild to moderate focal signs

Cerebrospinal fluid: appearance and related pathology

▶ Clear
  ▷ Normal
  ▷ Neurosyphilis
  ▷ Guillain-Barré syndrome
▶ Turbid
  ▷ Meningitis – bacterial, viral, tuberculosis (TB), or fungal
▶ Bloody
  ▷ Subarachnoid hemorrhage

Cerebrospinal fluid: whit blood cell (WBC) counts

▶ 0–4 – normal
▶ 5–50 – neurosyphilis, Guillain-Barré syndrome, both have wide variety, may be up to a few hundred
▶ 50+ – meningitis or hemorrhage
  ▷ Bacterial – up to 500 or more, mostly polymorphonuclear cells
  ▷ Viral – usually lower than bacterial, up to around 100
  ▷ TB or fungal – up to 500 or more, mostly lymphocytes
  ▷ Subarachnoid hemorrhage – approximately 1/1,000 of red cells, same as in blood

Herpes zoster

▶ Also known as shingles
▶ Pain and rash for days or weeks
▶ Antiviral treatment or prednisone – no clear evidence of benefits
▶ Pain management
  ▷ Analgesics
  ▷ Antiepileptics – gabapentin, carbamazepine

HIV associated dementia

▶ Also known as
  ▷ AIDS dementia complex
  ▷ HIV encephalopathy

▶ Progressive cognitive and behavioral decline
▶ Diffuse neurologic signs, extrapyramidal symptoms (EPS)
▶ Magnetic resonance imaging (MRI) or computer tomography (CT) shows
  ▷ Cerebral atrophy
  ▷ Deep white matter hyperintensities
▶ Subcortical disorder
▶ No evidence of primary neuronal infection
▶ Treatment – highly active antiretroviral therapy (HAART).

HIV meningitis

▶ Prevalence – 5% of HIV patients.
▶ May present at seroconversion, or later during illness
▶ Not considered AIDS, which refers to secondary infection
▶ The meningitis is benign and brief

HIV: serum test

▶ To detect the presence of anti-HIV antibodies in human serum
▶ Conventional test
  ▷ Uses blood
  ▷ Time to result 3–10 days
▶ Rapid test
  ▷ Uses an oral swab
  ▷ Time for result – 20 minutes
▶ Both tests are 99.9% sensitive and specific
▶ Seroconversion
  ▷ Most commonly occurs 6–12 weeks after infection
  ▷ In rare cases, 6–12 months

Lyme disease

▶ Ticks → human
▶ Subjects often unaware of the bite
▶ Early serologic diagnosis
▶ Cranial neuropathies common, particularly cranial nerve (CN) VII
▶ Treatment – doxycycline

Meningitis: causes

▶ Inflammation of meninges
▶ Infectious causes
  ▷ Viruses (most common)
  ▷ Bacteria (second most common)
  ▷ Fungi
  ▷ Parasites
▶ Noninfectious causes
  ▷ Physical injury
  ▷ Cancer

▷ Drugs
▷ Systemic lupus erythematosus
▶ Most common bacteria
  ▷ *Neisseria meningitidis* (Meningococcus)
  ▷ *Streptococcus pneumoniae* (Pneumococcus)

Meningitis: subacute or chronic

▶ Meningitis that lasts a month or longer
▶ Usually affects people with compromised immune system
▶ Risk factors
  ▷ AIDS
  ▷ Cancer
  ▷ Chemotherapy
  ▷ Long-term use of corticosteroid
  ▷ Partially treated acute meningitis
▶ Causes
  ▷ All pathogens of acute meningitis
  ▷ Cryptococcus fungus
  ▷ TB
  ▷ Syphilis
  ▷ Lyme disease
  ▷ Sarcoidosis
  ▷ Cancers
  ▷ Nonsteroidal antiinflammatory drug (NSAIDs)

Neurosyphilis: clinical features

▶ Rare in the post-penicillin era
▶ May rise among individuals with AIDS
▶ Classic neurological signs include
  ▷ Tremor
  ▷ Dysarthria
  ▷ Hyperreflexia
  ▷ Hypotonia
  ▷ Ataxia

Neurosyphilis: serum tests

▶ Venereal disease research laboratory (VDRL) – diagnostic if positive in CSF; however 25% negative
▶ Fluorescent treponemal antibody absorption (FTA-ABS) or microhemagglutination assay (MHA) – always positive in the blood

Progressive multifocal leukoencephalopathy

▶ John Cunningham (JC) virus (a papovarirus)
▶ Prevalence is 5% in AIDS
▶ Demyelinating disorder of the CNS
▶ Multifocal neurologic abnormalities

▶ White matter lesions without mass effect
▶ Diagnosis
▷ Plymerase chain reaction (PCR) in CSF positive for JC virus
▶ Treatment
▷ HAART, a combination of 3–4 antiviral agents

Syphilis: stages of infection

▶ Primary
▷ Vaginal, penile, or rectal lesions
▷ Positive blood VDRL in majority of patients
▶ Secondary
▷ Skin lesions, meningeal, and vascular signs
▷ Positive blood VDRL; however, may be negative with impaired immunity
▶ Tertiary
▷ CNS involvement – neurosyphilis
▷ Historical term – general paresis of the insane (GPI)
▷ Tabes dorsalis
▷ Argyll Robertson pupils
▷ Charcot joints
▷ Optic atrophy
▷ Nerve deafness

Toxoplasmosis in AIDS

▶ The most common infectious mass lesion in AIDS
▶ Headaches, seizures, focal deficits, and toxicity
▶ MRI or CT shows multiple ring-enhancing lesions
▶ Treatment
▷ Pyrimethamine
▷ Sulfadiazine
▷ Clindamycin

West Nile virus

▶ Mosquitoes → birds → human
▶ Encephalitis, myelitis, Guillain Barré syndromes
▶ Mental status changes
▶ No consensus treatment, but may use interferons and intravenous immunoglobulin (IVIG)

39 Seizure Disorders

Seizures are clinical phenomena of hypersynchronous electrical activities in the brain. Epilepsy refers to recurrent seizures. Common features of epileptic seizures include loss or alternation of consciousness, abnormal motor activity including sudden fall, abnormal sensory perceptions, and loss of bladder and bowel control. Psychiatric symptoms frequently appear before or after the seizure activity.

Seizure disorders are manifestations of underlying brain pathologies. Perinatal damages, inherited or familial conditions, head trauma, anoxic brain damage, infections, metabolic abnormalities, toxins, degenerative diseases of the central nervous system, tumors, and cerebral-vascular disorders are classical causes of seizure disorders. For each individual patient, more than one cause may appear.

There exist a number of classifications for seizure disorders. Owing to the complex of pathophysiology and anatomy, classifications based on clinical observation and electroencephalograph (EEG) are commonly accepted. The following is a general outline of classification for epileptic seizures

▶ Partial seizures (also known as focal seizures)
  ▷ Simple partial seizures – consciousness is not impaired
  ▷ Complex partial seizures – consciousness is impaired (also known as temporal lobe or psychomotor seizures)
  ▷ Partial seizures evolving to secondarily generalized seizures
▶ Generalized seizures
  ▷ Absence seizures (also known as petit mal)
  ▷ Myoclonic seizures
  ▷ Clonic seizures
  ▷ Tonic seizures
  ▷ Tonic-clonic seizures (also known as grand mal)
  ▷ Atonic seizures
▶ Unclassified epileptic seizures

Anticonvulsants, also know as antiepileptic drugs, are the mainstay of treatment. Surgery is reserved for refractory cases. Vagus nerve stimulation and other novel treatments are new alternatives with potential of wider acceptance. Patients with seizure disorders are prone to injuries, limited in normal daily activities, and often tend to adopt less than healthy life styles that may induce other problems in general health. Multidisciplinary support and counseling, including general medical care, mental health counseling, and social support, plays important role in the maintenance of the quality of life.

Absence seizure

▶ Also known as petit mal
▶ Begin at ages of 2–10 years and disappears in early adulthood
▶ May be precipitated by hyperventilation and phonic stimulation
▶ No aura
▶ Abrupt loss and resolution of consciousness
▶ Blinking, facial and finger automatisms
▶ Lasts for 1–10 seconds
▶ EEG – generalized 3 Hz spike-and-wave complexes
▶ Patient is unaware of episode; usually no postictal abnormal behavior
▶ Treatment
   ▷ Ethosuximide (first choice)
   ▷ Valproate

Antiepileptic drugs causing teratogenic defect

▶ Carbamazepine – neural tube defects
▶ Phenytoin
▶ Valproate
▶ High dose folate may reduce the risk

Antiepileptic drugs that do NOT block Na⁺ channel

▶ Ethosuximide – blocks T-type Ca^{++} channels
▶ Phenobarbital – enhances gamma-aminobutyric acid (GABA) activity
▶ Valproate – enhances GABA activity
▶ Levetiracetam – mechanism unknown

Antiepileptic drugs that induce hepatic metabolism of oral contraceptives

▶ Barbiturates
▶ Carbamazepine
▶ Lamotrigine
▶ Oxcarbazepine
▶ Phenytoin
▶ Topiramate

Antiepileptic drugs that may cause renal stones

▶ Topiramate
▶ Zonisamide
▶ Proper hydration may prevent renal stones

Antipsychotics that increase risk of seizures

▶ Clozapine (Clozaril)
▶ Chlorpromazine (Thorazine)
▶ Loxapine

Carbamazepine

▶ First line for partial seizures
▶ Na⁺ channel blocker
▶ Liver enzyme inducer
▶ Common side effects
  ▷ Drowsiness
  ▷ Diplopia
  ▷ Nystagmus
  ▷ Dizziness
  ▷ Rash
  ▷ Weight gain
▶ Uncommon side effects
  ▷ Bone marrow suppression
  ▷ Hyponatremia
  ▷ Stevens-Johnson syndrome
▶ Teratogenic – neural tube defects

Direction of eye deviation

▶ Eyes deviate to the direction of the excited neurons; therefore, eyes deviate toward the direction of the seizure focus during seizure, and away from the seizure focus postictally

Epidemiology of epilepsy

▶ One percent lifetime prevalence
▶ Sixty percent nonconvulsive seizures
▶ Complex partial seizures, often of temporal lobe or other limbic origin, are associated with a 6–12 fold increased risk of psychosis
▶ Depression occurs in over half of patients with epilepsy
▶ Suicide rate is five times that of the general public, in patients with temporal lobe epilepsy, 25-fold

Epilepsy and pregnancy

▶ Women suffers from epilepsy have higher rate of polycystic ovarian syndrome, and reduced fertility rate
▶ Seizure during pregnancy may cause fetal hypoxia
▶ Some antiepileptic drugs may have teratogenic effects

First line antiepileptic drugs

▶ Partial seizures – carbamazepine
▶ Absence epilepsy – ethosuximide
▶ Generalized epilepsies – valproate

Frontal lobe partial or focal seizures

▶ Primary motor cortex – contralateral motor seizures
▶ Supplementary motor cortex – complex bizarre automatisms (lip smacking, chewing, etc.)

Grand mal

▶ Most common type of generalized seizure
▶ First symptom – loss of conscious
▶ Eyes deviate upward (not to the right or left)
▶ Tonic-clonic movements are symmetrical
▶ Relative lack of trunk movement
▶ If longer than 7 minutes, status epilepticus

Interictal mood symptoms

▶ Less common than psychotic symptoms
▶ Often associated with nondominant temporal seizures
▶ May be associated with suicidal behaviors

Interictal psychotic symptoms

▶ Risk factors
  ▷ Female gender
  ▷ Left-handedness
  ▷ Puberty onset of seizures
  ▷ A left-sided lesion
▶ Usually proceeded by personality change
▶ Differentiation from schizophrenia
  ▷ Patients usually remain appropriate affect
  ▷ Common thought disorders are conceptualization and circumstantiality, while blocking and looseness are more common in schizophrenia

Lennox-Gastaut syndrome

William Lennox (1884–1960) was a U.S. neurologist.
Henri Gastaut (1915–1995) was a French neurologist.

▶ A form of childhood-onset epilepsy
▶ Ages 2–4 years
▶ Daily frequent seizures with different seizure types
▶ Slowed psychomotor development
▶ Characteristic slow spike-wave complexes appear on interictal EEG
▶ Causes
  ▷ Encephalopathy
  ▷ Tuberous sclerosis
  ▷ Infections – encephalitis, meningitis
  ▷ Hypoxia, ischemia
▶ Treatment
  ▷ Often treatment resistant
  ▷ Valproic acid and benzodiazepines are first line options
  ▷ Other anticonvulsants
  ▷ Vagus nerve stimulation
  ▷ Surgery – corpus callosotomy
  ▷ Ketogenic diet

Mechanisms of antiepileptic drugs

▶ Blocks Na⁺ channels
▶ Blocks of Ca⁺⁺ channels
▶ Enhances GABA activity
▶ Other unknown mechanisms
▶ Some agents may work with more than one mechanism

Occipital lobe partial or focal seizures

▶ Elementary visual hallucinations
▶ Blindness (ictal amaurosis)

Panic attacks vs. partial seizures

▶ Both may occur without trigger
▶ Both may present with hyperarousal, intense fear, perceptual distortion, and dissociative symptoms
▶ Both may respond to benzodiazepines
▶ Panic attacks have memory of the event intact

Parietal lobe partial or focal seizures

▶ Contralateral paresthesias or pain
▶ Gustatory hallucinations
▶ Language disturbances (dominant lobe)

Personality changes due to epilepsy

▶ Most commonly occurs in temporal lobe seizures
▶ Hyper religiosity
  ▷ Increased participation in religious activities
  ▷ Unusual preoccupation in moral and ethical issues
▶ Viscosity of personality
  ▷ Conversation – slow, overly detailed, circumstantial
  ▷ Viscosity in writing – hypergraphia, mirroring the characteristics of viscosity in speech
▶ Changes in sexual behavior
  ▷ Hyposexuality (most common)
  ▷ Hypersexuality
  ▷ Deviations in sexual interest – paraphilia

Postictal prolactin level

▶ The serum prolactin level usually rises following an epileptic seizure
▶ No elevation of prolactin after a nonepileptic seizure, or pseudo-seizure

Pregabalin

▶ Brand
  ▷ Lyrica

- ▶ Dosage
    - ▷ Up to 300 mg/day
- ▶ Indicated for
    - ▷ Partial seizures, adjunct
    - ▷ Diabetic neuropathy
    - ▷ Postherpatic neuralgia
    - ▷ Fibromyalgia
- ▶ Cautions
    - ▷ Dosage reduction if impaired renal function
    - ▷ May cause depression, behavior change, and rarely suicidality
- ▶ Metabolism
    - ▷ No significant hepatic metabolism
    - ▷ Mostly excreted unchanged in urine
- ▶ Mechanisms
    - ▷ A structural derivative of GABA but no direct binding to any GABA receptors
    - ▷ Binds to α-2-delta subunit of voltage-gated calcium channels
- ▶ Half-life – 6 hours

Suicide and epilepsy

- ▶ Higher risk of suicidality in epileptic population vs. general population
    - ▷ 5 × in all epileptic patients
    - ▷ 25 × in temporal lobe epilepsy
- ▶ Risk factors
    - ▷ Psychosis with paranoia and hallucinations
    - ▷ Ictal command hallucinations

Figure 39–1 Head CT of a 36 year old female who received a right anteromedial temporal resection. The right middle cranial fossa is filled with a porencephalic cyst.

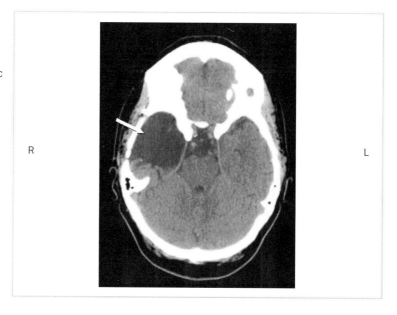

R

L

Surgical treatment for epilepsy (Figure 39–1)

▶ Criteria
  ▷ Failed sufficient trials of antiepileptic drugs
  ▷ Clinically judged to have a reasonable chance of benefiting from surgery
▶ Models of procedures
  ▷ Anteromedial temporal resection; indicated for mesial temporal lobe epilepsy; the most common procedure
  ▷ Corpus callosotomy; indicated for generalized epilepsy
  ▷ Multiple subpial transaction; a nonresective procedure that causes minimal lesion; indicated for seizure-producing cortex with indispensable functions

Temporal lobe focal seizures

▶ Often accompanied by psychiatric symptoms
  ▷ Auditory hallucinations
  ▷ Emotional disturbance – anger, fear, irritability
  ▷ Dissociative symptoms – Déjà vu, jamais vu, depersonalization

40 Strokes and Transient Ischemic Attacks

Cerebrovascular disease is one of the major causes of disability and death.

The primary risk factor is hypertension. The process of pathology starts from the sustained high blood pressure that damages the lining epithelium and exposes the underlying collagen. Platelets then aggregate at the damaged spot to start the process of repairing. Imperfect repair makes the site more vulnerable and inviting to new damage and new repair. Repeated damages and repairs change the architecture of the vessels and make them narrow, stiff, deformed, and uneven. These pathological changes cause double jeopardy – the abnormal cranial vascular system causes regional blood pressure fluctuation, and the vessels are vulnerable to blood pressure fluctuation. Episodes of lower blood pressure superimposed on already narrowed lumen may cause ischemic events, while episodes of higher blood pressure may tear apart the vessel wall and cause hemorrhagic strokes. Therefore, aggressive control of blood pressure is the single most important preventative measure for cerebrovascular accidents (CVAs).

Other conditions cause strokes and transient ischemic attacks (TIAs) include inflammatory disorders, cardiac arrhythmias, cardiac valve conditions, rheumatic heart disease, sickle cell disease, polycythemia, and hypercoagulable states.

Patients with cerebrovascular disorders were found to have higher rates of depression. Vascular dementia and disturbance in impulse control also call for psychiatric involvement. Another prominent psychiatric concern is drug interactions between psychotropics and other medicines, particularly with anticoagulants.

Anosognosia

▶ Unawareness of existing condition, e.g., a hemiplegic patient believes he has no problem in walking
▶ Appears following stroke or other brain injury, and usually resolves in weeks
▶ The term is also used to describe psychiatric patients without insight

Anterior cerebral artery stroke

▶ Unilateral
  ▷ Contralateral leg paresis
▶ Bilateral
  ▷ Motor impairments of both legs
  ▷ Pseudobulbar palsy
  ▷ Mutism
  ▷ Frontal lobe syndrome

Bulbar palsy vs. pseudobulbar palsy

▶ Bulb – medulla and lower portion of pons
▶ Bulbar cranial nerves (CNs)
  ▷ IX – glossopharyngeal
  ▷ X – vagus
  ▷ XI – accessory
  ▷ XII – hypoglossal
▶ Bulbar palsy
  ▷ Location – bulb
  ▷ Lower motor neuron injury
  ▷ Dysarthria and dysphagia
  ▷ Hypoactive jaw and gag reflexes
  ▷ Respiratory impairment
  ▷ No emotional lability and cognitive impairment
▶ Pseudobulbar palsy
  ▷ Location – frontal lobes or any location along the corticobulbar tract
  ▷ Upper motor neuron injury
  ▷ Dysarthria and dysphagia
  ▷ Hyperactive jaw and gag reflexes
  ▷ No respiratory impairment
  ▷ Emotional lability and cognitive impairment

Carotid artery TIAs

▶ Also known as anterior circulation TIAs
▶ Symptoms
  ▷ Aphasia
  ▷ Contralateral hemiparesis and hemisensory loss
  ▷ Ipsilateral amaurosis fugax
▶ Laboratory
  ▷ Carotid Doppler
  ▷ Magnetic resonance angiography (MRA)
  ▷ Cerebral arteriography
▶ Treatment
  ▷ Platelet inhibitors – Aspirin
  ▷ Carotid endarterectomy

Cerebellar hemorrhage

▶ Symptoms
  ▷ Occipital headache
  ▷ Ataxia
  ▷ Dysarthria
  ▷ Lethargy and loss of consciousness
▶ Treatment
  ▷ Immediate surgical evacuation

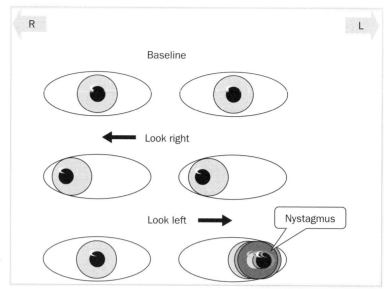

Figure 40–1 Schematic demonstration of right internuclear ophthalmoplegia.

Risk factors for cerebrovascular accidents

▶ Age
▶ Hypertension
▶ Cardiac condition
▶ Diabetes
▶ Cholesterol elevation
▶ Cigarette smoking
▶ Heavy alcohol use
▶ Physical inactivity
▶ Drug abuse
▶ Serologic markers – C-reactive protein elevation, homocysteine elevation

Internuclear ophthalmoplegia (Figure 40–1)

▶ Location – medial longitudinal fasciculus (MLF)
▶ Causes
  ▷ Unilateral – multiple sclerosis in younger patients, stroke in older patients
  ▷ Bilateral – multiple sclerosis
▶ Symptoms
  ▷ The eye ipsilateral to the lesion cannot turn medially across the midline
  ▷ No difficulty in looking to the direction ipsilateral to the lesion
  ▷ When attempted to look to the direction contralateral to the lesion, the eye ipsilateral to the lesion stops at midline, and the eye contralateral to the lesion turns laterally with nystagmus

Intracranial hemorrhage (Figure 40–2)

▶ Cause
  ▷ Hypertension (most common)

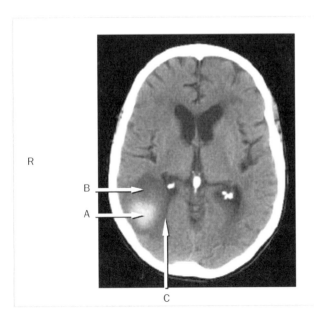

Figure 40-2 This head CT of a 50-year-old male shows an acute hemorrhage in the right temporal-parietal lobe (A) and the surrounding edema (B). There is an impression on the posterior horn of the right lateral ventricle (C).

▷ Head injury
▷ Vascular abnormality – berry aneurysm
▶ Symptoms
▷ Abrupt onset
▷ Headache
▷ Nausea and vomiting
▷ Loss of consciousness
▷ Symptoms of increased intracranial pressure and space occupation

Locked-in syndrome (See Figure 40–3 on page 308)

▶ Clinical presentation
▷ Mute
▷ Quadriplegia
▷ Intact cognition
▷ Communicate only by moving eyes
▷ Electroencephalogram (EEG) is normal
▷ May or may not affect peripheral nerves
▶ Location – ventral portion of pons and medulla
▶ Structural impairment
▷ Corticospinal tracts – quadriplegia
▷ CNs IX, X, XI, and XII – bulbar palsy
▶ Causes
▷ Infarction – occlusion of a branch of the basilar artery; no peripheral nerve symptoms
▷ Peripheral neuromuscular conditions – myasthenia gravis, Guillain-Barré syndrome, amyotrophic lateral sclerosis; with peripheral nervous symptoms

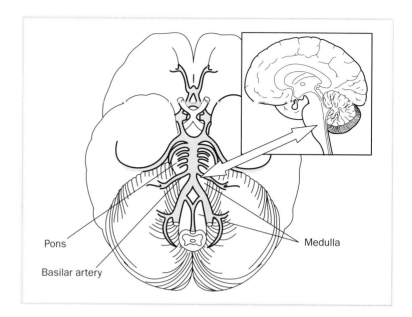

Figure 40-3 Locked-in syndrome. The double arrow indicates the location of lesion.

Pons

Basilar artery

Medulla

Middle cerebral artery stroke (Figure 40-4)

▶ Contralateral hemiparesis
▶ Contralateral hemisensory loss
▶ Aphasia (dominant hemisphere strokes)
▶ Hemi-inattention (nondominant hemisphere strokes)

Posterior cerebral artery stroke

▶ Contralateral homonymous hemianopsia
▶ Alexia without agraphia

Posterior circulation TIAs

▶ Originated in vertebral or basilar artery
▶ Symptoms
  ▷ Vertigo
  ▷ Nausea, vomiting
  ▷ Nystagmus
  ▷ Ataxia
  ▷ Diplopia
  ▷ Drop attacks
  ▷ Isolated hemianopsia or total blindness
▶ Laboratory
  ▷ Transcranial Doppler
  ▷ Magnetic resonance angiography
▶ Treatment – platelet inhibitors – Aspirin

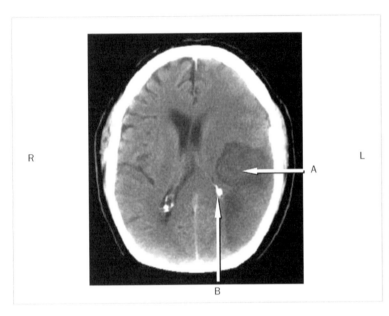

Figure 40–4 This head CT without contrast is of a 66-year-old male and shows extensive left middle cerebral artery infarct (A) and edema mass effect causing a right shift of midline and collapse of posterior horn of lateral ventricle (B).

Psychiatric conditions associated with strokes

▶ Vascular dementia
▶ Psychosis
  ▷ Acute delirium
  ▷ Auditory hallucination associated with temporal lobe strokes
  ▷ Visual hallucination associated with occipital lobe strokes
▶ Depression – appears in 30%–50% patients after strokes; DSM-IV-TR term – mood disorder due to a general medical condition
▶ Frontal lobe syndrome
  ▷ No strict connection of location and mental deficit
  ▷ Orbitofrontal lobe lesions are often associated with disinhibition and emotional lability
  ▷ Apathy may be associated with medial frontal lesions
  ▷ Depression may be associated with left frontal lesions
  ▷ Mania may be associated with right frontal lesions

Subarachnoid hemorrhage

▶ Usually due to a rupture of berry aneurysm
▶ Symptoms
  ▷ Excruciating headache
  ▷ Nuchal rigidity
▶ Diagnosis
  ▷ Computer tomography (CT) or magnetic resonance imaging (MRI)
  ▷ Lumbar puncture – bloody or xanthochromic
▶ Treatment
  ▷ Medical stabilization, most need intensive care unit (ICU) admission
  ▷ Structural correction for aneurysm – surgical clipping or endovascular coiling
  ▷ Urgent surgical evacuation if necessary

Tissue plasminogen activator (TPA)

▶ A thrombolytic agent
▶ Applied to ischemic strokes with expectation to dissolve cerebral arterial occlusions
▶ Potential risk of cerebral hemorrhage
▶ Administrated within 3 hours after stroke
▶ CT showing no hemorrhage

Transient global amnesia (TGA)

▶ Sudden onset of amnesia, lasting for 3–24 hours
▶ Usually affects only short-term memory
▶ Cause is believed to be transient ischemic status; most likely associated with basilar artery TIAs
▶ Though anxiety provoking, the prognosis is usually benign

TIA

▶ The most common cause – platelet emboli from major artery stenosis or ulceration
▶ Time – minutes to hours, by definition less than 24 hours
▶ May have mental and/or physical impairments
▶ CVAs follow TIAs
  ▷ Twelve percent in the first year
  ▷ Five percent yearly afterwards

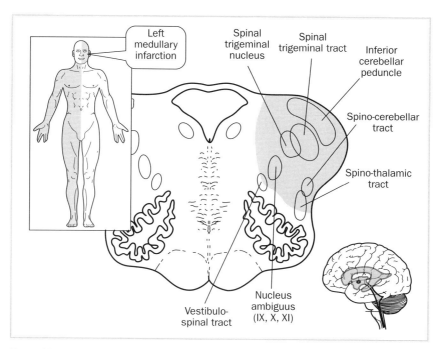

Figure 40–5 This upper medulla section shows territory of posterior inferior cerebellar artery (PICA) as shadowed area. The inset shows the most distinctive pattern of sensory signs – loss of pain and temperature sensation in ipsilateral face and contralateral body.

Wallenberg's syndrome (Figure 40–5)

Adolf Wallenberg (1862–1949) was a German neurologist.

▶ Lateral medullary infarction
▶ Caused by vertebral artery stroke, particularly posterior inferior cerebella artery (PICA)
▶ Owing to the structural complex of this area, the variety of clinical features is wide, depending on the extent of infarction; structures affected and the corresponding clinical features are
  ▷ Spinothalamic tract – contralateral deficits in pain and temperature sensation from body
  ▷ Spinal trigeminal nucleus and tracts – ipsilateral loss of pain and temperature sensation from face
  ▷ Vestibular system (CN VIII) – vertigo, nystagmus
  ▷ Inferior cerebellar peduncle – hemiataxia
  ▷ Descending sympathetic tract – ipsilateral Horner's syndrome
  ▷ Vagus nerve (CN X) – nausea, vomiting, dysphagia, hiccups, and hoarseness

41 Brain Tumors and Injuries

Both brain tumors and brain injuries initiate localized pathology. Brain tumors, either primary or secondary, often develop insidiously in patients with mood, thought, or cognitive disturbance without overt physical symptoms. Brain injuries usually have a clear onset following a traumatic incident; however, minor injuries may be omitted from prompt medical attention. Important and frequently mentioned conditions are discussed in this chapter. Acute and chronic cognitive change, personality change, and mood disturbance are frequent psychiatric concerns.

Acoustic neuroma

▶ Usually benign
▶ Originates from Schwann cell, not neurons
▶ Compression – trigeminal (V) and facial (VII) cranial nerves
▶ Symptoms
▶ Hearing impairment
▶ Tinnitus
▶ Imbalance
▶ Vertigo
▶ Facial sensory loss
▶ Facial muscle weakness
▶ Comorbidity – neurofibromatosis type 2 may arise with bilateral acoustic neuromas
▶ Test
  ▷ Gadolinium-enhanced magnetic resonance imaging (MRI)
  ▷ Auditory tests
  ▷ Brainstem auditory evoked responses (BAER)
▶ Treatment – surgical removal

Astrocytoma

▶ Common in children
▶ Location
  ▷ Children – cerebellum and brainstem
  ▷ Adult – cerebrum
▶ Prognosis
  ▷ Children – benign, often can be removed completely surgically
  ▷ Adult – guarded, usually infiltrates extensively, with more malignant growing
▶ Treatment – combination of surgery and radiotherapy

Brain tumors vs. meningiomas

▶ Brain tumors – diffuse symptoms
▶ Meningiomas – focal progressive symptoms

Coup and countercoup injuries

▶ Coup injury – damage of the underlying brain at the site of direct mechanical force
▶ Countercoup injury – head trauma that damages the opposite side of the brain
▶ Most significant impact on the frontal and temporal lobes

Epidural hematomas (Figure 41–1)

▶ Temporal bone fractures
▶ Middle meningeal artery lacerations
▶ Rapidly expanding of high-pressure masses of fresh blood
▶ May produce transtentorial herniation
▶ Requires immediate surgical evacuation

Glioblastoma

▶ Highly malignant glial tumor
▶ Grow rapidly in cerebrum, and cross corpus callosum
▶ Treatment is ineffective
  ▷ Surgery is rarely curative
  ▷ Radiotherapy and chemotherapy may provide brief survival. However, adverse effects of treatment, including radionecrosis, cause mental deterioration

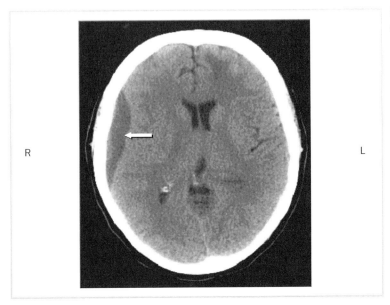

Figure 41–1 Right temporal epidural hematoma.

R

L

Meningiomas

▶ Develop only in adults
▶ Often associated with neurofibromatosis type 1
▶ Grow slowly, may compress or invade the underlying brain or spinal cord
▶ Treatment
  ▷ Small meningiomas may not need treatment
  ▷ Surgical removal

Metastatic tumors

▶ More common than primary brain tumors
▶ Clinical characteristics
  ▷ Multiple
  ▷ Surrounded by edema
  ▷ Rapidly growing
▶ Common original sites
  ▷ Lung
  ▷ Breast
  ▷ Kidney
  ▷ Skin
▶ Treatment
  ▷ Steroids to reduce the edema
  ▷ Radiotherapy
  ▷ Surgical removal of single metastasis

Pituitary adenoma

▶ Common types
  ▷ Prolactinomas – secrete prolactin
  ▷ Chromophobe adenomas – nonsecretory
▶ Symptoms
  ▷ Compression
  ▷ Hormonal effects
▶ Diagnosis
  ▷ MRI
  ▷ Hormone radioimmunoassay

Pseudotumor cerebri: clinical features

▶ Also known as
  ▷ Idiopathic intracranial hypertension (IIH)
▶ Increased intracranial pressure (ICP), in the absence of a tumor, meningitis, or other space occupying lesions
▶ Pathogenesis
  ▷ Increased production of cerebrospinal fluid (CSF)
  ▷ Reduced resorption
▶ Symptoms and signs
  ▷ Headache, worse in the morning
  ▷ Nausea

▷ Visual problems – double vision, loss of peripheral sight, blurring of vision
▷ Papilledema
▷ Absence of focal neurological findings

Pseudotumor cerebri: diagnosis

▶ History and symptoms
▶ CT and/or MRI – rules out mass lesions; may present "empty sella sign"
▶ Lumbar puncture

Pseudotumor cerebri: treatment

▶ Medications
  ▷ Adjust medication presumed to be offessive
  ▷ Carbonic anhydrase inhibitor acetazolamide
  ▷ Furosemide
  ▷ Topiramate
▶ Lumbar puncture
▶ Surgery
  ▷ Optic nerve sheath decompression
  ▷ Shunting – lumboperitoneal shunts, ventriculoatrial shunts
  ▷ Gastric bypass in case of severe obesity

Pseudotumor cerebri: risk factors

▶ Most likely in females of age 15–45 years
▶ May occur in any age and gender
▶ Obesity
▶ Medications
  ▷ Hormonal contraception
  ▷ Vitamin A
  ▷ Tetracycline antibiotics

Postconcussion memory impairment

▶ Usually mild and intermittent
▶ Accompanied by impairment in attention and slowed executive process
▶ Most common memory impairment is retrograde amnesia

Shaken baby syndrome

▶ Children bear vigorous shaking may develop raised intracranial pressure and intracranial bleeding
▶ Clinical findings
  ▷ Retinal hemorrhages
  ▷ Blood in the interhemispheric fissure
▶ Usually no fracture or obvious soft tissue injuries

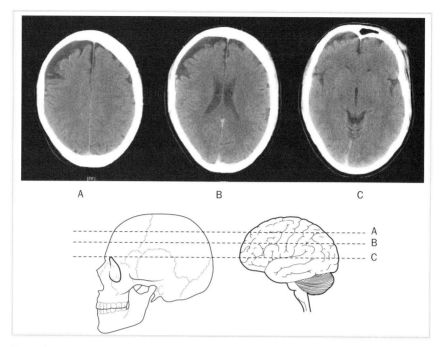

Figure 41–2 A fluid collection overlying the right frontal lobe is showed here in three sections of CT with no contrast. The fluid has the same radio density as CSF in ventricles, indicating old subdural hematoma. The patient is a 35-year-old male with alcohol history. He also has an old fracture of the right zygomatic arch, consistent with right side head injury.

Subdural hematomas (Figure 41–2)

▶ Bleeding from intracranial veins into subdural space
▶ Usually slow and nonfatal, and be arrested by the compression from the underlying brain
▶ If significantly compression developed against the brain, may develop transtentorial herniation
▶ Chronic subdural hematomas cause personality change and dementia, which are correctable with surgical evacuation

Traumatic brain injuries: pathological change (Figure 41–3)

▶ Direct penetrating injury (parenchyma destruction)
▶ Direct nonpenetrating injuries
  ▷ Coup injury
  ▷ Countercoup injury
▶ Diffuse axonal shearing
▶ Cerebral edema
▶ Herniation
▶ Foreign bodies that may cause
  ▷ Seizure
  ▷ Abscess

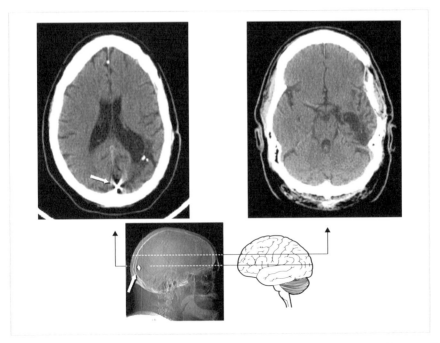

Figure 41–3 CT scan of a 47-year-old male who survived a gun shot wound at the left occipital area 2 years ago. The metallic bullet fragment can be seen at occipital lobe as indicated by arrow. There is encephalomalacia extended to the parenchyma of the left temporal lobe.

▶ Hematoma
   ▷ Epidural hematoma
   ▷ Subdural hematoma

Tumor at cerebellopontine angle

▶ Unilateral hearing loss
▶ Vertigo
▶ Unsteadiness
▶ Falls
▶ Headaches
▶ Mild facial weakness
▶ Ipsilateral limb ataxia

Tumor at temporal lobe

▶ Headache
▶ Mood swings
▶ Visual, tactile, and auditory hallucinations

42 Headache

Over 90% of Americans experience headache in each individual year. Over 90% of all headaches are not due to serious intracranial condition.

Not all the pains above the neck are headaches. Headache does not even have to be pain. Headache refers to a range of discomfort located in the region of the cranial vault. Facial pain, such as trigeminal neuralgia (tic douloureux), or pharyngeal pain, though relevant to headaches in diagnosis and treatment, is not usually considered headache.

History taking is the most important part of evaluation for headache. Essential information includes

▶ Quality of the pain
  ▷ Dull, pressure, stabbing, throbbing, etc.
▶ Intensity of the pain
  ▷ Subjective grading, functional impairment, sleep interruption, etc.
▶ Location of the pain
  ▷ Sharply localized, homolateral, etc.
▶ Mode of onset
  ▷ Abrupt attack, insidious onset, etc.
▶ Frequency and duration of the pain
▶ Precipitating factors

  Common types of headache are listed as below

▶ Migraine without aura (common migraine)
▶ Migraine with aura (classic migraine, neurologic migraine)
▶ Tension-type headache
▶ Cluster headache (histamine headache, migrainosus neuralgia)
▶ Headache due to meningeal irritation
  ▷ Meningitis
  ▷ Subarachnoid hemorrhage
▶ Intracranial space occupying lesion
  ▷ Brain tumor
▶ Other
  ▷ Posttraumatic (postconcussion)
  ▷ Pseudotumor cerebri
  ▷ Substance withdrawal
  ▷ Temporal arteritis

Treatment for headache should be planned according to the nature of the illness. A combination of several modalities is often needed, particularly for recurrent headaches. Narcotics should be avoided for chronic headaches. Options of treatment include

▶ Anticonvulsants
▶ β-blockers
▶ Calcium blockers
▶ Ergotamine
▶ Lithium
▶ Mannitol
▶ Nonsteroidal antiinflammatory agents (NSAIDs)
▶ Oxygen
▶ Steroids
▶ Tricyclic antidepressants

Cluster headache: clinical features

▶ Also known as
  ▷ Histamine headache
  ▷ Migrainous neuralgia
▶ More common in men
▶ Characteristics of headache
  ▷ Laterality – unilateral
  ▷ Location – periorbital or orbitotemporal
  ▷ Quality – stabbing, nonthrobbing
  ▷ Time – 1–2 hours after falling asleep
  ▷ Duration – attacks last from 20 minutes to 3 hours
  ▷ Frequency – nightly for several weeks; recurrence in months or years
▶ Accompanying symptoms
  ▷ Ptosis
  ▷ Miosis
  ▷ Lacrimation
  ▷ Rhinorrhea (runny nose)
  ▷ Nostril congestion

Cluster headache: treatment

▶ Before attack
  ▷ Ergotamine
▶ During attack
  ▷ Oxygen
  ▷ Triptans
▶ Prevention
  ▷ Corticosteroids
  ▷ Calcium blocker – verapamil
  ▷ Anticonvulsant – valproate
  ▷ Lithium
▶ Analgesics may not have time to take effect due to the short duration of symptoms

Demographics of headache

▶ Migraine with or without aura
  ▷ Adolescents and young adults
  ▷ More common in females

- Tension-type headache
  - Adults
  - Both sexes, somehow more common in females
- Cluster headache
  - Adolescents and adult
  - Mostly in males
- Meningeal irritation and intracranial space occupying lesion
  - Any age
  - Both sexes
- Pseudotumor cerebri
  - Females between 20 and 50 years of age
- Temporal arteritis
  - Over 50 years of age
  - Obesity
  - Both sexes

Ergotamine

- Available in combination with caffeine (Cafergot)
- Abortive therapy for migraine
- Mechanism
  - Nonselectively agonizes 5-HT1b, 5-HT1d, and other receptors
- More vasoconstrictive and more adverse effects than triptans

Headache due to intracranial space occupying lesion

- Often unilateral, but can be generalized
- Steady, nonthrobbing
- Progressive over days to weeks
- Often more severe in early morning, and awakening
- Accompanying symptoms
  - Papilledema
  - Seizures
  - Nausea and vomiting
  - May have focal signs
  - Cognitive impairment

Headache due to subarachnoid hemorrhage

- Sudden onset, very severe headache
- May have decreased level of consciousness
- Possible focal signs
  - Third cranial nerve (CN) palsy due to aneurysm of the posterior communicating artery
  - Hemiparesis due to aneurysm of the middle cerebral artery
  - Lethargy and paraparesis due to aneurysm of the anterior communicating artery

Headache with meningitis

▶ Acute headache
▶ Fever and chills
▶ Nuchal rigidity
▶ Photophobia
▶ Vomiting
▶ May have seizures and focal neurologic symptoms

Hemiplegic migraine

▶ A rare migraine variant
▶ Clinical features
   ▷ Unilateral weakness or hemiplegia precedes the headache
   ▷ May have language disturbance
   ▷ Neurologic deficit often resolves with the beginning of headache
▶ Familial disorder
   ▷ Autosomal dominant
   ▷ Mutation in the short arm of chromosome 19
▶ Sporadic hemiplegic migraine
   ▷ Migraine with motor weakness in the absence of family history

Migraine with aura (classic migraine): clinical features

▶ Location
   ▷ Mostly unilateral
   ▷ Frontotemporal
   ▷ Worse behind eye or ear
▶ Characteristics of headache
   ▷ Dull ache
   ▷ Moderate to severe intensity
   ▷ Throbbing
   ▷ Exacerbation with activity
▶ Time of onset – upon awakening or later in the day
▶ Duration – lasts 4–72 hours, mostly less than 24 hours
▶ Accompanying symptoms – at least one of the following
   ▷ Photophobia
   ▷ Phonophobia
   ▷ Nausea and vomiting
   ▷ Scalp sensitivity
▶ Aura
   ▷ Scintillating lights
   ▷ Visual loss
   ▷ Scotomas (blind spots in visional field)
   ▷ Unilateral paresthesias or weakness
   ▷ Dysphasia
   ▷ Vertigo

Migraine without aura

▶ Also known as common migraine
▶ Same symptoms as neurologic migraine, only without neurological symptoms preceding headache (aura)
▶ Often has family history

Migraine: pathophysiology

▶ 5-HT1b receptors are located on blood vessels; when activated, produces vasoconstriction
▶ 5-HT1d receptors are presynaptic nerve receptors; when activated, inhibits the release of vasoactive peptides, including substance P, histamine, bradykinins, etc.
▶ The assumed inherited central migraine generator is activated by environmental migraine triggers, and sends impulses through trigeminal nerve
▶ Vasoactive and inflammatory peptides are released through trigeminal nerve (CN V), and CN V then sends the pain message back to the brain

Migraine: status migrainosus

▶ Lasts longer than 3 days
▶ Prolonged vomiting with dehydration
▶ Treatment
  ▷ Hydration
  ▷ Antiemetics
  ▷ Opioids
  ▷ Steroids

Migraines: treatment

▶ Prophylactic
  ▷ β-blockers
  ▷ Calcium channel blockers
  ▷ Antiepileptics
  ▷ Tricyclic antidepressants
▶ Abortive
  ▷ Triptans
  ▷ Ergotamine
▶ Symptomatic
  ▷ NSAIDs
  ▷ Antiemetics
  ▷ Sedatives
  ▷ Analgesics

Provoking factors of headache

▶ Migraine with or without aura
  ▷ Bright light
  ▷ Noise
  ▷ Alcohol

▶ Tension-type headache
  ▷ Fatigue
  ▷ Mental stress
  ▷ Analgesic abuse
▶ Cluster headache
  ▷ Alcohol (in some cases)
▶ Meningeal irritation and intracranial space occupying lesion
  ▷ Significant provoking factors – none
▶ Temporal arteritis
  ▷ Significant provoking factors – none

Pseudotumor cerebri

▶ Also known as
  ▷ Idiopathic intracranial hypertension
▶ Characteristics of headache
  ▷ Headache and papilledema
  ▷ May cause blindness and empty sella syndrome
▶ Increased intracranial pressure
▶ Lumbar puncture is diagnostic and therapeutic

Signs of secondary headache requiring neuroimaging

▶ New onset severe headache
▶ Change in character of headache
▶ Focal neurological sign

Temporal arteritis (See Figure 42–1 on page 324)

▶ Also known as giant cell arteritis
▶ Age – over 55 years
▶ More common in Caucasian women
▶ Symptoms
  ▷ Headache
  ▷ Jaw claudication
  ▷ Local tenderness and swelling
  ▷ Delayed treatment may result in ischemic optic neuritis and loss of vision
▶ Pathophysiology
  ▷ A cell-mediated immune response directed toward elastic tissue component of the arterial wall
  ▷ Comorbidity with polymyalgia rheumatica is approximately 20%
▶ Treatment
  ▷ Emergency room treatment is crucial
  ▷ High-dose prednisone
  ▷ Alternative – intravenous methylprednisolone (Medrol)

Tension headache

▶ The most common type of headache
▶ Location – generalized (holocephalic), or frontal and occipital

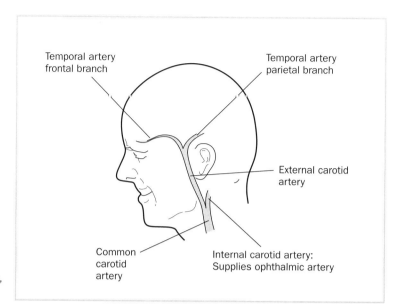

Temporal artery
frontal branch

Temporal artery
parietal branch

External carotid
artery

Common
carotid
artery

Internal carotid artery:
Supplies ophthalmic artery

Figure 42-1 Temporal arteritis, also known as giant cell arteritis.

- ▶ Characteristics of headache
  - ▷ Pressure, tightness
  - ▷ Nonthrobbing
  - ▷ Continuous with variable intensity
- ▶ Duration
  - ▷ Episode lasts days to months
- ▶ Treatment
  - ▷ Anxiolytics
  - ▷ Antidepressants
  - ▷ Symptomatic

Trigeminal neuralgia: clinical features

- ▶ Also known as tic duoloureus
- ▶ Age – usually after 50 years
- ▶ Characteristics of pain
  - ▷ Recurrent attacks of unilateral pain in trigeminal area
  - ▷ Triggered by activities touching the area
  - ▷ Stabbing, shocking, burning, often debilitating
  - ▷ Lasts seconds to hours per attack
  - ▷ Frequent attacks for days
  - ▷ Remission may last for months to years
  - ▷ Atypical cases may have migraine like headache in addition to facial pain

Trigeminal neuralgia: pathology

- ▶ Pathology
  - ▷ Often idiopathic
  - ▷ Compression of CNV by superior cerebella artery or other vessels, aneurysm, or tumor

▷ Traumatic injury such as accident in driving or sports, tongue piercing
▷ Multiple sclerosis
▷ Shingles

Trigeminal neuralgia: treatment

▶ Medicinal treatment
  ▷ Anticonvulsant
  ▷ Analgesics including long-acting narcotics
  ▷ Tricyclic antidepressants
▶ Procedural treatment
  ▷ Botulinum toxin injection
  ▷ Surgical decompression
  ▷ Stereotactic radiation therapy

Triptans

▶ Drugs
  ▷ Naratriptan (Amerge)
  ▷ Almotriptan (Axert)
  ▷ Frovatriptan (Frova)
  ▷ Sumatriptan (Imitrex, Imitrex Nasal)
  ▷ Rizatriptan (Maxalt, Maxalt MLT)
  ▷ Eletriptan (Relpax)
  ▷ Zolmitriptan (Zomig, Zomig Nasal, Zomig ZMT)
▶ Mechanism
  ▷ Selectively agonize 5-HT1b and 5-HT1d and produce vasoconstriction
  ▷ Inhibit the release of vasoactive neuropeptides presynaptically, e.g., substance P
▶ Use for headache treatment
  ▷ Abortive therapy for migraines
▶ Risks
  ▷ Theoretical risk of cardiac vasoconstriction and serotonin syndrome

43 Spinal Cord Anatomy and Related Conditions

Spinal cord is an extension of the brain, or the medulla oblongata, to be more precise. In contrast to the complexity of the brain, the function of spinal cord is rather focused. Spinal cord provides physical pathways for the transmission of neuronal signals between the brain and the peripheral nervous system.

The anatomy of spinal cord is relatively straight forward, and usually reveals clear and intriguing clue of pathology when injuries or diseases occur. Besides vertebral column, the intervertebral discs, the facet joints between vertebra, the ligaments and muscles surrounding the vertebral column are all crucial structures of an integrate system to protect the spinal cord. Injuries and diseases in these structures often give direct impact on the spinal cord.

Brown-Séquard syndrome (Figure 43–1)

Charles Brown-Séquard (1817–1896) was a British neurologist.

▶ Lateral hemitransection of spinal cord
▶ Motor
  ▷ Interruption of corticospinal tract
  ▷ Ipsilateral upper motor neuron paresis
  ▷ Ipsilateral hyperactive deep tendon responses and Babinski sign
▶ Sensory
  ▷ Interruption of dorsal columns and spinothalamic tract
  ▷ Ipsilateral – position and vibratory sense loss (dorsal columns)
  ▷ Contralateral – pain and temperature sense loss (spinothalamic tract)

Cauda equina syndrome (Figure 43–2)

▶ The sections of spinal cord are shorter than their corresponding vertebra, which results in the termination of spinal cord at the second lumber vertebrae
▶ Injuries occur below the L2 vertebrae may cause cauda equina (from Latin, horse tail) syndrome
▶ Symptoms
  ▷ Pain in legs and lower back
  ▷ Flaccid areflexic paraparesis
  ▷ Incontinence

Cerebrospinal fluid: glucose level

▶ Normal – 60–100 mg/dL; Guillain-Barré syndrome has normal glucose
▶ Mildly low – 40–80 mg/dL, seen in neurosyphilis, tuberculosis (TB), and fungal meningitis
▶ Significantly low – 0–60 mg/dL, seen in bacterial and viral meningitis

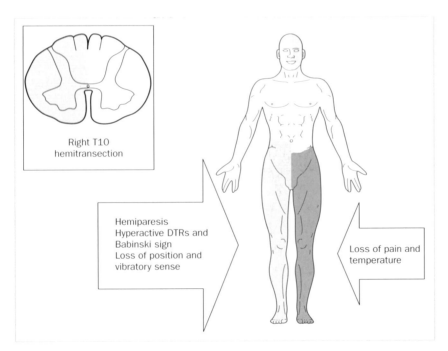

Figure 43-1 Brown-Sequard syndrome, depicted as right T10 hemitransection. Notice the pain and temperature sensory deficits are 1-2 segments caudal to the lesion. This is because the central process of primary neurons in the spinal ganglion ascends in Lissauer's fasciculus before entering the posterior horn.
DTR, deep tendon reflex.

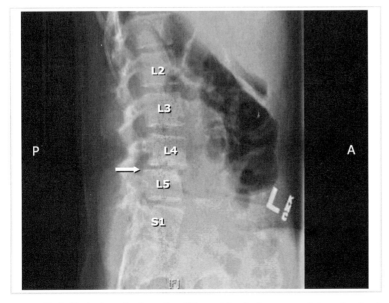

Figure 43-2 This lumbar spine X-ray of a middle-aged female shows severe degenerative disc disease between the fourth and fifth lumbar vertebral bodies. The patient suffers from severe chronic lower back pain and lower body weakness.

Cervical radiculopathy (Figure 43–3)

▶ Causes – nerve root compression due to
  ▷ Inflammation
  ▷ Disk herniation
  ▷ Degenerative changes about the neural foramen
  ▷ Most common at C5 to C7
▶ Clinical presentations
  ▷ Pain and numbness
  ▷ Reduced range of movement
  ▷ Muscle weakness
  ▷ Reduced deep tendon reflexes
▶ Treatment
  ▷ Physical therapy – icing, rest, traction, isokinetic exercises
  ▷ Nonsteroidal antiinflammatory drugs (NSAIDs), tricyclic antidepressants
  ▷ Oral steroids
  ▷ Epidural steroids
  ▷ Surgical intervention

Combined system disease

▶ Vitamin B12 deficiency
▶ Most common cause – antibodies to intrinsic factor blocks the absorption of vitamin B12, and cause pernicious anemia
▶ Other causes
  ▷ Malabsorption
  ▷ Vegetarian diet

Figure 43-3 Cervical radiculopathy. Sagittal MRI cut shows at C5-C6 level a posterior disc osteophyte complex which effaces the ventral subarachnoid space.

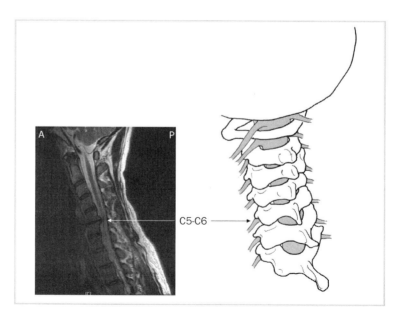

▶ Clinical features
  ▷ Anemia
  ▷ Dementia
  ▷ Spinal cord impairment – loss of lateral (corticospinal tract) and posterior columns
▶ Labs
  ▷ Serum homocysteine elevated
  ▷ Serum methylmalonic acid elevated
  ▷ Intrinsic factor antibodies
  ▷ Schilling test
▶ Treatment – vitamin B12 injection

Dermatones (Figure 43–4)

▶ Each dermatome is supplied by a single spinal nerve
▶ Neighboring dermatomes overlap
▶ There is no C1 dermatome, because C1 has no sensory root

Lateral spinothalamic tracts (See Figure 43–5 on page 330)

▶ Ascending in anterolateral portion of spinal cord
▶ Sensory – pain and temperature from contralateral body
▶ Primary neurons
  ▷ In the spinal ganglion
  ▷ Central processes enter Lissauer's fasciculus, ascend 1–2 segments, and enter the posterior horn

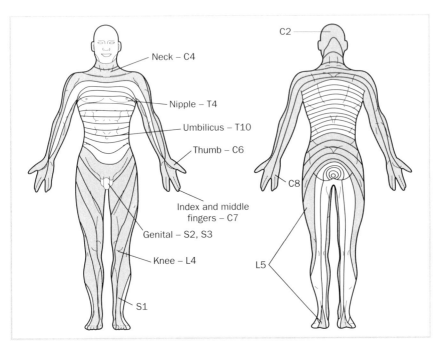

Figure 43–4 Dermatomal landmarks. Cervical and lumbar sections are shaded.

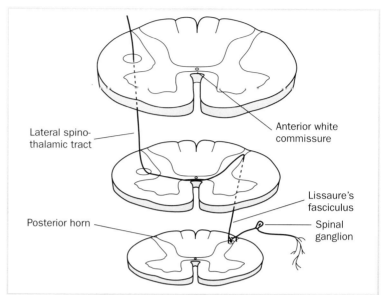

Figure 43-5 Lateral spinothalamic tract and associated structures.

▶ Secondary neurons
   ▷ In the posterior horn
   ▷ Synapse with the central processes of primary neurons
   ▷ Axons cross the midline in the anterior white commissure and ascend as the lateral spinothalamic tract
▶ Tertiary neuron
   ▷ In thalamus
   ▷ Project to ipsilateral sensory cortex

Lower back pain

John Sarno (1923–) is a U.S. physician of rehabilitation medicine.

▶ Causes
   ▷ Physiological – ruptured disk, fracture, congenital defects, ligamentous muscle strain
   ▷ Psychosomatic
▶ Conventional treatment
   ▷ Analgesics
   ▷ Muscle relaxants
   ▷ Physical therapy
▶ Psychoeducational treatment, developed by John Sarno
   ▷ Proper medical evaluation concluded no structural abnormality account for symptoms
   ▷ Educating patients about physiological and psychological components of the symptoms
   ▷ Resuming physical activities with minimal mandatory physical therapy

Meningocele and meningomyelocele

▶ Neural tube closure defects
▶ Congenital defect
▶ Risk factors
  ▷ Valproate
  ▷ Carbamazepine
  ▷ Arnold-Chiari malformation
▶ Symptoms
  ▷ Flaccid areflexic paraplegia
  ▷ Impotence
  ▷ Incontinence
▶ Testing
  ▷ Maternal serum or amniotic fluid α-fetoprotein
  ▷ Ultrasound
▶ Prevention – possible benefit from folate treatment for pregnant mothers

Posterior column

▶ Fasciculi gracilis and cuneatus
▶ Ascending tracts
▶ Sensory
  ▷ Position
  ▷ Vibration
  ▷ Stereognosis

Spinocerebellar ataxias (SCAs)

▶ Trinucleotide repeats expansion on different chromosomes
▶ Autosomal recessive or dominant
▶ Loss of myelin in posterior columns and spinocerebellar tracts
▶ Motor – ataxia
▶ Sensory
  ▷ Loss of vibration and position sense
  ▷ Pes cavus (foot deformity with abnormally high arch)

Spinocerebellar tracts

▶ Ascending
▶ Lateral periphery
▶ Feedback to cerebellum

Syringomyelia

▶ Cavities in spinal cord
▶ Spinothalamic tract damage
▶ Loss of pain and temperature, but preserved position sensation

Tabes dorsalis

▶ Manifestation of neurosyphilis
▶ Sensory impairment
  ▷ Pains
  ▷ Position sense loss – steppage gate (high stepping to allow the drooping foot to clear the ground)
  ▷ Romberg's sign
  ▷ Argyll Robertson pupils – pupils accommodate but do not react

Upper motor neuron vs. lower motor neuron damages

▶ Upper motor neuron (UMN) damage
  ▷ Hyperactive deep tendon reflex
  ▷ Babinski sign positive (plantar reflex is extensor)
▶ Lower motor neuron (LMN) damage
  ▷ Hypoactive deep tendon reflex
  ▷ Lack of plantar reflex

Wallerian degeneration

Augustus Waller (1816–1870) was a British neurophysiologist.

▶ Demyelination of nerve tracts distal from the injury
▶ Motor tracts
  ▷ Descending demyelination
▶ Sensory tracts
  ▷ Ascending demyelination

44 Movement Disorders

Movement disorders consist of a group of neurological conditions that affect the speed, frequency, quality, and control of movement. Movement disorders call for special attention in psychiatry because

▶ Psychiatric disorders may have movement symptoms
  ▷ Disorders in cognition and mood spectrum often present with, mimic, or overshadow certain movement symptoms
▶ Movement disorders may have psychiatric symptoms
  ▷ Psychosis, depression, and dementia may appear in movement disorders
  ▷ Movement disorder may cause secondary mood symptoms
▶ Medications for movement may cause psychiatric symptoms
  ▷ Some therapeutic agents for movement disorders may induce psychosis and other psychiatric symptoms
▶ Psychiatric medications may cause movement symptoms
  ▷ Antipsychotics and some other psychiatric medications may cause movement disorders

Most categories of DSM-IV-TR have the diagnoses of psychiatric disorder due to general medical condition that may be specified as movement disorders. DSM-IV-TR also allows diagnoses of medication-induced movement disorders as the following

▶ Neuroleptic-induced Parkinsonism
▶ Neuroleptic malignant syndrome
▶ Neuroleptic-induced acute dystonia
▶ Neuroleptic-induced acute akathisia
▶ Neuroleptic-induced tardive dyskinesia
▶ Medication-induced postural tremor
▶ Medication-induced movement disorder not otherwise specified (NOS)

This chapter reviews commonly encountered movement disorders. The anatomy and physiology of the basal ganglia play important roles in many movement disorders, and therefore reference to Chapters 1 and 3 is recommended.

Athetosis: pathology

▶ Injury of basal ganglia
▶ Usually from jaundice (kernicterus), anoxia, and prematurity

Botulinum toxin

▶ Botulinum toxin prevents the release of acetylcholine vesicles from presynaptic nerve terminals, and therefore reduces muscle spasm
▶ Botulinum toxin is effective in the treatment of
  ▷ Blepharospasm
  ▷ Dystonic dysphonia
  ▷ Torticollis
  ▷ Other muscle spasm disorders

Dementia with Lewy body vs. Parkinson's disease

▶ Both have Lewy bodies, but different distributions
▶ Dementia with Lewy body – cortex, brainstem, and hypothalamus
▶ Parkinson's disease – substantia nigra
▶ Dementia with Lewy body has rapid onset of dementia, and extrapyramidal symptoms (EPS)

Dopa-responsive dystonia

▶ Dystonia onset in childhood, more frequently in females
▶ Diurnal fluctuation – asymptomatic in morning and dystonia or Parkinsonism in evening
▶ Responds dramatically to L-dopa
▶ Autosomal dominant defect on chromosome 14q
▶ Deficient guanosine triphosphate (GTP); GTP is required for the synthesis of tetrahydrobiopterin, which is a cofactor in tyrosine hydroxylase synthesis

Early onset primary dystonia

▶ Also known as dystonia musculorum deformans
▶ Most common in Ashkenazi Jews
▶ Onset age 8–14 years
▶ Autosomal dominant, chromosome 9, CAG deletion
▶ Treatment – pallidotomy, deep brain stimulation (DBS)

Extrapyramidal system

▶ Pathways among basal ganglia and other nervous system
▶ Regulation of involuntary movement
▶ When impaired, may present with
  ▷ Akathisia
  ▷ Athetosis
  ▷ Ballism
  ▷ Chorea
  ▷ Dystonia
  ▷ Myoclonus
  ▷ Tremor

Hemiballismus

▶ Infarction in contralateral subthalamic nucleus – the corpus of Luysii
▶ Flinging movements of unilateral extremities and shoulder

Huntington's disease

George Huntington (1850–1916) was a U.S. physician.

▶ Also known as Huntington's chorea
▶ Onset age 30–50 years
▶ Pathophysiology
  ▷ Autosomal dominant disease, carried on chromosome 4
  ▷ Expansion of CAG trinucleotide – $N \geq 36 \rightarrow$ Huntington's disease; $N \geq 60 \rightarrow$ juvenile Huntington's disease
▶ Clinical features
  ▷ Chorea – rapid, jerky motions of trunk and limbs
  ▷ Dementia appears within 1 year of onset of chorea
▶ Brain images
  ▷ Atrophy of cerebral cortex and head of the caudate nuclei
  ▷ Bat-wing ventricles – compensatory enlargement of lateral ventricles

Illnesses with expansion of trinucleotide repeats

▶ Huntington's disease
▶ Myotonic dystrophy
▶ Fragile X syndrome
▶ Spinobulbar muscular atrophy
▶ Spinocerebellar ataxia type 1
▶ Machado-Joseph disease

Movement disorders with vs. without dementia

▶ Movement disorders with dementia
  ▷ Huntington's disease
  ▷ Wilson's disease
  ▷ Parkinson's disease
▶ Movement disorders without dementia
  ▷ Sydenham's chorea
  ▷ Hemiballismus
  ▷ Dopa-responsive dystonia

Parkinson's disease: etiology

James Parkinson (1730–1813) was an English physician.

▶ Toxins
  ▷ Mn^{++}
  ▷ MPTP
  ▷ Free radicals
  ▷ Rotenone

▶ Age-related changes
▶ Mitochondrial failure – oxidative stress
▶ Mutations – parkin, synuclein

Parkinson's disease: pathology

▶ Impaired dopamine synthesis in the nigrostriatal tract
▶ Loss of pigment in
  ▷ Substantia nigra
  ▷ Locus ceruleus
  ▷ Dorsal motor cranial nerve (CN) X nucleus
▶ Lewy bodies – eosinophilic intraneuronal inclusions in substantia nigra; Lewy bodies stain for α-synuclein

Parkinson's disease: symptoms

▶ Tremor – pill rolling, resting, 3–5 Hz
▶ Rigidity
▶ Bradykinesia and akinesia
▶ Festinating gait – small accelerating steps
▶ Postural reflex abnormalities
▶ Micrographic
▶ Depression
▶ Dementia
▶ Psychosis

Parkinson's disease: treatment

▶ Dopamine precursors – L-dopa (usually with dopa decarboxylase inhibitor, carbidopa)
▶ Dopamine agonists – pramipexole, ropinirole, apomorphine
▶ Monoamine oxidase B (MAO-B)
▶ COMT inhibitor – entacapone
▶ Surgery – pallidotomy or thalamotomy
▶ DBS

Pyramidal system

▶ Precisely demarcated pathways from cortex to muscle
▶ Voluntary movements
▶ When impaired, may present with paralysis, paresis, hyperreflexia, and spasticity

Sydenham's chorea

Thomas Sydenham (1624–1689) was an English physician.

▶ A manifestation of rheumatic fever following infection via group A β-hemolytic streptococcus
▶ Onset in childhood
▶ Symptoms
  ▷ Rapid, irregular, and aimless involuntary movements of the arms and legs, trunk, and facial muscles

▷ Uncoordinated movements including difficulty in writing
▷ Muscular weakness
▷ Slurred speech
▷ Emotional instability
▶ Treatment
  ▷ No specific treatment
  ▷ Sedative drugs, such as benzodiazepines, as needed
  ▷ Anticonvulsants such as valproic acid may be tried
  ▷ Treatment for rheumatic fever – antibiotics
▶ Prognosis
  ▷ Most recover completely in 3–6 weeks
  ▷ A small number of cases have persistent chorea despite treatment
  ▷ Endocarditis may occur in a small minority of patients
  ▷ In a third of the children recurrent attack may appear in 1–2 years
▶ PANDAS
  ▷ Pediatric autoimmune neuropsychiatric disorder associated with streptococcal infections (PANDAS)
  ▷ Patients with previous Sydenham's chorea may have abrupt onset forms of obsessive-compulsive disorder, attention deficit/hyperactivity disorder, tic disorders, and autism
  ▷ The attribution of etiology is a controversial concept and requires further study

Tardive dyskinesia: specific types

▶ Orofacial dyskinesia
▶ Tardive akathisia
▶ Tardive blepharospasm
▶ Tardive dystonia
▶ Tardive myoclonus
▶ Tardive Tourettism
▶ Tardive tremor

Wilson's disease: clinical features

Samuel Wilson (1878–1937) was a British neurologist.

▶ Onset age 15–45 years, average 16 years
▶ Hepatic cirrhosis
▶ Kayser-Fleischer ring
▶ Movement symptoms
  ▷ A variety of involuntary movements
  ▷ Asterixis – flapping tremor of hands, some called it "wing-beating tremor," as though the patient was attempting to fly
  ▷ Rigidity, dystonia, bradykinesia or akinesia
  ▷ Parkinsonian symptoms
  ▷ Dysarthria
▶ Psychiatric symptoms
  ▷ Dementia – early onset, may begin before the movement symptoms
  ▷ Personality changes, mood disturbances, disinhibition

Wilson's disease: diagnosis

▶ Suppressed ceruloplasmin level
▶ Copper level in blood and 24 hours urine
▶ Liver biopsy
▶ Kayser-Fleischer rings

Wilson's disease: pathophysiology

▶ Also known as hepatolenticular degeneration
▶ Autosomal-recessive inheritance
▶ Mutation of ATP7B gene on chromosome 13
▶ Accumulation of copper in tissues
  ▷ Inhibited copper transportation to bile results in accumulation of copper in liver
  ▷ Copper deposits in the basal ganglia, particularly in the lenticular nucleus (putamen and globus pallidus)

Wilson's disease: treatment

▶ Chelating agents – D-penicillamine
▶ British anti-lewisite agent (BAL, dimercaprol)
▶ Low copper diet
▶ Zinc
▶ Liver transplant

45 Language Impairment

Language sets humans apart from the rest of the animal world. While preliminary forms of communication through prearranged signals exist in many social animals, there are no comparison to the complication, sophistication, and efficiency of human language. The evolution of a rationally organized cortical center for linguistic reason and communication took estimated one million years. The most paramount form of language is speech. However, the brain's capacity of using language is not limited to speech. A deaf and mute individual may reason with unspoken language and use signal language to communicate.

Language impairment is devastating. It may be caused by diseases in relatively small portion of the brain. With the exception of the most global and massive injuries, brain damages usually do not destroy all forms of linguistic communication. Researchers in neurology have studied anatomic and physiologic correlations of language, and developed rather elegant and logistic tests for language-related disorders.

Although adult-onset language impairment is not a diagnostic category in DSM-IV-TR, its interaction with cognition, behavior, and emotion deserves close attention in psychiatric evaluation and treatment.

Alexia without agraphia

▶ Symptoms
  ▷ Impaired reading
  ▷ Preserved writing
▶ Anatomy
  ▷ Dominant visual cortex damage
▶ Pathology
  ▷ Infarction of the left posterior cerebral artery

Aphagia and dysphagia

▶ Aphagia
  ▷ Inability of swallowing
▶ Dysphagia
  ▷ Difficulty in swallowing

Conduction aphasia

▶ Fluent, with impaired repeat
▶ Caused by focal lesions at posterior temporal lobe, where the arcuate fasciculus locate

Fluent aphasia: clinical characteristics

▶ Fluent aphasia is also known as
  ▷ Receptive aphasia
  ▷ Sensory aphasia
  ▷ Wernicke's aphasia
  ▷ Posterior aphasia
▶ Language symptoms
  ▷ Normal articulation
  ▷ Paraphasias
  ▷ >100 words per minute
  ▷ Impaired in all formal language testing
▶ Associated symptoms
  ▷ Hemianopsia (blindness in one half of the visual field)
  ▷ Hemisensory loss
  ▷ Minimal hemiparesis

Fluent aphasia: pathology

▶ Discrete structural lesions or diffuse cerebral injury
▶ Location – temporoparietal region
▶ Causes
  ▷ Strokes
  ▷ Trauma
  ▷ Frontotemporal dementia
  ▷ Alzheimer's disease
  ▷ Cerebral anoxia
  ▷ Metabolic disturbances

Formal language testing

▶ Speaking, reading, and writing tests in the following area
  ▷ Comprehension
  ▷ Naming
  ▷ Repetition

Gerstmann syndrome

Josef Gerstmann (1887–1969) was an Austrian-born American neuropsychiatrist.

▶ Agraphia accompanied by
  ▷ Acalculia
  ▷ Finger agnosia
  ▷ Left/right confusion
▶ Location of lesion
  ▷ Angular gyrus of the dominant parietal lobe

Global aphasia

▶ An extreme form of nonfluent aphasia
▶ Language symptoms

 ▷ Lack of intelligible communication
 ▷ Mute
▶ Behavioral symptoms
 ▷ Behavioral withdrawal
 ▷ Emotionally unresponsive
▶ Physical deficits
 ▷ Right hemiplegia
 ▷ Right homonymous hemianopsia
 ▷ Conjugate deviation of the eyes toward the left
▶ Causes
 ▷ Left internal carotid occlusions
 ▷ Left middle cerebral artery occlusions
 ▷ Left cerebral hemorrhages
 ▷ Left cerebral penetrating injuries

Language forms and relevant hemisphere

▶ Dominant hemisphere
 ▷ Speaking
 ▷ Writing
 ▷ Listening
 ▷ Reading
 ▷ Sign language
 ▷ Hieroglyphics (using pictorial symbols to represent meaning or sounds)
▶ Nondominant hemisphere
 ▷ Singing
 ▷ Prosody (tone of speaking)
 ▷ Gestures (body language)
 ▷ Cursing
 ▷ Music

Nonfluent aphasia: clinical characteristics

Pierre Broca (1824–1880) was a French anatomist.

▶ Also known as
 ▷ Expressive aphasia
 ▷ Motor aphasia
 ▷ Broca's aphasia
 ▷ Anterior aphasia
▶ Language symptoms
 ▷ Slow language output, usually <50 words per minute
 ▷ Dysarthria
 ▷ Impaired naming and repeating
 ▷ Preserved comprehension
▶ Associated symptoms
 ▷ Right-sided hemiparesis

Nonfluent aphasia: pathology

▶ Usually discrete structural lesion
▶ Location of lesion
  ▷ Frontal lobe, in or near Broca's area
  ▷ Left middle cerebral artery distribution
▶ Lesions often involve nearby motor and sensory cortex, and underlying white matters

Paraphasias

▶ Also known as paragrammatism
▶ Using substituted words and inappropriate grammar to produce a fluent but meaningless speech
  ▷ Phonological paraphasia – using phonologically similar words to substitute the target words
  ▷ Neologistic paraphasia – new words created
  ▷ Verbal paraphasia – using categorically related words to similar words to substitute the target words

Pathways of language

Richard Heschl (1824–1881) was an Austrian anatomist.
Carl Wernicke (1848–1905) was a German physician.
Franciscus Sylvius (1614–1672) was a German-Dutch physician and anatomist.

▶ Verbal input – CN VIII → lateral lemniscus → medial geniculate body → Heschl's gyri → Wernicke's area
▶ Visual input – CN II → Occipital cortex → visual association area in left parietal cortex (right occipital signal via corpus callosum) → Wernicke's area
▶ Perisylvian language arc – Wernicke's area → arcuate fasciculus → Broca's area
▶ Motor output (speaking or writing) – Broca's area → motor cortex

Transcortical aphasia

▶ Also known as isolation aphasia
▶ Fluent with echolalia – can only repeat
▶ Isolates language arc from the remaining cortex
▶ Preserved areas surrounding perisylvian arc
▶ Usually associated with anoxia, CO poisoning, and Alzheimer's disease

46 Neuromuscular Disorders and Peripheral Nerve Disorders

Neuromuscular disorders cover a wide range of conditions that affect the control of voluntary muscles. The pathological nature may be nervous, muscular, or junctional. The symptoms are prominently weakness and muscular atrophy. Associated symptoms are cramps, muscle tenderness, stiffness, and fasciculations. Muscle breakdown may cause myoglobinuria, rhabdomyolysis, and acute renal failure.

The peripheral nervous system refers to the parts of the nervous system outside brain and spinal cord. Dysfunction of peripheral nerves may result from damage to axon, body of the neuron, or myelin sheath. Peripheral nerve disorders may be motor, sensory, or both. Considered sometimes part of neuromuscular disorders, the symptoms of peripheral nervous disorders are usually anatomically more focused.

Patients with neuromuscular disorders and peripheral nerve disorders usually maintain intact cognition. The decline of physical ability and severe sensory suffer almost inadvertently lead to emotional distress. Clinical anxiety and depression are common call for psychiatric consult.

Selected conditions reviewed in this chapter are

▶ Muscle diseases
  ▷ Becker's muscular dystrophy
  ▷ Duchenne vs muscular dystrophy
  ▷ Mitochondrial respiratory chain diseases
▶ Neuromuscular junction diseases
  ▷ Myasthenia gravis
  ▷ Tetanus
  ▷ Eaton-Lambert syndrome
▶ Other neuromuscular disorders
  ▷ Amyotrophic lateral sclerosis
  ▷ Guillain-Barré syndrome
▶ Peripheral nerve diseases
  ▷ Carpal tunnel syndrome
  ▷ Femoral nerve injury
  ▷ Radial nerve injury
  ▷ Sciatica
  ▷ Ulnar nerve injury

Amyotrophic lateral sclerosis (ALS)

▶ Motor neuron disease – both upper and lower neuron degeneration
▶ Onset age – over 70 years
▶ Clinical features

▷ Asymmetric paresis
▷ Atrophy with fasciculation
▷ Both bulbar and pseudobulbar palsy
▷ No direct mental impairment
▷ No sensation change
▷ No ocular motility change
▶ Treatment
▷ Riluzole blocks Na$^+$, Ca^{++}, and N-methyl-D-aspartate (NMDA) receptors
▷ Supportive
▶ Prognosis
▷ Progressive and fatal
▷ Average survival time is 3–5 years
▷ The most common cause of death is respiratory failure

Becker's muscular dystrophy

Peter Becker (1908–2000) was a German geneticist.

▶ Also known as benign pseudohypertrophic muscular dystrophy
▶ X-linked recessive inheritance
▶ Clinically similar to Duchenne's, but relatively benign
▶ Onset in teens; slowly progressive muscle weakness of lower extremities and pelvis
▶ No mental retardation
▶ Tests
▷ Creatine phosphokinase (CPK) elevation
▷ Electromyography (EMG)
▷ Muscle biopsy
▷ Genetic study
▶ Treatment – symptomatic and supportive

Botulism

▶ *Clostridium botulinum* toxin inhibits release of acetylcholine at the neuromuscular junction
▶ Causes ocular, papillary, facial, and bulbar palsy
▶ Respiratory paralysis

Carpal tunnel syndrome: clinical features

Jules Tinel (1879–1952) was a French neurologist.
George Phalen (1911–1998) was an American orthopaedist.

▶ Tinel's sign
▷ Also known as distal tingling on percussion
▷ Painful paresthesias when flexor surface of the wrist is tapped
▶ Phalen's sign
▷ Also known as Phalen's maneuver or Phalen's test
▷ Painful paresthesias when wrist is hyperflexed

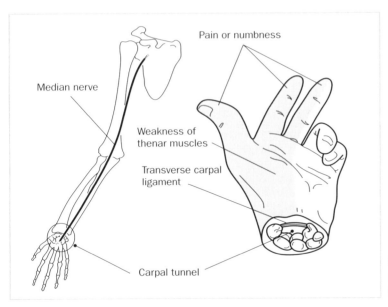

Figure 46–1 Carpal tunnel anatomy and carpal tunnel syndrome.

Carpal tunnel syndrome: pathophysiology (Figure 46–1)

▶ Compression of the median nerve
▶ Symptoms
  ▷ Pain and/or loss of sensation in the wrist, thumb, and index and middle fingers
  ▷ Weakness of the thenar muscles
▶ Causes – repetitive stress injuries, such as
  ▷ Typing
  ▷ Using screwdrivers
  ▷ Prolonged driving
  ▷ Fluid retention
  ▷ Pregnancy

Carpal tunnel syndrome: treatment

▶ Splints
▶ Steroid injections
▶ Surgery – unroof the tunnel

Causes of general weakness

▶ Myasthenia gravis
▶ Myopathy
▶ Lyme disease
▶ Chronic fatigue syndrome
▶ Amyotrophic lateral sclerosis

Duchenne's muscular dystrophy

Guillaume Duchenne (1806–1875) was a French neurologist.
Sir William Gowers (1845–1915) was a British neurologist.

▶ Sex-linked recessive inheritance
▶ Childhood onset
▶ The most common muscular dystrophy of childhood
▶ Loss of dystrophin, a muscle membrane protein
▶ Proximal weakness
▶ Gower's maneuver – requires arms' support to arise from chair or floor
▶ Pseudohypertrophy – muscles enlarged but weak, from fat infiltration
▶ Mental retardation in one-third of cases
▶ Elevated CPK and aldolase

Eaton-Lambert syndrome

Lealdes Eaton (1905–1958) was a U.S. neurologist.
Edward Lambert (1905–) is a U.S. neurophysiologist.

▶ Also known as Lambert-Eaton myasthenic syndrome (LEMS)
▶ A paraneoplastic disorder, associated with small-cell lung cancer
▶ Pathology
  ▷ Antibodies to presynaptic voltage-gated calcium channels
  ▷ Impairs release of acetylcholine from the presynaptic neuromuscular membrane
▶ Symptoms
  ▷ Progressive weakness that usually involves minimally the respiratory muscles and the muscles of the face
  ▷ The proximal parts of the legs and arms are predominantly affected; reflexes are usually reduced or absent
  ▷ Other symptoms – dry mouth, impotence
▶ Treatment – efficacy is limited
  ▷ Corticosteroids
  ▷ Immunosuppressants – azathioprine
  ▷ 3, 4-Diaminopyridine
  ▷ Plasma exchange
  ▷ Intravenous immunoglobulin

Femoral nerve injury

▶ Paresis of knee extensors
▶ Impaired quadriceps deep tendon reflex (DTR)
▶ Sensory loss in the areas of anterior thigh and medial calf

Guillain-Barré syndrome

Georges Guillain (1876–1961) and Jean-Alexandre Barré (1880–1967) were French neurologists.

▶ Also known as
  ▷ Inflammatory polyradiculoneuropathy
  ▷ Acute inflammatory demyelinating polyneuropathy (AIDP)
▶ Preceding gastrointestinal tract (GI) or respiratory infections

▶ Symptoms develop over 1–2 weeks, and resolve over several months; may relapse chronically
▶ Severe weakness – quadriplegia, respiratory paralysis, even locked-in syndrome
▶ No direct mental changes
▶ Cerebrospinal fluid (CSF) – elevated protein, no cellular increase, termed "albumino-cytologic dissociation"
▶ Treatment
  ▷ Plasmapheresis
  ▷ Intravenous immunoglobulins
  ▷ Supportive care

Mitochondrial respiratory chain diseases

▶ Maternal inheritance – the ovum supplies all the zygote's mtDNA
▶ Most involve brain and skeletal muscles
▶ Prevalence 1/10,000
▶ Examples
  ▷ MERRF – myoclonic epilepsy with ragged red fibers; cytochrome c oxidase activity is absent
  ▷ MELAS – mitochondrial encephalopathy, lactic acidosis, and strokelike episodes
  ▷ PEO – progressive external ophthalmoplegia

Myasthenia gravis: clinical symptoms

▶ Ptosis
▶ Ocular paresis with diplopia
▶ Dysarthria
▶ Dysphagia
▶ DTRs are preserved
▶ Fatigue and weakness
▶ No mental change

Myasthenia gravis: diagnosis

▶ Characteristic clinical features
▶ Acetylcholine receptor antibodies
▶ Edrophonium test – edrophonium, a short-acting acetylcholinesterase inhibitor, can temporally reduce the weakness
▶ EMG – abnormal response to repetitive stimulation
▶ Thyroid dysfunction – 50% have thyroid hyperplasia, 10% have thymomas

Myasthenia gravis: treatment

▶ Anticholinesterase agents
▶ Steroids
▶ Plasmapheresis
▶ Thymectomy
▶ Human intravenous immunoglobulin – HIG or IVIG
▶ Immunosuppressant
  ▷ Azathioprine
  ▷ Mycophenolate

Myopathy vs. neuropathy

▶ In myopathy, proximal weakness is more prominent, while in neuropathy, distal weakness

▶ In myopathy, DTR loss is due to loss of muscle strength, which is proportional to weakness; in neuropathy, DTR is lost early

▶ Neuropathy causes anesthesia, while in myopathy, sensation is intact

▶ Autonomic nervous system is often impaired in neuropathy, but normal in myopathy

Myotonic dystrophy

▶ Autosomal dominant inheritance, on chromosome 19

▶ Trinucleotide expansion

▶ Onset in late childhood to young adult

▶ A multisystem disorder – neurologic and nonneurologic changes

▶ Neurologic symptoms
  ▷ Distal and proximal weakness and atrophy
  ▷ Facial muscle atrophy
  ▷ Baldness
  ▷ Myotonia – increased muscle contractility with impaired relaxation
  ▷ DTRs normal or decreased

▶ Psychiatric features
  ▷ Mental retardation
  ▷ Dementia
  ▷ Personality disorders

▶ Other physical symptoms
  ▷ Endocrine organ failure
  ▷ Cardiac abnormalities
  ▷ Subcapsular cataracts

Figure 46–2 Radial nerve anatomy and radial nerve injury.

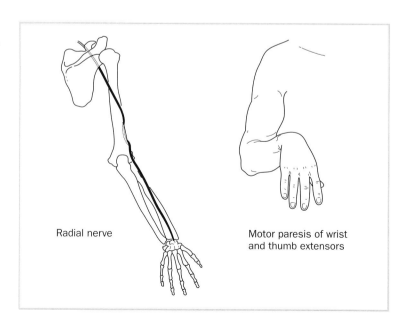

Radial nerve

Motor paresis of wrist and thumb extensors

Radial nerve injury (Figure 46–2)

► Peripheral injury
  ▷ Wrist drop – paresis of wrist and thumb extensor
  ▷ Sensory loss at dorsum of hand
  ▷ Often due to prolonged compression of arm
► Central injury
  ▷ All the above plus loss of DTR
  ▷ Often due to brain abscesses, acquired immunodeficiency syndrome (AIDS), and cerebrovascular accidents
  ▷ If right arm is involved, aphasia may present

Sciatica

► Motor paresis of ankle dorsiflexors and plantar flexors
► Impairment of Achilles tendon reflex
► Sensory loss and pain in the areas of buttock, lateral calf, and foot

Tetanus

► Pathogen is *Clostridium tetani* toxin
► Interferes with inhibitory neurotransmitters
  ▷ gamma-aminobutyric acid (GABA)
  ▷ Glycine
► Sustained muscle spasms
  ▷ Trismus (lockjaw)
  ▷ Rigidity
  ▷ Stimulus-sensitive spasms

Ulnar nerve injury

► Causes
  ▷ Blunt injuries
  ▷ Compression
  ▷ Diabetes
► Clinical features
  ▷ Paresis of finger and thumb adduction
  ▷ Fourth and fifth fingers sensory loss

47 Suicide and Violence

Violent behaviors toward self or others are among the primary concerns in psychiatric practice.

There exists a wide variety of historical and cultural views on suicide. Debates regarding suicide are usually focused on the meaning of suicide in religious, cultural, legal, and medical spheres. In most religious traditions, suicide is seen as a sign of disbelief or offense toward God. In some jurisdictions, suicide, even an incomplete attempt, is considered to be a crime.

The consensual view of modern medicine is that suicide is a serious medical problem, and is almost always associated with mental illness. Medically assisted suicide (euthanasia) is yet another controversial issue. The "right to die" is often defended when facing severe physical suffer of conditions with hope of improvement beyond any possibility. No matter under what circumstance, suicidal behavior has significant impact on the victim's immediate and extended family, friends, and the community. Suicidal behavior also represents a huge cost to the family and the society.

In cases of suicide and violence, crisis intervention is necessary. Continuous psychiatric treatment should focus on improving impulse control, stress management, and hope restoration.

Antipsychotics for acute agitation: oral concentrate vs. injections

▶ Oral concentrate
  ▷ Decreases the patient's feeling of helplessness
▶ Injections
  ▷ Have more predictable absorption
  ▷ Eliminate the need for hepatic metabolism

Date Rape

▶ Also known as acquaintance rape
▶ The rapist is known to the victim, and often romantically involved
▶ Statistics
  ▷ Male students – 11% reported had committed date rape
  ▷ Female students – 16% reported were date raped
▶ Mental health issues
  ▷ Posttraumatic stress disorder (PTSD) symptoms
  ▷ Self-blaming for poor judgment or for provoking the rapist

Depression and suicide

- Hopelessness predicts long-term suicidal risk
- High risk when recovering from depression
- A suicide attempt may fulfill the psychological need for punishment, and sometimes improves depression

Emergency restraints

- Material – leather is the safest type
- Team – at least four staffs should be used
- Psychological support
  - Explain to the patient the purpose of restraining
  - A staff member should always be visible
  - Reassurance should be continued through the process
- Safety
  - At least two restraints should be used
  - The patient's head is raised slightly
  - The restraints should be checked periodically
  - When agitation improved, remove one restraint at a time at 5-minute intervals
- Documentation
  - The reason for the restraints
  - The course of treatment
  - The patient's response

Interview with psychotic patients

- Communication should be straightforward
- Clinical interventions should be explained
- Interview should be structured and modified according to the situation
- Interview should be ready to be terminated if necessary

Parasuicide

- Self-mutilation without wish to die
- Fifty times more common in psychiatric patients than in the general population
- Epidemiology
  - Four percent in psychiatric-hospital patients
  - Thirty percent of oral substances abusers
  - Ten percent of intravenous substances abusers
  - Gender – female to male = 3 to 1
  - Prevalence in psychiatric patients is at least 50 times higher than general population
- The cut
  - Usually delicate, not coarse
  - Usually done in private
- The cutters
  - Most in their 20s
  - Most claim to experience no pain
  - Often give reasons, such as anger, relief of tension, and the wish to die

▶ Mental health considerations
  ▷ Personality disorders
  ▷ Alcohol and substance abuse
  ▷ Introverted anger and tension
  ▷ Unconscious wish to punish self or an introjected object

Psychotherapy in emergency setting

▶ Goal
  ▷ To help patients' self-esteem
▶ Techniques
  ▷ Listen – when don't know what to say
  ▷ Respect – support wounded self-esteem
  ▷ Empathy – as in any psychotherapy
  ▷ Conceptualization – help clarify the history and feeling

Rape of men

▶ Legal concept
  ▷ Sodomy – unnatural intercourse, such as anal intercourse or oral sex; sodomy is often used as a legal term for male rape
  ▷ Rape – classically refers to nonconsensual penile penetration of the vagina; in some states the definition of rape has been changed to wider spectrum of nonconsensual sexual activity and not limited to man-to-woman act
  ▷ Sexual assault – a more general term, sometimes refers to nonvaginal sexual activities
▶ Most common form is man-to-man anal intercourse
▶ Most often happens in prisons or other close institutions
▶ The perpetrator
  ▷ May be heterosexual, bisexual, or homosexual
  ▷ Seeks for discharge of aggression
  ▷ Has emotional gratitude of being a victor or conqueror
▶ The victim
  ▷ Is usually smaller, weaker, and passive
  ▷ Has similar traumatic experience as female victims of rape, including PTSD
  ▷ Some victims fear that they may become homosexual after being man-raped

Rape of women: principles of support and care for the victims

▶ Immediate support and opportunity to ventilate the fear and rage to
  ▷ Family members
  ▷ Physicians
  ▷ Law enforcement officials
▶ Assurance of knowing that she has socially acceptable means of recourse, such as the arrest and conviction of the rapist, can help a rape victim
▶ Individual therapy
  ▷ Usually starts with a supportive approach
  ▷ Restores the victim's sense of adequacy
  ▷ Encourages the sense of control over her life
  ▷ Relieves feelings of helplessness, dependence, and obsession with the assault
  ▷ Group therapy with other rape victims is often very helpful

Rape: epidemiology

▶ Annual prevalence – 0.7–1.5 million
▶ Lifetime chance of being victimized – 1/8

Rape: psychological trip of the victims

▶ Rape is often a life-threatening situation to the victims
▶ During the rape
  ▷ Shock, fright, panic
  ▷ Desperate desire to stay alive
▶ After a rape
  ▷ Shame, humiliation
  ▷ Confusion
  ▷ Fear
  ▷ Rage
  ▷ Symptoms of PTSD
  ▷ Phobia about sexual interaction

Rape: statistics of rapists

▶ Age – 25 to 44 years
▶ Races – 51% white, 47% black, 2% others
▶ Rapists and their victims tend to be from the same ethnic group
▶ Alcohol is involved in 34% rape cases
▶ Gang rape – 10% of cases

Rape: statistics of victims

▶ Age – wide variety, from 15 months to 85 years
▶ Women of 16–24 years are at highest risk
▶ Most common location of rape – near or inside the victim's home
▶ Approximately half of the victims are known to the rapists previously

Risk factors for homicide and aggressive behavior

▶ Upbringing
  ▷ Poor parental model
  ▷ Experience of violence in early childhood
  ▷ Poor education
▶ Life style
  ▷ No significant others available
  ▷ Unstable life style
  ▷ Isolated from social life
▶ Economic and legal situations
  ▷ Low socioeconomic status
  ▷ Unable to use resources of help
  ▷ Multiple arrest history
▶ Psychiatric condition
  ▷ Chronic drug and alcohol use

▷ History of psychiatric hospitalization
▷ History of violence or impulsive behavior
▷ Depression and anxiety
▶ Other
  ▷ Specific plan
  ▷ Available weapon

Suicidal ideas: assessment

▶ All patients must be assessed about suicidal thoughts
▶ Assessment includes
  ▷ Intent
  ▷ Plans
  ▷ Means
  ▷ Perceived consequences
  ▷ Personal history of suicide
  ▷ Family history of suicide
▶ Asking about suicide does NOT increase the risk of suicide

Suicidal prevention contracts

▶ Not recommended for
  ▷ Patients under influence
  ▷ New patients with whom no therapeutic alliance is established yet
  ▷ Emergency settings
  ▷ Psychotic or volatile patients
▶ Be cautious when using suicidal prevention contracts, and not to falsely lower clinical vigilance
▶ Provide no legal protection for the clinicians

Suicidal risk in ethnic groups

▶ In descending order
  ▷ Caucasians, with highest risk in elderly white males
  ▷ Native Americans
  ▷ African-Americans
  ▷ Hispanic Americans
  ▷ Asian-Americans

Suicidal risks in patients with schizophrenia

▶ Young
▶ Male
▶ High premorbid functioning
▶ Akathisia
▶ Abrupt neuroleptic discontinuation
▶ Depression following the resolution of psychotic symptoms
▶ Commanding hallucinations

Suicidality and mental illness

▶ Most people who commit suicide have a diagnosed mental disorder
▶ Any mental disorder – 95%
▶ Mood disorders – 80%, where highest risk is in bipolar mixed state
▶ Alcohol dependence – 25%
▶ Schizophrenia – 10%
▶ Delirium and/or dementia – 5%

Suicide: biological factors

▶ Decreased serotonin in the central nervous system
  ▷ Low level of 5-hydroxyindoleacetic acid (5-HIAA), a serotonin metabolite, in the lumbar cerebrospinal fluid (CSF)
  ▷ Changes in serotonin binding sites in suicide victims
▶ Genetic factors
  ▷ Twin studies and adoption studies provided evidence of genetic impact on suicidal behavior
  ▷ Polymorphism in the gene of tryptophan hydroxylase (TPH) – TPH is involved in the synthesis of serotonin; two alleles, U and L, were identified in human *TPH* gene; the presence of the L allele was associated with a reduced capacity to synthesize serotonin, and an increased risk of suicide attempts

Suicide: biological therapeutics

▶ Antidepressants
  ▷ Treatment for depression may reduce suicidal ideations
  ▷ However, there were reports of induction of suicidal ideations in short term
▶ Lithium
  ▷ Maintenance treatment for bipolar and unipolar depression
▶ Antipsychotics
  ▷ Clozapine – proved to reduce suicidality
  ▷ Other second-generation antipsychotics may also reduce suicidal rate
▶ Electroconvulsive therapy – may reduce suicidal ideation for short term

Suicide: characteristics of completed and uncompleted

▶ Completed suicide
  ▷ Male
  ▷ Greater rate in Caucasian population
  ▷ Over 60 years of age
  ▷ Usually precipitated by a loss
  ▷ Lethal method – firearms, hanging
▶ Uncompleted suicide
  ▷ Female
  ▷ Under age of 35 years
  ▷ Low lethality of method – overdose, wrist cut
  ▷ Ten percent will finally be successful

Suicide: chronological risks

▶ Within 3 months of the onset of a major depressive episode
▶ Previous attempt
▶ The risk of a second attempt is highest within 3 months of the first attempt

Suicide: Durkheim's theory

Emile Durkheim (1858–1917) was a French sociologist.

▶ Three social categories of suicide – egoistic, altruistic, and anomic
▶ Egoistic suicide
  ▷ Socially isolated individuals
  ▷ Lack of sense of social involvement and integration
▶ Altruistic suicide
  ▷ Individuals with excessive integration into a social group
▶ Anomic suicide
  ▷ Socially integrated individuals
▶ Distressed because of change of social stability, or the individual shifting to a different socioeconomic level where the customary norm is no longer familiar to him or her

Suicide: epidemiology

▶ In the United States
  ▷ Annual mortality is 30,000, or 12.5 per 100,000
  ▷ Increased rate in adolescent and elderly in recent years
  ▷ Ranked the 8th in the overall cause of death
▶ Countries with high suicide rate (suicide belt)
  ▷ Scandinavia, Switzerland, Germany, Austria, the eastern European countries, and Japan
  ▷ Suicide rates are more than 25 per 100,000
▶ Countries with low suicide rate
  ▷ Spain, Italy, Ireland, Egypt, and the Netherlands
  ▷ Lower than 10 per 100,000

Suicide: medical conditions that increase the risk

▶ Multiple sclerosis
▶ Huntington's disease
▶ Seizure disorders
▶ Spinal cord injury
▶ Cancers
▶ Human immunodeficiency virus (HIV) and acquired immunodeficiency syndrome (AIDS)
▶ Chronic obstructive pulmonary disease
▶ Systemic lupus erythematosus
▶ Pain syndromes
▶ Peptic ulcer disease

Suicide: National Strategy for Suicide Prevention

- ▶ Established in 2001 in National Institutes of Health (NIH)
- ▶ A framework for suicide prevention for the nation
- ▶ Primary goals
  - ▷ Promote awareness of suicide as a public health problem
  - ▷ Develop support and reduce stigma
  - ▷ Develop suicide prevention programs
  - ▷ Reduce access to lethal means
  - ▷ Improve access to mental health services
  - ▷ Improve surveillance system

Suicide: physicians

- ▶ Physicians have a higher suicide rate than general population
- ▶ Female physicians are at higher risk
- ▶ Physicians who commit suicide
  - ▷ Have a mental disorder, most often depressive disorder, substance dependence, or both
  - ▷ More often by substance overdoses and less often by firearms than general population
- ▶ Physician specialties
  - ▷ Psychiatrists are at greatest risk
  - ▷ Ophthalmologists the second
  - ▷ Anesthesiologists the third

Suicide: psychiatric evaluation

- ▶ Current psychiatric symptoms
- ▶ Past suicidal and self-injurious behavior
- ▶ Past treatment history, particularly therapeutic relationships
- ▶ Family history
- ▶ Current psychosocial situation
- ▶ Psychosocial strengths and vulnerabilities

Suicide: psychosocial protective factors

- ▶ Children in the home
- ▶ Being pregnant
- ▶ Religiosity
- ▶ Positive social support
- ▶ Positive therapeutic relationship
- ▶ Reality test ability

Suicide: psychosocial risk factors

- ▶ Unemployment
- ▶ Living alone
- ▶ Lack of social support
- ▶ Domestic violence
- ▶ Recent deterioration in socioeconomic status
- ▶ Recent life stressors

Suicide: psychological theories

▶ Sigmund Freud's theory
  ▷ Suicide is an introjected, emotionally charged form of aggression
  ▷ Probably a repressed desire of homicide
▶ Karl Menninger's theory
  ▷ Suicide is an inverted desire of homicide
  ▷ Described self-directed Thanatos (death instinct, a Freudian concept)
  ▷ Described three components of hostility in suicide – the wishes to kill, to be killed, and to die
▶ Contemporary theories
  ▷ Act on fantasies and wishes for what may happen after suicide – revenge, punishment, sacrifice, escape, rebirth, reunion with the dead, etc.
  ▷ Overwhelming affects (rage, guilt)
  ▷ Identification with a suicide victim
  ▷ Group dynamics – may be associated with mass suicides

Violent behavior: differential diagnosis

▶ Substance induced
  ▷ Alcohol idiosyncratic intoxication
▶ Personality disorder
  ▷ Antisocial
  ▷ Paranoid
  ▷ Obsessive compulsive
▶ Schizophrenia
  ▷ Catatonic
  ▷ Disorganized
▶ Infections
▶ Cerebral neoplasms
▶ Dissociative disorders
▶ Impulse control disorders
▶ Temporal lobe epilepsy, bipolar disorder
▶ Uncontrollable violence secondary to interpersonal stress

48 Abuse and Neglect

Abuse and neglect are harmful acts toward individuals who are vulnerable to maltreatment or dependent on others' support and care. Both abuse and neglect are usually not frank assaults that are severe enough to be imminently life threatening. Victims often tolerate the maltreatment over significant periods without reporting or seeking for help. The accumulated psychological and physical impairment through repeated abuse and neglect can be profound and irreversible at times.

Battered children

▶ Children vulnerable to abuse are often
  ▷ Premature
  ▷ Mentally retarded
  ▷ Physically disabled
  ▷ "Difficult" – cry excessively, demanding, hyperactive

Child abuse and neglect: socioeconomic risks

▶ Overcrowded housing
▶ Poverty
▶ Social isolation
▶ Unemployment
▶ Lack of a support system

Child abuse: characteristics of abusive parents

▶ Abusive parents were often abused in their own childhood, or were exposed to violent home lives for a long term with harsh punishment and cruel treatment
▶ Abusive parents often have substance abuse and mental health problems
▶ Mothers are often the physical abusers, while fathers are often the sexual abusers or mixed physical and sexual abusers
▶ Eighty percent abusers live with the abused children
▶ Eighty percent abused children live with married parents
▶ Abusive parents have inappropriate expectations of their children, with a reversal of dependence needs; parents treat an abused child as if the child were older than the parents
▶ Abusive parents often have inappropriate dependence needs, such as turning to children for reassurance, nurturing, and comfort

Domestic violence: risk factors for abusers

- ▶ Male
- ▶ Antisocial personality disorder
- ▶ History of depression
- ▶ Abuse alcohol or drugs
- ▶ Young
- ▶ Low socioeconomic status
- ▶ Low educational level

Domestic violence: risk factors for victims

- ▶ Female
- ▶ Single, separated, or divorced
- ▶ Aged between 17 and 28 years
- ▶ Low socioeconomic status
- ▶ Abuses alcohol or drugs
- ▶ Has been abused before

Incest relations

- ▶ Sexual relations between close blood relatives, or other social kinship bond that is culturally regarded as formal family relations
- ▶ Incest is a taboo prohibited in almost all cultures, only with different formalities
- ▶ Biological factors
  - ▷ Inbreeding raises risk of unmasking genes that are pathological and recessive
- ▶ Older male–younger female incest
  - ▷ Father–daughter is the most common form (75% of reported cases)
  - ▷ Stepfathers, uncles, and older siblings are also common perpetrators
  - ▷ The mother in the house is often weak, sick, or absent
  - ▷ The daughter in the incest relation often takes on the role of the weak mother
- ▶ Mother–son incest
  - ▷ The rarest form of incest
  - ▷ Often indicates severe psychopathology
- ▶ Father–son and mother–daughter incest
  - ▷ Rarely reported
  - ▷ The family is usually severely disturbed, with violence, alcohol problem, and antisocial behavior

Incest: socioeconomic consideration

- ▶ Reported more frequently among families of low socioeconomic status
- ▶ Often hidden by families of high socioeconomic status
- ▶ Incestuous behavior has been associated with
  - ▷ Alcohol abuse
  - ▷ Mental disorders
  - ▷ Intellectual deficiencies
  - ▷ Overcrowding that provides increased physical proximity
  - ▷ Rural or isolative environment

Neglect of child: parents

▶ Parents who neglect their children often are
  ▷ Young and inexperienced
  ▷ Socially isolated
  ▷ Lacking knowledge
  ▷ Impoverished
  ▷ Unemployed
  ▷ From single-parent family
  ▷ From chaotic, abusive, and neglectful homes
  ▷ Emotionally stressed and depressed
  ▷ Abusing substance
  ▷ Resentful and paranoid

Neglect of child: signs of a neglected child

▶ Psychosocial signs of neglect
  ▷ Lack of appropriate social interaction
  ▷ Being indiscriminately affectionate or socially withdrawn
  ▷ Being irritable
  ▷ Symptoms of conduct disorder
  ▷ Binge eating or bizarre eating behaviors such as pica
▶ Physical signs of neglect
  ▷ Failure to thrive
  ▷ Malnutrition
  ▷ Poor skin hygiene
  ▷ Chronic infections
  ▷ Reversible endocrinological changes – decreased growth hormone

Sexual harassment

▶ Refers to behavior of a sexual nature that is unwelcomed by the victim
▶ Examples
  ▷ Abusive language
  ▷ Requests for sexual favors
  ▷ Sexual jokes
  ▷ Staring
  ▷ Ogling
  ▷ Giving massages
▶ Gender
  ▷ Man harassing woman – the most common
  ▷ Man harassing man – reported
  ▷ Woman harassing man – rare
▶ Policies to reduce sexual harassment at workplace
  ▷ Distribution of educational material
  ▷ Employers are obligated to investigate every complaint
  ▷ Appropriate organizational responses to confirmed cases

Stalking

▶ Stalking is a form of harassment by obsessively following, observing, or contacting the victim; often suggesting potential violence
▶ Gender
  ▷ Most stalkers are males
  ▷ Stalkers of both genders are likely to act out violently toward the victims
▶ Best deterrent
  ▷ Report to law enforcement agencies

49 Legal and Ethical Issues

Psychiatry and the law intersect and converge over the history. Issues of medical matters in the past may become legal matters today. Some interactions between psychiatrists and patients that were accepted by the society or even believed therapeutic in the past may now considered unethical or even illegal. The consensus of the society and medical profession has experienced significant evolution over the past century. This chapter reviews important issues of contemporary legal and ethical concerns in psychiatry. After all, the very best core of psychiatry as a profession is that to always put the patients' safety and health at first.

Basic bioethics

▶ Autonomy
   ▷ Patients are not coerced, and are given adequate information to make decisions
▶ Beneficence
   ▷ Fiduciary responsibility to patients, acting in the patient's best interests
▶ Nonmaleficence
   ▷ Do no harm
▶ Justice
   ▷ Nondiscrimination, equitable distribution of resources and benefits

Breaching the confidentiality

▶ Under the following circumstances, breaching the confidentiality may be appropriate
   ▷ Patient waiver
   ▷ Emergency situation
   ▷ Reportable disease
   ▷ Commitment proceeding
   ▷ Incompetence proceeding

Competency vs. capacity

▶ Competency is a legal status declared only by a judge, not a physician
▶ A physician may perform clinical assessment on capacity of decision making
▶ Capacity evaluation is used as evidence in legal proceedings, and in practice often indicates the likely outcome of legal proceedings
▶ Capacity evaluation should be task specific, unless the patient is found to be globally incapable

▶ Most common clinical capacity evaluation is regarding treatment decision making; a patient is capable of making treatment decision if he/she has
  ▷ Factual understanding of the information
  ▷ Appreciation of consequences of accepting or rejecting treatment
  ▷ Ability to manipulate the information rationally and to come to a decision logically
  ▷ Ability to communicate of a preference

Confidentiality in the court

▶ Psychiatrists have an ongoing obligation to treatment confidentiality
▶ A patient's right to exclude certain material from judicial settings testimony, e.g., information revealed by psychiatrist or counselor; this is called "testimonial privilege"
▶ Exceptions to testimonial privilege
  ▷ Military court
  ▷ Child abuse case
  ▷ Civil commitment
  ▷ Court-ordered examinations
  ▷ Competency proceedings
  ▷ Malpractice case brought by the patient
  ▷ Situation in which patient enters mental condition into proceedings, e.g., not guilty due to insanity

Confidentiality regarding human immunovirus infection

▶ Human immunovirus (HIV) test should not be given without informed consent
▶ The results of an HIV test should be shared with no one except members of a medical team and potential victims, such as potential and past sexual or intravenous (IV) substance use partners
▶ The patient should be advised against disclosing the results of HIV testing to people to avoid discrimination
▶ Physicians responsibility of protection
▶ A treating physician knows that an HIV infected patient is putting another person at risk should act on protection, including involuntary hospitalization or to notify the potential victim

Ethical justification of randomization in medical research

▶ Equipoise – equal degree of doubt about which intervention is more efficacious, or has fewer side effects, or both
  ▷ Theoretical equipoise – the equipoise accepted within the scientific community
  ▷ Clinical equipoise – the equipoise accepted within the expert treating community

Four Ds in malpractice

▶ Four Ds are required proof of allegation in malpractice cases
  ▷ Duty to care, i.e., has established doctor–patient relationship
  ▷ Deviation from the accepted standard of care
  ▷ Damage happened to the patient
  ▷ Damage was directly caused by the deviation

Guilty but mentally ill

▶ A plead essentially similar to the verdict of guilty
▶ The intention of this plead is usually seeking to ensure access to treatment

Informed Consent

▶ To assure an effective informed consent, the patient should be provided sufficient information to make decision, which include the following
  ▷ Indications for treatment
  ▷ The nature of the proposed treatment
  ▷ The possible risks and adverse effects of the treatment
  ▷ The inability to predict the results of treatment
  ▷ Alternative treatments available, including no treatment
  ▷ Risks of not having treatment

Involuntary hospitalization

▶ The doctrine of *parens patriae* (father of his country) allows the state to act as surrogate parent
▶ Involuntary hospitalization does not preclude the patient's competency in refusing medication
▶ Right to refuse medication is overridden in emergency situations

Irresistible impulse

▶ Also known as "policeman-at-the elbow law"
▶ A defense states that the defendant should not be held liable because of the inability of controlling the act, as if the accused would have committed the act even if a policeman had been at the accused's elbow
▶ Often associated with some forms of mental disturbance
▶ Distinguished from "not guilty due to insanity" in that it may plead only diminished responsibility and probable milder punishment

M'Naghten rule

In an 1843 British court, Daniel M'Naghten was found not guilty by the reason of insanity due to his delusions of persecution when committing the crime of murder.

▶ A rule by the British courts granted not guilty by the reason of insanity
▶ Commonly known as "the right-wrong test"
▶ According to M'Naghten rule, to establish a defense of the ground of insanity, clear evidence is required that at the time of committing the act, the defender
  ▷ Suffered from disease of the mind
  ▷ Did not know the nature of the act he was doing
  ▷ Did not know what he was doing was wrong

Management of seductive patient

▶ First, the therapist should examine his/her own behavior for possible countertransference
▶ Consider exploring the meaning of the patient's behavior

▶ Observe the professional ethical code and boundary
▶ Assess the potential harmfulness to the therapeutic alliance

Negligent prescription practices

▶ Common negligent prescription issues
  ▷ Prescribing out of indications
  ▷ Exceeding recommended dosages
  ▷ Failing to adjust the medication level to therapeutic levels
  ▷ Inappropriate mixing of drugs
  ▷ Failing to disclose adverse effects
  ▷ Failure to recognize and treat adverse effects
  ▷ Failure to monitor a patient's compliance
  ▷ Prescribing addictive drugs to vulnerable patients
  ▷ Failure to refer for expert consultation
  ▷ Negligent withdrawal of treatment
▶ Informed consent
  ▷ Substitute health care decision maker for cognitively incompetent patients
  ▷ Informed consent on each time of medication change
▶ Frequency of visits
  ▷ According to their clinical needs
  ▷ The longer the time interval between visits, the greater the chance of adverse reactions
  ▷ Recommended longest interval – 6 months
  ▷ The psychiatrist is duty bound to provide appropriate treatment, regardless of managed care or other payment policies

Not guilty due to insanity

▶ At the time an act was committed, due to the defect of mind, the individual did not have the ability to
  ▷ Know that the nature of the act was wrong
  ▷ Control over impulse/behavior

O'Connor vs. Donaldson

K. Donaldson was a psychotic patient who was involuntarily confined for 15 years in Florida State Hospital. J. O'Connor was a treating psychiatrist.

▶ A landmark decision in mental health law. The 1976 case established the legal doctrine of right to refuse treatment
▶ The Supreme Court ruled that
  ▷ Harmless mentally ill patients cannot be confined against their will
  ▷ Mental illness alone cannot justify a hospitalization against the patient's will
  ▷ Involuntarily confined patients must be considered dangerous to themselves or others, or unable to care for themselves

Physician-assisted suicide

▶ Highly controversial issues under debate
▶ Currently, no legal or professional codes support euthanasia or assisted suicide

▶ Psychiatrists view suicide as an irrational behavior and almost always influenced by mental illness, usually depression
▶ Evaluation upon request for suicide
  ▷ Depression and other psychiatric conditions
  ▷ Decision-making competence
▶ Treatment and management upon request for suicide
  ▷ Discuss with patient about the option of treatment, including removal of unwanted treatment
  ▷ Consultation with other professionals
  ▷ Explain why physician-assisted suicide is not compatible with the principle of care protocol

Privacy Rule and Security Rule in HIPAA

▶ HIPAA – Health Insurance Portability and Accountability Act of 1996
▶ Privacy Rule applies to all protected health information in all forms
▶ Mandatory disclosures are
  ▷ To patients
  ▷ To U.S. Department of Health and Human Service (HHS)
▶ Privacy Rule preempts state law unless
  ▷ HHS determines contrary state law is not preempted
  ▷ State law covers mandatory reporting
  ▷ State law is more stringent than Privacy Rule
▶ Security Rule applies only to electronic data that contains protected health information

Professional boundaries

▶ The physician is obligated to put the best interests of the patient ahead of the physician's interest
▶ Any behavior that blurs the physician's interest with the patient's interest may cause boundary violations
▶ It is the physician's responsibility, not the patient's, to maintain appropriate boundaries
▶ Commonly concerned violation of boundaries
  ▷ Sexual contact between a current patient and a physician of any specialty, or former patient and a psychiatrist
  ▷ Business dealings and avoidable social contact between doctor and patient

Reporting duties

▶ The list of conditions mandate report has been growing in recent years; reporting duties vary from state to state, but in general may include the following
  ▷ Abuse and neglect – child, elderly, disabled
  ▷ Impaired driving ability
  ▷ Sexually transmitted diseases and other communicable diseases
  ▷ Impaired health-care professional
▶ The patient should be informed of the reporting requirement and the content of the report

Seclusion and restraint

▶ Seclusion and restraint require
  ▷ Written order from medical authority (usually physician)
  ▷ Regular reevaluation of clinical condition and necessity of extension
▶ Indications for restraint
  ▷ To prevent imminent harm
  ▷ To prevent damage
  ▷ As part of ongoing behavioral modification
▶ Indications for seclusion
  ▷ Indications for restraints when applicable
  ▷ To avoid sensory stimulation
  ▷ At patient's request
▶ Contraindications for seclusion and restraints
  ▷ Destabilized medical and psychiatric conditions
  ▷ As discretionary punishment
  ▷ Only to meet staff needs

Standard of care in malpractice cases

▶ Usually the standard of care is established by
  ▷ Expert witnesses
  ▷ Reference to journal articles and professional textbooks
  ▷ Practice guidelines by professional organizations

Statutory rape

▶ Having sexual intercourse with a person under the age of consent is considered unlawful
▶ Forcible behavior is not required; sexual relation may otherwise be considered legal except the age
▶ Age of consent refers to the mental age, not the chronological age; therefore a mentally retarded adult may be considered under age of consent.
▶ Qualified circumstances where sex with under aged is not a crime
  ▷ Both parties are minors
  ▷ The parties are married
  ▷ The parties are close in age (Romeo and Juliet laws)

Tarasoff I and II

▶ Tatiana Tarasoff was the victim in the case of Tarasoff vs. Regents of the University of California (1976). The perpetrator was a patient treated at UC Berkeley's Cowell Memorial Hospital, and the intent of killing was confided to his psychologist a few months before the murder occured.
▶ Tarasoff I (1974)
  ▷ Duty to warn the intended victims of dangerous patients
▶ Tarasoff II (1976)
  ▷ Duty to warn the intended victims of dangerous patients
  ▷ Duty to take steps to protect the intended victims, such as notifying police, warning the intended victim, and/or committing the patient to inpatient treatment

Worker's compensation

▶ The assumption
  ▷ The stresses at work cause or worsen mental illnesses, which result in disability
  ▷ Patients are entitled to compensation for job-related disabilities
▶ The burden to the evaluating psychiatrist
  ▷ Seeking to establish the causal relationship between the illness and the work related occurrence
▶ The caution
  ▷ Malingerers may seek financial gain for purported psychological injury
  ▷ The evaluation may be seen as an integrate part of treatment; unfavorable results may impair therapeutic alliance

50 Cultural and Social Psychiatry

Cultural psychiatry, sometimes also termed cross-cultural psychiatry, studies the cultural and ethnic context of mental disorder. Issues of interest include epidemiology and clinical presentations of mental disorders in different cultures, the study of migrant populations and ethnic diversity within countries, and the appropriateness of psychiatric classifications to different cultures and ethnic groups.

The early concerns of cultural psychiatry were initiated from Colonial interest. Today, the process of globalization may encourage or even force people to adapt to the change of cultural norm and social acceptance to their traditional pattern of thoughts and behavior. The flexibility and strategy of adaption may play a crucial role in the manifestation and prognosis of mental illness.

Culture-bound syndromes are recurrent, culture- or locality-specific pattern of abnormality in inner experience and behavior. DSM-IV-TR provides an outline for cultural formulation and description of 25 culture-bound syndromes. Frequently mentioned culture-bound syndromes include

▶ Amafufanyane
▶ Amok
▶ Ataque de nervios
▶ Bilis and colera
▶ Boufée delirante
▶ Brain fag
▶ Dhat
▶ Falling-out or blacking out
▶ Ghost sickness
▶ Koro
▶ Latah
▶ Mal de ojo
▶ Pibloktoq
▶ Shenjing shuairuo
▶ Shen-k'uei or shenkui
▶ Susto
▶ Taijin kyofusho
▶ Zar

Social psychiatry refers to mental health in the context of communities and societies. Studies in social psychiatry concern the contribution of social factors to the development of illness, the social consequences of mental disorders, and the use of social resource for treatment and preventive measures. Cultural psychiatry is often considered a branch of social psychiatry. In the era of evidence-based paradigm, epidemiology has taken an ever centralized role in social psychiatry.

Altruism

▶ A behavior that increases the reproductive success of the group at the cost of sacrificing the initiator
▶ Occurs in mammals as well as humans
▶ Theories
  ▷ Darwinian theory – altruistic traits may be selected against and finally disappear
  ▷ Evolution in group selection – altruistic groups survive over the selfish groups

Amafufanyane (Figure 50-1)

▶ A culture-bound syndrome occurs in Zulu population of southern Africa.
▶ Clinical features
  ▷ Sleep paralysis
  ▷ Abdominal pain
  ▷ Blindness
  ▷ Shouting and sobbing
  ▷ Amnesia
  ▷ Pseudoseizure
▶ Often occurs in young females, influenced by witchcraft, contains sexual content

Amok (Figure 50-2)

From Malay – amuk, mad with rage

▶ A culture-bound syndrome occurs in population of Malaysia, Indonesia, Laos, and Philippines

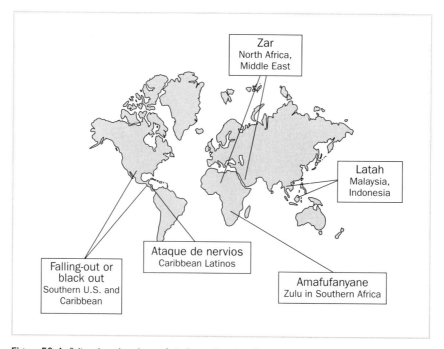

Figure 50-1 Culture-bound syndromes featuring panic or hysteric attacks – approximate geographic distributions.

▶ Clinical features
  ▷ Sudden outburst of rage
  ▷ Running out
  ▷ Aggressive and violent behavior toward people and self
▶ May be precipitated by demon possession, or running out of a shameful situation

Asian patients

▶ Tend to have more somatic complaints
▶ Often expect rapid relief of symptoms
▶ Are cautious about potential side effects by western medicine
▶ Typically believe polypharmacy is more effective
▶ May use herbal medicines
▶ May respond to lower doses of tricyclic antidepressants, clozapine, and lithium
▶ More likely to have extrapyramidal symptoms

Ataque de nervios (Figure 50–1)

From Spanish – attack of nerves

▶ A culture-bound syndrome occurs among Latinos from the Caribbean
▶ Clinical features
  ▷ Uncontrollable shouting
  ▷ Crying episodes
  ▷ Trembling

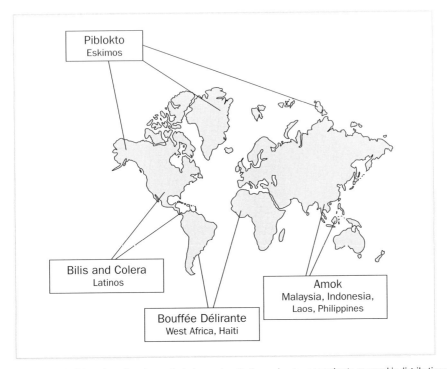

Figure 50–2 Culture-bound syndromes featuring acute agitation and rage – approximate geographic distributions.

▷ Sense of heat rising from chest moving toward head
▷ Amnesia of the episode

Bilis and colera (See Figure 50–2 on page 373)

▶ A culture-bound syndrome among Latinos
▶ Anger, rage, tension, headache, screaming, trembling, stomach disturbances

Bouffée délirante (See Figure 50–2 on page 373)

Originally an old French diagnosis; also translated as "acute delusional psychosis"

▶ A culture-bound syndrome found in West Africa and Haiti
▶ Clinical symptoms
  ▷ Sudden outburst of agitation
  ▷ Aggressive behavior
  ▷ Confusion

Brain fag (Figure 50–3)

"Fag" – to droop, decline; from Middle English

▶ A syndrome encountered mostly in West Africa
▶ Symptoms
  ▷ Depressed mood
  ▷ Difficulty in concentration

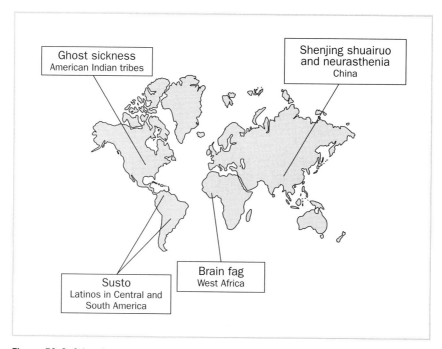

Figure 50-3 Culture-bound syndromes featuring chronic depression and somatoform symptoms – approximate geographic distributions.

▷ Vague somatic symptoms
▷ Fatigue
▶ Generally believed to be a depression-anxiety spectrum condition

Chicago study

▶ A clinical study examined admissions in psychiatric hospitals in Chicago between 1922 and 1934
▶ The study found that first hospital admissions for schizophrenia were highest among persons from the lowest socioeconomic group
▶ Concepts developed based on the findings
▷ Social causation theory – low socioeconomic status causes mental illness
▷ Social selection theory and drift hypothesis – mental illness makes a person "drift" downward in socioeconomic status

Cultural determinism: history and current consensus

Abraham Kardiner (1891–1981) was a U.S. psychoanalyst.
Bronislaw Malinowski (1884–1942) was a Polish anthropologist.
Margaret Mead (1901–1978) was a U.S. anthropologist, known for her research on Samoa culture that became a theoretical foundation of cultural determinism as well as sexual revolution in 1960s.

▶ Sigmund Freud and Carl Jung
▷ Traced human behaviors back to early human artifacts
▷ However, in large they believed adult personality is determined during childhood
▶ Abraham Kardiner
▷ Each culture is associated with a common personality structure, or national character
▷ His theory was, however, used to foster political and discriminatory attitude
▶ Bronislaw Malinowski
▷ Challenged the universality of the Oedipus complex
▶ Margaret Mead
▷ Mead believed that a society can create deviance by encouraging or condemning certain behavior patterns
▷ Mead argued that the general casualness of the whole society may make personality maturation easier and healthier; by this she referred mainly to the societal acceptance of open, nonpossessive sexual relationship
▷ Research has shown, however, that Mead's methodology was flawed, and her conclusions were questionable
▶ Current consensus
▷ A clinically meaningful prediction about personality cannot be made on the basis of cultural background alone
▷ Personality may reflect a culture's configuration as people tend to assume a society's expected behavior pattern

Cultural formulation

▶ The formulation of a cultural assessment for diagnosis and care is recommended in DSM-IV-TR

▶ Cultural identity
  ▷ Ethnicity
  ▷ Involvement with original and host cultures
▶ Cultural explanation
  ▷ Explanations and idioms used in the culture in regarding symptoms and illness
▶ Cultural factors impacting patients' psychosocial functioning
▶ Cultural differences between the patient and clinician; this may cause problems in
  ▷ Communicating and negotiating a patient–clinician relationship
  ▷ Distinguishing between normal and pathological behaviors

Death in ethnic groups: leading causes of death associated with behavioral concerns

▶ Homicide
  ▷ Ranked first in Black males of ages 15–34
▶ Suicide
  ▷ Ranked second in all non-Blacks and Black females of ages 15–34
▶ Human immunovirus (HIV)
  ▷ Ranked second in Black males of ages 35–44

Dhat (Figure 50–4)

According to old Hindu tradition, it takes forty drops of blood to create a drop of bone marrow and forty drops of bone marrow to create a drop of sperm.

▶ Found in the Indian and Pakistani cultures
▶ Male patients suffer from premature ejaculation or impotence, and passing whitish fluid, which is believed to be semen, in the urine
▶ Symptoms
  ▷ Guilt associated with excessive masturbation
  ▷ Anxiety and dysphoria
  ▷ Weakness and fatigue
  ▷ Palpitations
  ▷ Insomnia
  ▷ Subjective feeling of shortening of penis
▶ Some called it "semen-loss anxiety" comparible to shen-k'uei
▶ Treatment
  ▷ Cognitive-behavior therapy
  ▷ Treatment for comorbid conditions

Downward drift hypothesis

▶ A hypothetic theory offered explanation for the finding that schizophrenic victims, differing from normal patterns, have a lower socioeconomic status than their parents
▶ It proposes that the functional impairment due to the illness leads to a downward drift in socioeconomic status

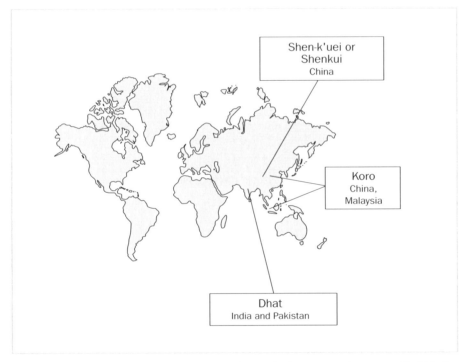

Figure 50–4 Culture-bound syndromes featuring anxiety of genital disturbance – approximate geographic distributions.

Falling-out or blacking out (See Figure 50–1 on page 372)

▶ Occurs primarily in southern United States and Caribbean population
▶ Symptoms
  ▷ Sudden collapse
  ▷ Dizziness
  ▷ Pseudo-neurologic symptoms
▶ May correspond to conversion disorder or dissociative disorder

Gender and mental illness

▶ More popular in females
  ▷ Major depression
  ▷ Borderline personality disorder
  ▷ Panic disorder
▶ More popular in males
  ▷ Substance related disorders
  ▷ Antisocial personality disorder.
▶ No gender preference
  ▷ Schizophrenia
  ▷ Bipolar disorders

Ghost sickness (See Figure 50–3 on page 374)

▶ Occurs in American-Indian tribes
▶ Symptoms
  ▷ Bad dreams
  ▷ Weakness
  ▷ Loss of appetite
  ▷ Fainting and dizziness
  ▷ Fear and anxiety
  ▷ Confusion
  ▷ Loss of consciousness
▶ Attributed to preoccupation with death and the deceased; may be associated with witchcraft

Koro (See Figure 50–4 on page 377)

From Malay – head of a turtle

▶ A culture-bound syndrome found in males of China and Malaysia
▶ Symptoms
  ▷ Intense anxiety
  ▷ Senses as if genital retracted back into the body
▶ Some patients use devices to attach the genital to the wall to prevent such retraction

Landmark psychiatric therapeutics: the initial introductions

Though fluoxetine is popularly believed to be the first serotonin selective reuptake inhibitor (SSRI), fluvoxamine was launched in 1984 in Switzerland and was not approved by Food and Drug Association (FDA) until 1997.

▶ Electroconvulsive treatment
  ▷ The first biological therapy
  ▷ Introduced in 1938
▶ Lithium
  ▷ The first psychotropic agent
  ▷ Introduced in 1949
▶ Chlorpromazine (Thorazine)
  ▷ The first antipsychotic
  ▷ FDA approved in 1954
  ▷ Some divided the field of psychiatry as "pre-" and "post-Thorazine era"
▶ Imipramine (Tofranil)
  ▷ The first tricyclic antidepressant and the first antidepressant
  ▷ Introduced in 1957
▶ Fluoxetine (Prozac, Sarafem)
  ▷ Arguably the first SSRI
  ▷ FDA approved in 1987

Latah (See Figure 50–1 on page 372)

▶ A culture-bound syndrome occurs in Malaysia and Indonesia
▶ It is more frequent in middle-aged women

▶ Symptoms
  ▷ Startle response
  ▷ Intense light reactions
  ▷ Echolalia and echopraxis
▶ Dissociative or trancelike behavior

Levels of prevention

▶ Primary prevention
  ▷ Preventative treatment before the onset of a disease
  ▷ Reduces incidence by removing causative agents, enhancing host resistance, and blocking the transmission
  ▷ Example – immunizations, iodine in salt, public education for healthy life style
▶ Secondary prevention
  ▷ Treatment at the early stage of illness
  ▷ Reduces prevalence by shortening the duration of illness
▶ Tertiary prevention
  ▷ Maintenance treatment and rehabilitation
  ▷ Reduces prevalence of disability
  ▷ Enables chronic patients to attain best potential of functioning

Mal de ojo

From Spanish – evil eye

▶ A culture-bound syndrome in Mediterranean cultures
▶ Symptoms
  ▷ Crying without a reason
  ▷ Vomiting
  ▷ Diarrhea
▶ Often occurs in children

Midtown Manhattan study

▶ A study sampled from New York City in 1954
▶ The objective was to determine the effects of demographic and social factors on mental health
▶ Socioeconomic status was the single most significant variable affecting mental illness

National Alliance for the Mentally III (NAMI)

▶ The largest grassroots mental health organization
▶ Mission – to improving the lives of persons with mental illness
▶ Members – usually families and relatives of patients
▶ Main activities
  ▷ Public education and information providing
  ▷ Peer support activities for patients and families
  ▷ Advocacy on the federal level for public visibility, and lobbying for service improvement

National Institute of Mental Health Epidemiologic Catchment Area Survey (NIMH-ECA)

▶ Major findings
  ▷ Approximately 15% of the population of the United States is affected by mental disorders
  ▷ The majority of mental health conditions are treated by primary care physicians; only one-fifth of those persons received specialty care
  ▷ Prevalence of depression is twice as high for females
  ▷ Males are more likely to have alcohol dependence
  ▷ Substance abuse is more common in persons under age 30 years
▶ Significance comparing to previous studies
  ▷ Reliable diagnosis through better diagnostic tools and more specific criteria
  ▷ Much larger samples are used than in the previously described studies

New Haven study

▶ Findings
  ▷ Neurosis was associated with high socioeconomic status
  ▷ Psychosis was associated with low socioeconomic status
  ▷ Low socioeconomic status and downward drift were associated with psychiatric disability

Piblokto (See Figure 50–2 on page 372)

▶ A culture-bound syndrome in Eskimos
▶ Symptoms
  ▷ Screaming
  ▷ Tearing off clothing
  ▷ Running out in the snow
  ▷ Hysterical seizures
  ▷ Echo phenomena
  ▷ Amnesia

Prevalence of mental illness in the United States (all listed in approximate number)

▶ All mental illness – one-fourth of adult population have at least one condition; among them about half have more than one condition
▶ Depression – 10%
▶ Bipolar disorder – 3%
▶ Schizophrenia – 1%
▶ All anxiety disorders – 1/5 (20%)
▶ Panic disorders – 3%
▶ Obsessive-compulsive disorder (OCD) – 1%
▶ Suicide – 1/10,000 died of suicide

Shenjing shuairuo and neurasthenia (See Figure 50–3 on page 374)

From Chinese – nerve weakness
George Beard (1939–1983) was a U.S. neurologist

▶ Shenjing shuairuo is a culture-bound syndromes found in China
▶ Shenjing shuairuo has also been translated as "neurasthenia"
▶ Neurasthenia, however, when originally coined by George Beard, was meant to be a culture-bound condition that appeared in Americans, and typically upper class with sedentary jobs
▶ The two are indeed very similar, with common symptoms include
  ▷ Chronic fatigue
  ▷ Dizziness and headaches
  ▷ Sleep difficulties
  ▷ Nonspecific, multiple somatic complaints
▶ These conditions are likely related to depression, anxiety, fibromyalgia, chronic fatigue and irritable bowel syndromes

Shen-k'uei or shenkui (See Figure 50–4 on page 377)

Literally "kidney weakness"; according to traditional Chinese medical theory, kidneys carry the essence of sexual and masculine power

▶ Occurs in Chinese culture
▶ Symptoms
  ▷ Anxiety
  ▷ Dizziness
  ▷ Fatigability
  ▷ Backache
  ▷ Insomnia
  ▷ Sexual dysfunction
▶ Attributed to excessive semen loss from frequent intercourse and masturbation
▶ Comparable to Dhat, another form of "semen-loss anxiety"

Susto (See Figure 50–3 on page 374)

Spanish and Portuguese – fright

▶ Occurs in Latinos population in Central and South America
▶ A frightening event that causes the soul to leave the body
▶ Symptoms
  ▷ Appetite disturbances and gastrointestinal tract (GI) discomfort
  ▷ Sleep disturbance, dreams
  ▷ Sadness
  ▷ Lack of motivation
  ▷ Feelings of low self-worth
  ▷ Muscle aches and pains
  ▷ Headache
▶ May be related to depression, posttraumatic stress disorder, and somatoform disorders

Taijin kyofusho

Literally "people phobia"

▶ Found in Japanese culture
▶ Symptoms
　▷ Fear of offending others by blushing, having foul body odor, or bodily deficiency
　▷ Debilitating self-examination
　▷ Avoidance of eye contact and other forms of social contact
▶ Has some similarity to society anxiety disorder and body dysmorphic disorder; however, the fear is not of being embarrassed or judged, but of offending others

Twin studies: intelligence quotient

▶ Correlation rate of intelligence quotient (IQ) between twins reared apart
　▷ Identical twins – 0.75
　▷ Nonidentical twins – 0.38
▶ Similarities in IQ are not significantly influenced by
　▷ Access to educational material
　▷ Parental education
　▷ Socioeconomic status
　▷ Characteristics of parenting behavior
▶ Conclusion
　▷ Overall, IQ is determined roughly 2/3 by nature and 1/3 by nurture

Twin studies: personality and behavior patterns

▶ Similarities in Minnesota Multiphasic Personality Inventory (MMPI) test scores
　▷ Strong genetic influence through all MMPI scales
▶ Similarities in behavior traits
　▷ Alcohol use
　▷ Substance abuse
　▷ Antisocial behavior
　▷ Visuomotor skills
　▷ Religious interests
　▷ Job satisfaction
　▷ Social attitudes
　▷ Vocational interests
　▷ Work values
▶ Similarities in electroencephalogram (EEG) pattern and skin conductance in response to
　▷ Music
　▷ Voices
　▷ Sudden noises
　▷ Other perceptional stimulations

Zar (Figure 50–1)

▶ Appears in North African and Middle Eastern countries
▶ Dissociative symptoms include shouting, laughing, hitting the head against the wall
▶ It is believed to be associated with possession by a spirit
▶ Often not considered pathological locally

Questions

1. A 27-year-old black male was brought to the hospital for evaluation after a "crazy" episode while taking a walk with his girlfriend in a park. He was witnessed to be suddenly very horrified, threw himself to the ground seeking for cover. During the interview he appeared quite coherent. He said he saw an attacking helicopter in the air and he was trying to rescue himself. He is an Iraq veteran who was honorably discharged 14 months ago after his 1-year service in Iraq. His live-in girlfriend reported that he had no known psychiatric history before his service in Iraq, and no apparent difficulties in returning to civilian life after the discharge. However, she had noticed that he was reluctant to talk about his military experience. In the past 4 months, he experienced depression, insomnia, and flashbacks of his wartime experience. He also became preoccupied with news stories about Iraq. He began to have difficulty sleeping, and often woke up in the midst of nightmare. The "visual hallucinations" of his wartime experience had appeared several times but usually were very brief. He said this was the first time that he became "crazy." What is the most likely diagnosis?

   A. Major depressive disorder
   B. Panic disorder with agoraphobia
   C. Psychotic disorder due to head injury with hallucinations
   D. Posttraumatic stress disorder
   E. Nightmare disorder

2. The brain structures basal ganglia, limbic system and perceptual cortices are involved in the type of memory that deals with skills, habits, and nonassociative learning. This type of memory does not require conscious awareness and concentration, and usually remains intact after brain injury. This type of memory is called

   A. Implicit memory
   B. Declarative memory
   C. Eidetic memory
   D. Explicit memory
   E. Working memory

3. The following are characteristic for central pontine myelinolysis **EXCEPT**

   A. Disturbances of affect, behavior, and consciousness
   B. Hypernatremia and its inappropriate correction play central role in the etiology
   C. Damage in the corticobulbar and corticospinal tracts
   D. Neurological signs may include pseudobulbar palsy, dysarthria, dysphagia, and tetraparesis
   E. CT and MRI may find hypodense areas within the central pons

4. Which of the following factors have NOT been found to be associated with incestuous behavior

    A. Alcohol abuse
    B. Mental disorders
    C. Intellectual deficiencies
    D. Overcrowding that provides increased physical proximity
    E. Inner city environment

5. Which of the following proves are **NOT** required to confirm the allegation in malpractice cases

    A. There is an established doctor–patient relationship
    B. There is deviation from the accepted standard of care
    C. There is a known intention to deviate from the accepted standard of care
    D. There is damage happened to the patient
    E. The damage was directly caused by the deviation

6. Which of the following eye-related symptoms is paired correctly with the addictive substances

    A. Lacrimation – opioid intoxication
    B. Pupillary constriction – intoxication of hallucinogen
    C. Pupillary dilation – intoxication of cocaine
    D. Conjunctival injection – intoxication of alcohol
    E. Nystagmus – cannabis intoxication

7. A 25-year-old male was brought to the emergency room unconsciously. Family reported history of heavy drinking, and recurrent fall. Blood alcohol level was 312. Head CT scan is shown on page 385. The patient was under supportive therapy. He woke up in 2 hours, appeared confused, with no focal signs. What is the most likely cause of his loss of conscious? *(Figure Q7)*

    A. Epidural hemorrhage
    B. Subdural hemorrhage
    C. Scalp hematoma
    D. Alcohol intoxication
    E. Alcohol withdrawal

8. The following statements are correct regarding assessment of suicidal risk **EXCEPT**

    A. All patients, even those in apparent low risk, must be assessed about suicidal thoughts
    B. Assessment should include the patient's intent, plans, and perceived consequences
    C. If the patient is judged to be at high risk, query of potential means should be delayed so to avoid giving ideas that may increase the risk of suicide
    D. Personal history of suicide is the most relevant predictive factor for future suicidal behavior.
    E. Family history of suicide is a factor of increased suicidal risk

9. When asked what the fifth month of a year is, a patient answered "July." When asked what are the colors of the national flag, this patient answered "Blue, yellow, and orange." What is his symptom?

    A. Abulia
    B. Circumstantiality

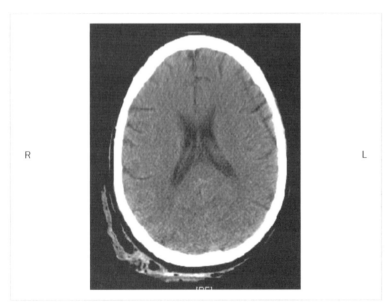

Figure Q7.

C. Capgras syndrome
D. Ganser syndrome
E. Paramnesia

10. La belle indifference is

A. Meaningless repetition of words or phrases
B. Inability to articulate the individual's thoughts by forgetting key words, phrases, or names in conversation
C. The patient exhibits a persisting response to a previous stimulus after a new stimulus has been presented
D. Inability to have goal-directed thoughts or conversation; often seen in demented patients
E. Inappropriately lack of concern about the deficit or disability

11. The symptom of inability to be aware of or express one's own mood and feeling is

A. Abulia
B. Blocking
C. Lethologica
D. Alexithymia
E. Paramnesia

12. The following statements are true regarding reparative therapy **EXCEPT**

A. It is psychotherapeutic approaches aimed at changing homosexual people's sexual orientations
B. Behavior modification and aversion therapy are the major techniques used in reparative therapy
C. Psychoanalysis played a role in reparative therapy
D. Reparative therapy is moderately effective at changing sexual orientation
E. American Psychiatric Association has held the position that homosexuality is a non-pathologic human behavior rather than a disorder

13. The most appropriate description for executive function is

   A. The capacity of analysis and problem solving
   B. The capacity of controlling emotion and impulse
   C. The capacity of accomplishing goal-directed behavior
   D. The capacity of purposefully applying one's physical skill
   E. The capacity to identify stimuli on the basis of recent experience with the same stimuli

14. The following are correct regarding the completed suicides among elderly people in the United States, **EXCEPT**

   A. The completed suicide rate in elderly is higher than in the general population
   B. The completed suicide rate in elderly is greater in the African-American population
   C. The completed suicide rate in elderly is greater in the Asian population
   D. The completed suicide is usually accomplished by violent means
   E. The completed suicide rate in elderly is greater in the Caucasian population

15. To evaluate whether a test measures what it purports to measure, one should examine the following aspects, **EXCEPT**

   A. Theoretical grounds
   B. Correlations from numerous studies using the test
   C. Correlation of the measure with variables that are known to be related to the construct purpose
   D. Whether the test reproduces consistent result when used at different times and by different raters
   E. Correlations that fit the expected pattern contribute

16. A 29-year-old male salesperson traveled to a town where he had never visited. He could not recall why he came here. He could not remember where he was from. He started to get worried about the situation. However, when he walked out of the train station, he suddenly felt the street looked familiar to him, though he could not recall in any detail. He had the symptom termed

   A. Jamais vu
   B. Déjà vu
   C. Folie à deux
   D. Dissociative identity disorder
   E. Déjà pense

17. To detect underlying subtle thought processes, bizarre ideation, particularly psychotic thought disorders, one may use the following projective tests, **EXCEPT**

   A. Thematic apperception test (TAT)
   B. Y-BOCS
   C. Draw-A-Person test
   D. Rorschach test
   E. Sentence completion test

18. In clinical studies, it is essential to select subjects under strict and consistent diagnostic criteria. What is the most reliable instrument to make clinical diagnosis according to DSM criteria?

   A. SCID
   B. AIM

C. BPRS

D. MMPI-2

E. PANNS

19. Amygdala has output to the following locations **EXCEPT**

   A. Hypothalamus

   B. Nuclei of the trigeminal nerve (CN V)

   C. Nuclei of the facial nerve (CN VII)

   D. Ventral tegmental area (VTA)

   E. Nuclei of the vagus nerve (CN X)

20. The following tests are designed to be administered by clinicians, **EXCEPT**

   A. Brief psychotic rating scale

   B. Clinical global improvement scale

   C. Beck depression inventory

   D. Hamilton rating scale for depression

   E. Millon clinical multiaxial inventory

21. According to Lawrence Kohlberg, the principle of conventional morality is

   A. To avoid punishment

   B. To rely more on intuitive sense in decision making, rather than rules and reasoning

   C. To gain approval from others

   D. To assure resources and security from the caregiver or provider

   E. To stand for ethical principles

22. Which of the following is correct regarding pseudobulbar palsy

   A. It is associated with lesions at or near nuclei of cranial nerves IX to XII

   B. Hypoactive jaw and gag reflexes often appear

   C. Respiratory impairment is a prominent concern in pseudobulbar palsy

   D. It often has emotional lability and cognitive impairment

   E. The prefix "pseudo-" implies the fact that dysarthria and dysphagia are psychogenic

23. Some children receive contradictory parental demands about their behavior, where they are not possibly able to fulfill both. Repeated exposure to this difficult situation may cause confusion and frustration in children. This was originally proposed as a cause of schizophrenia. But this causal relationship has not been validated. Nonetheless, this is generally viewed as a negative factor in mental development. What is the right term for this situation, and who originally conceptualized it?

   A. Basic trust, Eric Erikson

   B. Self-object function, Heinz Kohut

   C. Learned helplessness, Martin Seligman

   D. Double bind, Gregory Bateson

   E. Strange situation, Mary Ainsworth

24. "Ethnicity" is a preferred term by cross-cultural researchers in denoting human groupings. It is defined by the following **EXCEPT**

   A. Ancestry

   B. Belief

   C. History

   D. Sense of common identity

   E. Biological measurement

25. A patient was unsatisfied at her male therapist. She told him the therapy had not been effective because he disliked her, he hated women, that he was mean, that he lacked sympathy, and that he bound not to be a successful therapist. In return, the therapist stated – "Well, you should think about why you are not liked. If all my patients are women like you, I won't have a chance to be successful."

The interaction between this patient and the therapist is an example of which of the following defense mechanisms?

A. Splitting
B. Projective identification
C. Sublimation
D. Suppression
E. Passive aggression

26. According to Eric Erikson's life cycle theory, what is the primary task at the age of 40–65 years?

A. Intimacy vs. self-absorption or isolation
B. Industry vs. inferiority
C. Generativity vs. stagnation
D. Repression vs. suppression
E. Initiative vs. guilt

27. A dog usually salivates when served with food. After repeated exposure to bell sound paired with food, the dog salivates upon bell sound alone without food. However, after a long while of being given bell sound without food, the dog gradually reduced, and finally stopped, salivating. According to Pavlov's classical conditioning, which of the following is the conditioned stimulus?

A. Dog
B. Saliva
C. Food
D. Bell sound
E. Both saliva and bell sound

28. A 7-year-old boy has developed rational and logical thought. He understands water in a tall cup has the same volume as in a bowl. He also is able to understand someone else's point of view. According to Jean Piaget, which developmental stage is this boy in?

A. Phallic stage
B. Sensorimotor stage
C. Concrete operational stage
D. Rapprochement stage
E. Formal operational stage

29. Regarding clinical capacity evaluation, which of the following is correct

A. Capacity is the medical equivalence to competency; both declare the patient's legal privileges to make decision
B. Factual understanding of the information is required for a patient to make treatment decision
C. If the patient can not speak, he/she has no capacity of making decision
D. The ability to manipulate information rationally is required for decision making, therefore all psychotic patients with thought disorder are considered incapable of decision making

E. To be capable of decision making, a patient must appreciate the possible consequences of accepting treatment, but not necessarily the consequences of rejecting treatment

30. The following statements regarding caudate nucleus is correct **EXCEPT**

A. Together with putamen, caudate nucleus forms the dorsal striatum, which forms part of basal ganglia

B. Caudate nucleus is an important part of learning and memory system

C. Caudate nucleus is highly innervated by dopamine neurons

D. Dopamine neurons project to caudate originate mainly from hypothalamus

E. Caudate nucleus is separated from the lenticular nucleus by the internal capsule

31. The following are appropriate situations to start ECT **EXCEPT**

A. History of adequate response to ECT

B. No adequate trial of psychotropics nor psychotherapy, but a rapid response is desired due to the psychosocial situation

C. The patient's medical condition imposes higher risk from less intrusive treatment

D. The patient prefers ECT rather than other forms of psychiatric treatment

E. The treating physician is highly trained and experienced in ECT

32. Succinylcholine is commonly used as a muscle relaxant in preparation for ECT. The major specific concern of giving succinylcholine to a patient with undetected pseudocholinesterase deficiency is

A. Muscle soreness due to fasciculation

B. Polarization of the neuromuscular junction that may cause prolonged apnea

C. Prolonged apnea due to slowed succinylcholine metabolism

D. Elevated extracellular potassium that may suppress the cardiac conductivity

E. Increased intracranial pressure due to rapid induction of seizure

33. The following statements regarding biological changes in posttraumatic stress disorder are true **EXCEPT**

A. Abnormalities of hypothalamus-pituitary-adrenal (HPA) axis

B. Physiological arousal after exposure to cues in individuals with PTSD

C. Increase in norepinephrine turnover in the locus coeruleus

D. Suppressed reactivity in amygdala, hippocampus, and anterior cingulated cortex

E. Increased norepinephrine activity in limbic regions and cerebral cortex

34. Apoptosis is a process of cell death with the following characteristics

A. Involves expression of specific genes

B. Follows acute insult or injury

C. Has inflammatory response

D. May be enhanced by neurotrophins under certain conditions

E. Usually triggered by external damage

35. Clinical effects of histamine blockade include the following **EXCEPT**

A. Allergy relief

B. Hypertension

C. Sedation

D. Weight gain

E. Decreased gastric acid production

36. A 31-year-old female complains of inability to experience orgasm. She reports emotionally attached to her husband, and feels erotic pleasure during lovemaking. However, she has never been able to reach the climax. What should be the next step in treatment?

A. Pubococcygeal exercise focusing on strengthening the pelvic diaphragm
B. Sensate focus exercises, with assistance of masturbation, and using of vibrator
C. Evaluation on possible medication side effects and neurologic impairments
D. Trial of bupropion and SE5 inhibitors
E. Evaluation on anxiety and relationship problems

37. Regarding direct-coupled ion channels, the following are correct **EXCEPT**

A. No second messengers are involved
B. Typically constructed with single unit that has 4–5 transmembrane domains
C. Fast in response to neurotransmitter activities
D. Nicotinic cholinergic receptors are direct-coupled ion channels
E. Ion channels are part of the receptors

38. The following dopaminergic neuronal locations are associated with the correct neurological functions **EXCEPT**

A. Dopaminergic neurons at substantia nigra are associated with extrapyramidal side effects
B. Dopaminergic neurons at ventral tegmental area are associated with antipsychotic effect
C. Dopaminergic neurons at raphe nuclei are associated with antiemetic effects
D. Dopaminergic neurons at ventral tegmental area are associated with the rewarding system
E. Dopaminergic neurons at hypothalamus are associated with prolactin regulation

39. Action potential is an important cellular mechanism in neuronal functioning. Which of the following statements regarding action potential is correct?

A. Na-K-ATPase pump moves Na^+ in and K^+ out against their concentration gradient, and maintains the resting potential
B. Depolarization is the process to reduce the cytosol negative charge, makes the cell membrane ready to have action potential
C. The action potential starts with depolarization by rapid influx of Cl^-
D. Ca^{++} involves in many cytosol activities, also activates repolarization by outward Na^+ current
E. The outward K^+ current causes depolarization, and transiently decreases cell membrane excitability after an action potential

40. Which of the following factors implies the organic cause for anxiety symptoms

A. Onset of symptoms before the age of 25 years
B. Significant anticipatory anxiety
C. Presence of avoidance behavior
D. Family history of anxiety disorders
E. Poor response to anxiolytic agents

41. Melatonin system is essential in sleep-wake cycle. Which of the following statements is **INCORRECT?**

A. Melatonin is secreted by neurons at caudal locus ceruleus
B. Melatonin synapses and receptors are concentrated at suprachiasmatic nucleus (SCN) of the hypothalamus

C. Melatonin plays an important role in circadian regulation

D. Melatonin neurons receive positive feedback from increased sleep drive in the evening

E. Melatonin neurons receive negative feedback from the retinohypothalamic tract

42. Which of the following statements regarding monoamine oxidase is correct?

A. MAO-B breaks down tyramine from food in the intestine

B. When MAO-A is induced, tyramine-rich food can cause surge of tyramine in blood

C. Hypertensive crisis may occur with the surge of serum tyramine level due to the induction of MAO-A

D. Both MAO-A and MAO-B appear in the central nervous system

E. MAO-B appears in the central nervous system as well as blood vessel walls, liver, and intestine

43. Which of the following statements regarding NMDA receptor is correct?

A. NMDA receptor is one of the five major types of glutamate receptors, and plays a key role in learning and memory

B. When activated by 2 molecules of glutamate and 1 of glycine, NMDA receptor opens the integrated Ca^{++} channel to allow influx of calcium

C. NMDA receptor may be blocked by Mg^{++}

D. Down regulation of NMDA receptor may cause psychosis

E. Acamprosate, atomoxetine, and phencyclidine are drugs bind to NMDA receptor

44. The following are correct regarding serotonin receptor distribution and proposed clinical relevance **EXCEPT**

A. Serotonin receptors in brainstem are associated with sexual side effects of SSRIs

B. Serotonin receptors at basal ganglia are associated with agitation, and akathisia

C. Serotonin receptors at gastrointestinal system are associated with nausea and vomiting

D. Serotonin receptors at limbic system are associated with sedation and insomnia

E. Serotonin receptors at cranial vasculature are associated with migraine

45. Trinucleotide repeat expansion may cause change in cellular structure and function, and is an important mechanism of the following neurological conditions **EXCEPT**

A. Fragile X syndrome

B. Myotonic dystrophy

C. Spinocerebellar ataxia type 1

D. Machado-Joseph disease

E. Parkinson's disease

46. The following descriptions of levels of prevention are correct **EXCEPT**

A. Detection and treatment of disease belong to the secondary prevention

B. Rehabilitation is part of tertiary prevention

C. Immunization is considered primary prevention

D. Continuous treatment to enable chronic patients to attain best potential of functioning is an important part of secondary prevention

E. Primary prevention is the most effective step in all levels of prevention

47. Headache associated with pseudotumor cerebri has the following characteristics **EXCEPT**

A. Headache accompanied with papilledema

B. Usually appears in young obese women

    C. Increased intracranial pressure

    D. Lumbar puncture is diagnostic but not therapeutic

    E. May cause blindness and empty sella syndrome

48. A 47-year-old engineer complains of headache focused in the left temporal area for 1 month. The headache has been progressively worse. In the past 2 weeks he was awakened in early morning with severe headache. What is the most likely nature of his headache?

    A. Migraine

    B. Cluster headache

    C. Meningitis

    D. Space occupying lesion

    E. Subarachnoid hemorrhage

49. Prophylactic treatment for migraine including the following **EXCEPT**

    A. β-blockers

    B. Calcium channel blockers

    C. Antiepileptic drugs

    D. Tricyclic antidepressants

    E. Triptans

50. The following statements regarding migraine pathophysiology are correct **EXCEPT**

    A. Activated 5-HT1b receptors on blood vessels produce vasodilation

    B. Activated presynaptic 5-HT1d receptors inhibit the release of vasoactive peptides

    C. The central migraine generator is activated by environmental migraine triggers, and sends impulses through trigeminal nerve

    D. Vasoactive and algogenic peptides are released through CN-V (trigeminal)

    E. Trigeminal nerve sends the pain message back to the brain

51. The so called "irritable heart" syndrome during the civil war closely resembles the modern diagnosis of

    A. Atrial fibrillation

    B. Effort syndrome

    C. Borderline personality disorder

    D. Posttraumatic stress disorder

    E. Panic disorder

52. A 40-year-old Chinese male complains of chronic fatigue for 2 years. He also complains of dizziness, headache, disturbance in sleep, aches and pains all over the body, indigestion, and impotence. He presents with the typical features of which of the following culture-bond syndromes?

    A. Shenjing shuairuo

    B. Mal de mojo

    C. Koro

    D. Amafufanyane

    E. Ataque de nervios

53. Which of the following is **NOT** a risk factor of child abuse

    A. Having a parent who was abused

    B. Being behaviorally disordered.

C. Being a handicapped child
D. Low birth weight
E. Poverty

54. The following symptoms imply possible organic etiology of anxiety **EXCEPT**

A. Onset of symptoms after the age of 35 years
B. Lack of avoidance behavior
C. Significant anticipatory anxiety
D. Poor response to anxiolytic agents
E. Lack of personal or family history of anxiety disorders

55. Which of the following statements regarding fluent aphasia is **INCORRECT**

A. The location of injury is at temporal or parietal lobe
B. Word speed is over 100 words per minute
C. Normal articulation but with paraphasia
D. Impaired in all formal language testing
E. Often accompanied with hemiparesis

56. Which one of the following was the first introduced biological remedy for mental illness that has been proved effective and is still in active clinical use today

A. Lithium
B. Chlorpromazine
C. ECT
D. Imipramine
E. Fluoxetine

57. The following are culture-bond syndromes appearing mainly in Asian countries **EXCEPT**

A. Shenjing shuairuo
B. Koro
C. Latah
D. Boufee delirante
E. Amok

58. The following statements regarding nonfluent aphasia are correct **EXCEPT**

A. Dysarthria
B. Slow language output, usually <50 word per minute
C. Often associated with right-sided hemiparesis
D. Impaired comprehension
E. Impaired naming and repeating

59. According to Kurt Schneider, the following are fundamental symptoms of schizophrenia, or "first rank symptoms," **EXCEPT**

A. Audible thoughts
B. Emotional impoverishment
C. Delusional perceptions
D. Voices arguing or discussing
E. Somatic passivity experiences

60. Recent researches have found volume reduction in several regions of the brain in schizophrenic patients. Which of the following has **NOT** been found to have volume reduction in schizophrenic individuals?

A. Prefrontal cortex
B. Thalamus
C. Hippocampus
D. Occipital cortex
E. Superior temporal cortex

61. According to DSM-IV-TR, which of the following is correct regarding delusional disorder

A. Nonbizarre delusions for at least 6 months
B. Clinically significant impairment of social and occupational functioning
C. Never met symptomatic criteria for schizophrenia
D. May have olfactory and tactile hallucinations congruent with delusional theme
E. Identified subtypes include grandiose, persecutory, and nihilistic

62. A 20-year-old male is brought to the office for evaluation of behavior problem. The patient has difficulty in socialization. He has found people often aggravate him and don't understand him. He becomes angry easily and has involved in physical altercation with family and coworkers several times, though no significant injury has occurred. He feels anxious and jittery inside all the time. Though the formal test found he has normal intellectual quotient, and he had an average school performance, he has not been able to hold a job for longer than 3 months. The patient complains people are difficult to work with. Physical examination showed he is tall, mildly obese, with weakened male habitus. Otherwise he is fairly well developed. The patient is likely to have which of the following congenital conditions?

A. Sturge-Weber syndrome
B. Seckel syndrome
C. Klinefelter's syndrome
D. Turner's syndrome
E. William's Syndrome

63. The following are good prognostic factors for schizophrenia **EXCEPT**

A. Later age of onset
B. Married status
C. Acute onset
D. Predominance of positive symptoms
E. Lack of precipitating factors

64. The language function of the dominant hemisphere is associated with which of the following forms of language

A. Hieroglyphics
B. Singing
C. Prosody
D. Body language
E. Cursing

65. The following cerebral structures are components of verbal language input pathway, **EXCEPT**

    A. Lateral lemniscus

    B. Medial geniculate body

    C. Heschl's gyri

    D. Occipital cortex

    E. Wernicke's area

66. The following statements regarding pseudobulbar palsy are correct **EXCEPT**

    A. Location of lesion is at medulla and lower portion of pons

    B. Upper motor neuron injury

    C. Dysarthria and dysphagia, but no respiratory impairment

    D. Hyperactive jaw and gag reflexes

    E. Associated with emotional lability and cognitive impairment

67. Which of the following medicines is least likely to cause sexual dysfunction

    A. Amitriptyline

    B. Sertraline

    C. Propranolol

    D. Prednisone

    E. Mirtazapine

68. Which of the statements regarding transcortical aphasia is **INCORRECT**

    A. It is usually associated with anoxia, CO poisoning, and Alzheimer's disease

    B. It is a fluent aphasia with preserved repeating ability

    C. It is also known as global aphasia

    D. The pathological change isolates language arc from the remaining cortex

    E. Areas surrounding the perisylvian arc are preserved

69. An EEG shows frequency of 8–12 Hz, with the amplitude slightly higher on the dominant side. Assume this is from a healthy individual, which stage is the subject in

    A. Awake, relaxed, with eyes closed

    B. Drowsy or in stage 1 sleep

    C. Stage 2 sleep

    D. Stages 3 and 4 sleep

    E. Rapid eye movement sleep

70. Phalen's test is applied for

    A. Eaton-Lambert syndrome

    B. Carpel tunnel syndrome

    C. Guillain-Barré syndrome

    D. Locked-in syndrome

    E. Cauda equine syndrome

71. Common side effects of phenelzine include the following **EXCEPT**

    A. Insomnia

    B. Sedation

    C. Weight gain

    D. Hypertension

    E. Sexual dysfunction

72. Which of the following statements regarding memantine is **INCREECT**?

    A. Memantine enhances the physiological function of Mg^{++}
    B. By reducing the calcium influx, memantine blocks neuronal toxicity yet allows normal function necessary for memory and other cognitive function
    C. Memantine is approved for moderate to advanced dementia of Alzheimer's type
    D. Memantine's metabolism is nonhepatic, therefore has minimal drug interactions
    E. Memantine is a competitive NMDA receptor antagonist with moderate affinity to NMDA receptor

73. Lewy bodies eosinophilic neuronal inclusions are composed of the following components **EXCEPT**

    A. α-synuclein
    B. Ubiquitin
    C. β amyloid
    D. Neurofilament protein
    E. α B crystallin

74. A 35-year-old male complains of chronic sleep disturbance. For the past 2 years, he has been drinking excessively in the evening to help sleep. He recently was charged for driving while intoxicated. Facing the risk of more severe loss in his career and family life, he is eager to receive psychiatric help. During the assessment of his sleep problem, you are likely to find the following **EXCEPT**

    A. Increased sleep latency
    B. Decreased total sleep time
    C. REM is increased over all the night
    D. Sleep fragmentation
    E. Reduction of restful sleep and day time fatigue

75. Which of the following is **NOT** a risk factor for cerebrovascular accident?

    A. Advanced age
    B. Malnutrition
    C. Hypertension and cardiac condition
    D. Diabetes mellitus
    E. Cigarette smoking and/or heavy alcohol use

76. Brain volume reduction is found in individuals with chronic schizophrenia. The following are locations of volume reduction **EXCEPT**

    A. Prefrontal cortex
    B. Thalamus
    C. Hippocampus
    D. Superior temporal cortex
    E. Lateral and third ventricles

77. St. John's wort is commonly used in folk medicine that has been popular in Europe for hundreds of years. Some study showed its possible efficacy for mild to moderate depression and anxiety. The following statements are correct regarding St. John's wort **EXCEPT**

    A. It is an inducer of CYP 3A4
    B. It may decrease blood levels of protease inhibitors
    C. It may mildly enhance the antidepressive effect when combined with SSRIs
    D. Combination with MAOIs should be avoided
    E. It should be discontinued 5 days before surgery

78. Which of the following over the counter medicines is safe to be used with phenelzine (Nardil)

    A. Robitussin DM

    B. Sudafed

    C. Sudafed PE

    D. Robitussin

    E. Afrin

79. The purpose of Wada test is to

    A. Confirm cerebral dominance

    B. Detect the location of lesion

    C. Evaluate the residual cognitive function

    D. Clarify the personality traits

    E. Test subtle psychotic symptoms

80. Locked-in syndrome has a remarkable clinical presentation with a combination of mute, quadriplegia, with intact cognition, and communication only through moving eyes. EEG is usually normal. Which of the following statements regarding the structural impairment is **INCORRECT**?

    A. Cranial nerves IX (glossopharyngeal) and X (vagus) are impaired

    B. It is associated with occlusion of a branch of the internal carotid artery

    C. Location of lesion is at the ventral portion of pons and medulla

    D. Impairment of corticospinal tracts causes quadriplegia

    E. Cranial XI (accessory) and XII (hypoglossal) are impaired

81. Besides treating hypertension, propranolol has been used for the following conditions **EXCEPT**

    A. Migraine headache

    B. Pheochromocytoma

    C. Serotonin syndrome

    D. Posttraumatic stress disorder

    E. Restless leg syndrome

82. The following psychotropic medicines have minimum protein-binding **EXCEPT**

    A. Gabapentin

    B. Valproate

    C. Oxcarbazine

    D. Topiramate

    E. Venlafaxine

83. A 15-year-old girl presented with swallowing and breathing difficulties. The symptoms started subtly in the past 3 years, and became more dibilitating in the past 6 months. She also complains of headache, neck pain, dizziness, general fatigue, and muscle weakness. Physical examination found an afebrile girl with impaired fine motor skills. MRI found the cerebellar tonsils are elongated and pushed down through foramen magnum. What is likely the recommended treatment?

    A. Conservative observation

    B. Decompression surgery

    C. Lumber puncture to reduce intracranial pressure

    D. Ventriculoperitoneal shunt

    E. IV antibiotics

84. Combined system disease, or pernicious anemia is a severe form of vitamin B12 deficiency. Most common cause is a disturbance of immunology system – antibodies are produced to intrinsic factor, and therefore block the absorption of vitamin B_{12}. It may also be caused by severe malabsorption and strict vegetarian diet. The following statement regarding combined system disease is true **EXCEPT**

A. Clinical features include anemia and dementia
B. Schilling test is diagnostic
C. Loss of lateral and posterior columns may occur
D. Serum homocysteine is decreased
E. Serum methylmalonic acid elevated

85. A 20-year-old female complains of sudden onset of paresthesias and numbness in the fingers and toes 2 days ago. She had diarrhea last week that lasted for 2 days and that resolved without any intervene. The symptoms quickly moved up to legs, hands, and arms. The second day after admission, she started to have shortness of breath, and difficulty in opening the eyes and speaking. The most likely CSF profile is

A. Clear, WBC 15, protein 150, glucose 90
B. Clear, WBC 0, protein 40, glucose 90
C. Turbid, WBC 380, protein 150, glucose 20
D. Turbid, WBC 80, protein 90, glucose 60
E. Bloody, WBC 80, protein 90, glucose 90

86. For an individual with complaint of sexual desire disorder, the following are potentially attributed **EXCEPT**

A. Low testosterone
B. Low prolactin
C. Thyroid disturbance
D. Adrenal insufficiency
E. Exogenous corticosteroids

87. A 16-year-old boy has mild mental retardation. He has a long face with the jaw projecting markedly. He has large ears. Examination of the mouth found he has high-arched palate. His upper and lower teeth have difficulty in closing. Physical examination found moderated developed breasts, enlarged testicles, decreased muscle tones, flat feet, and abnormally forwarded curvature of the lumbar spine. What is the likely finding in chromosome examination?

A. Mutation on the long arm of X chromosome
B. Abnormality on short arm of chromosome 5
C. Extra X chromosome, i.e., XXY
D. Deletions in chromosome 15
E. Monosomy X, i.e., 45 X

88. Which of the following is wrong regarding frontal lobe syndrome

A. No strict connection of location and mental deficit
B. Orbitofrontal lobe lesions are often associated with disinhibition
C. Emotional lability may be associated with medial frontal lesions
D. Depression may be associated with left frontal lesions
E. Mania may be associated with right frontal lesions

89. The most common defense mechanism appearing in depressive disorders is

    A. Projection

    B. Suppression

    C. Sublimation

    D. Introjection

    E. Repression

90. Which of the following is not a part of the basal ganglia?

    A. Putamen

    B. Nucleus accumbens

    C. Subthalamic nucleus

    D. Ventral tegmental area

    E. Substantia nigra

91. Which of the following is correct regarding dopa-responsive dystonia

    A. Dystonia onset in early adulthood

    B. More prevalent in males

    C. Dystonia and Parkinsonism appear more severely in the morning, and improve in the evening

    D. Autosomal dominant defect on chromosome 14q

    E. Deficient adenosine triphosphate (ATP)

92. A 45-year-old woman complains of rapid jerky motions of the trunk, arms, and legs. The family reports she has had this condition for over a year. The symptoms have been gradually getting worse. In the past 3 months, her memory had significantly declined. She now needs assistance to balance her checking account and to pay her bills. Head CT scan showed atrophy of cerebral cortex. MRI found atrophy of cortex and particularly the head of the caudate nuclei. Her lateral ventricles are enlarged with a pattern of bat-wing. This patient suffers from a condition with the pathophysiology of

    A. Accumulation of copper in tissues

    B. Expansion of CAG trinucleotide

    C. Eosinophilic neuronal inclusions found scattered in cortex, which composed of α-synuclein.

    D. High normal level of intracranial pressure

    E. Senile plaques with β amyloid in center and neurofibrillary tangles with tau protein.

93. Regarding suicide among physicians, which of the following statements is correct?

    A. Physician has lower suicide rate than general population

    B. Male physicians are at higher risk

    C. Physicians of psychiatry, ophthalmology, and anesthesiology have greater risk of suicide than other specialties

    D. Physicians who commit suicide usually suffer from mental disorder, most often psychotic disorder

    E. Firearms and other violent suicide measures are more often used by physicians than general population

94. Consensus of expert opinion agreed that a seizure that has good opportunity to produce superior clinical efficacy should possess the following quality **EXCEPT**

    A. Symmetrical

    B. With at least 60 second sustained seizure duration

   C. With high interhemispheric coherence
   D. With marked postictal suppression
   E. Accompanied by a prominent tachycardia response

95. The tasks of bereavement in children with deceased parents include

   A. Accepting the reality of loss
   B. Resisting the pain of loss
   C. Relocating to a new environment in which the deceased is not missed
   D. Finding ways to forget the deceased
   E. Learning to manage the most difficult task, that is to deal with a prior dependent relationship between the child and the deceased parent

96. The following statements regarding Down's syndrome are correct **EXCEPT**

   A. The prevalence is approximately 1/1,000
   B. Single transverse palmar crease and epicanthic fold of the eyelid are characteristic physical features
   C. Larger than normal space is found between the big and the second toes
   D. Individuals with Down's syndrome have higher risk for congenital renal defects
   E. High incidence of Alzheimer's dementia is observed in Down's syndrome population

97. During the process of the fourth revision on DSM, a work model was established that designated to guide the future revision. This work model include the following **EXCEPT**

   A. Designate work groups on each category
   B. Conduct extensive review of published literature
   C. Reanalyze the research data, including unpublished data provided by researchers
   D. Conduct issue-focused field trials
   E. Conduct treatment trials to help verify the assumed etiology

98. When drunk, people with chronic alcohol consumption have the following change in sleep pattern **EXCEPT**

   A. Decreased sleep latency
   B. Increased slow-wave sleep in early part of the night, but decreased overall slow-wave sleep
   C. Increased REM sleep in the early morning, but decreased overall REM sleep
   D. Sleep fragmentation
   E. Sleep disturbances may continue even with prolonged abstinence

99. Depression is associated with which of the following sleep changes

   A. Prolonged REM latency
   B. Increased REM frequency
   C. Delayed morning awakening due to extensive dreaming
   D. Increased REM density
   E. Increased sleep efficiency

100. Regarding melatonin, the following statements are correct **EXCEPT**

   A. Melatonin synthesis receives negative feedback from the retinohypothalamic tract
   B. Tryptophan, serotonin, and 5-HIAA are precursors of melatonin in biosynthesis
   C. Antipsychotics inhibit the synthesis of melatonin
   D. Melatonin is synthesized in the pineal gland
   E. Antidepressants promote the synthesis of melatonin

101. Regarding orexins, the following statements are correct **EXCEPT**

    A. Orexins are inhibitory neuropeptides
    B. Hypocretins are metabolites of orexins
    C. Orexins are produced in hypothalamus
    D. Orexin receptors are direct-coupled ion channels
    E. Orexins' potential medical use is under investigation

102. Chronic schizophrenia is associated with brain volume reduction in which of the following locations

    A. Prefrontal cortex
    B. Basal ganglia
    C. Lateral ventricles
    D. Inferior temporal cortex
    E. The third ventricle

103. Adolf Meyer believed that schizophrenia is a condition resulted from personality dysfunction, and endorsed the following term

    A. Dementia precox
    B. Schizophrenic reaction
    C. Manic-depressive psychosis
    D. Ego disintegration
    E. Paraphrenia

104. Amphetamine intoxication may have the following symptoms **EXCEPT**

    A. Tachycardia
    B. Bradycardia
    C. Fatigue
    D. Pupillary dilation
    E. Weigh loss

105. Which of the following statement regarding the endogenous marijuana system is correct

    A. Cannabinoid receptors are direct-coupled ion channels
    B. Activation of cannabinoid receptor CB1 causes increase of calcium influx
    C. Cannabinoid receptor CB1 may also modulate potassium channels
    D. Delta-9-tetrahydrocannabinol (THC) is one of the endocannabinoids
    E. Endocannabinoids are peptides that bind to cannabinoid receptors

106. Cocaine can transmit through the placenta rapidly. Cocaine use during pregnancy may be associated with the following problems **EXCEPT**

    A. Hypoperfusion of the fetal brain
    B. Fetal growth retardation
    C. Decreased birth weight
    D. Malformations of the urogenital system of the newborn
    E. Present in breast milk may increase blood pressure, rapid heart rate, and miosis in the newborn

107. Which of the following statements regarding the neurophysiology of anxiety is correct?

    A. Blockade of locus coeruleus may generate panic attacks
    B. Structures in the limbic system mediate anxiety response

    C. GABAergic system is involved in modulating noradrenergic and serotonergic systems

    D. GABAergic system is widely distributed with highest density at the frontal cortex

    E. Benzodiazepines can bind to GABA receptors and induce anxiety

108. Dementia of Alzheimer's type has the following neuropathologic changes **EXCEPT**

    A. Senile plaques are quantitatively correlated with the severity of the dementia

    B. Senile plaques are composed of amyloid beta (Aβ), astrocytes, dystrophic neuronal processes, and microglia.

    C. Neurofibrillary tangles are cytoskeletal elements including phosphorylated tau protein

    D. Granulovascular degeneration of the neurons, neuronal loss, and synaptic loss appear in the cortex and the hippocampus

    E. Increased neuronal projections from the nucleus basalis of Meynert

109. The options of treatment for conversion disorder include the following **EXCEPT**

    A. The most important issue is to maintain a therapeutic relationship with the patient

    B. Interview with assistance of amobarbital often reveal reliable history regarding the motivation of faking the symptoms

    C. Psychotherapy should focus on stress and coping

    D. Hypnosis may be effective in some cases

    E. Anxiolytics may be effective in some cases

110. Uncompleted suicide has which of the following characteristics

    A. Female

    B. Under age of 35 years

    C. Low lethality of method

    D. Approximately 10% of uncompleted suicide will finally be successful

    E. Greater rate in Caucasian population

111. A 35-year-old male patient carries HIV positivity for over 10 years. In the past 6 months he has slowly progressing tiredness and dizziness. He is cognitively lucid and afebrile. Physical examination found no prominent focal signs, nor abnormal movements. Head CT scan found multiple enhancing lesions with ring pattern. SPECT found hot lesions. CSF is normal. What is the most likely diagnosis

    A. Toxoplasmosis

    B. Lymphoma

    C. HIV meningitis

    D. Cryptococcus

    E. Neurosyphilis

112. The following are psychosocial risk factors for suicide **EXCEPT**

    A. Unemployment

    B. Living alone

    C. Lack of social support

    D. Children in the home

    E. Recent deterioration in socioeconomic status

113. Which of the following represents the ethnic risk of suicide in descending order

    A. African-Americans, Caucasians, Native Americans, Hispanic Americans, and Asian-Americans

B. Caucasians, Native Americans, African-Americans, Hispanic Americans, and Asian-Americans

C. Asian-Americans, Native Americans, African-Americans, Hispanic Americans, and Caucasians

D. African-Americans, Hispanic Americans, Caucasians, Native Americans, and Asian-Americans

E. Caucasians, African-Americans, Asian-Americans, Hispanic Americans, and Native Americans

114. For which of the following antidepressants, animal reproduction studies have shown an adverse effect on the fetus, but there are no adequate and well-controlled studies in humans?

A. Paroxetine

B. Imipramine

C. Desipramine

D. Maprotiline

E. Bupropion

115. Nondeclarative memory refers to the type of memory that

A. Deals with skills, habits, and nonassociative learning

B. Is also known as explicit memory

C. Requires conscious awareness and concentration

D. Is usually impaired after brain injury

E. Involves brain structures including hippocampus, orbitofrontal cortex, and parahippocampal gyrus

116. The following are important aspects of medical treatment for anorexia nervosa **EXCEPT**

A. Primary medical goal is weight restoration

B. Encourage pregnancy as this may relieve the body image disturbance

C. Correction of electrolyte disturbance, particularly hypokalemia

D. Vitamin supplementation

E. Inpatient care for patients with severe weight loss and electrolyte imbalance

117. Which of the following substances is a serotonin reuptake blocker?

A. Lysergic acid diethylamide (LSD)

B. Marijuana

C. Ecstasy

D. Phencyclidine (PCP)

E. Heroin

118. In the development of DSM system, there was a major revision known as "neo-Kraepelinian." This revision labeled the transition of the field from the original dominance by psychodynamic theories to the new focus on scientific reliability of psychiatric diagnosis. Between which two editions did this historical revision occur?

A. DSM-I and DSM-II

B. DSM-II and DSM-III

C. DSM-III and DSM-III-R

D. DSM-III-R and DSM-IV

E. DSM-IV and DSM-IV-TR

119. Which of the following is not the correct milestone of language development?

    A. Vowel sounds – 2–6 month

    B. Word production – 11–13 month

    C. Word comprehension – 18 month

    D. Word combination – 20–24 month

    E. Grammar – 2–3 year

120. Inhibition of which CYP isozyme can elevate the serum level of tricyclic antidepressant and reduce the effect of codeine

    A. CYP 1A2

    B. CYP 3A4

    C. CYP 2E1

    D. CYP 2D6

    E. CYP 2C19

121. The following drugs can cause elevation of lithium plasma level **EXCEPT**

    A. Theophylline

    B. Angiotensin converting enzyme inhibitors

    C. Fluoxetine

    D. Ibuprofen

    E. Thiazide diuretics

122. Which of the following describes the function of ego

    A. It is dominated by primary process

    B. It dictates moral conscience and value

    C. It functions largely unconsciously

    D. It spans over unconscious, preconscious, and conscious

    E. It lacks the capacity to delay or modify the instinctual drives

123. Regarding the cultural influence on individual personality, some theorists believed that each culture is associated with a common personality structure, or "national character." This theoretical view, however, was at times used to foster political and discriminatory attitude. Which theorist presented this idea first?

    A. Bronislaw Malinowski

    B. Margaret Mead

    C. Abraham Kardiner

    D. Sigmund Freud

    E. Carl Jung

124. Shen-k'uei, or shenkui, refers to which of the following culture-bound syndromes?

    A. It occurs in Chinese culture. It presents with symptoms of anxiety, dizziness, fatigability, insomnia, and sexual dysfunction. It was believed to be caused by excessive semen loss from frequent intercourse and masturbation.

    B. It is found in China and Malaysia. The symptoms are focused on intense anxiety on the retraction of genital back into the body.

    C. It is found in India and Pakistan, where male patients suffer from premature ejaculation and impotence. Some patients complain of passing whitish fluid that is believed to be semen. Accompanied symptoms include anxiety, guilt about excessive masturbation, feelings of weakness, fatigue, palpitation, and subjective feeling of shortening of genital.

D. It is found in China, with similar condition also found in the United States. Main symptoms are chronic fatigue, dizziness and headaches, sleep difficulties, and nonspecific somatic complaints. It may be clinically related to chronic fatigue, fibromyalgia, and depression.

E. It is found in Latinos population in Central and South America. It is believed to be associated with loss of soul due to a frightening event. Symptoms include gastrointestinal tract (GI) disturbance, sleep disturbance, frightening dreams, sadness, lack of motivation, aches and pains, feelings of low self-worth.

125. The following factors imply good prognosis for schizophrenia **EXCEPT**

    A. Paranoid subtype
    B. High IQ
    C. Affective symptoms
    D. Insidious onset
    E. Confusion or other organic symptoms

126. Which of the following benzodiazepines is relatively safe when prescribed for patients with liver function impairment

    A. Alprazolam (Xanax)
    B. Oxazepam (Serax)
    C. Triazolam (Halcion)
    D. Midazolam (Versed)
    E. Chlordiazepoxide (Librium)

127. A 3-year-old boy presents in a neurology clinic with chief complaint of recurrent "spells." The symptom started approximately 2 months ago. He has frequent spells of brief loss of attention, daze, or loss of conscious. He had several incidences of sudden fall. Fortunately there has not been any significant head injury. During several of these spells he had tremor and muscle spasms. The boy had high fever approximately 3 months ago and was treated with IV drugs in another hospital. Medical record is not available. Electroencephalograph shows slow spike-wave complexes. What is the most likely first line of treatment

    A. Phenytoin
    B. Vagus nerve stimulation
    C. Corpus callosotomy
    D. Ketogenic diet
    E. Valproic acid

128. Patients with epileptic disorders may sometimes have interictal thought disorders mimicking psychotic disorders. The following are characteristics of interictal psychosis **EXCEPT**

    A. Usually proceeded by personality change
    B. Patients usually remain appropriate affect
    C. More frequent in male patients
    D. Circumstantiality is more common while blocking and looseness are rare
    E. More frequent in left-handed patients

129. Which of the following anticonvulsants has the highest probability to cause renal stones

    A. Carbamazepine
    B. Lamotrigine

    C. Oxcarbazepine

    D. Topiramate

    E. Phenytoin

130. The following states regarding seizure disorders and pregnancy are true **EXCEPT**

    A. Women suffering from epilepsy have higher rate of polycystic ovarian syndrome

    B. Women with epileptic disorders have reduced fertility rate

    C. Seizure during pregnancy may cause fetal hypoxia

    D. Carbamazepine, phenytoin, and valproic acid carry certain risk of causing fetal developmental defects

    E. High-dose vitamin D may reduce the risk of neural tube defects induced by antiepileptic drugs

131. In patients with anorexia nervosa, the following laboratory changes are usually found **EXCEPT**

    A. Hypokalemic alkalosis

    B. Lowered levels of protein and albumin

    C. Leukopenia with relative lymphocytosis

    D. Hypersecretion of corticotrophin-releasing hormone (CRH)

    E. Elevated β-carotene

132. An 81-year-old female was brought to the hospital for new onset lower back pain worsened for 2 weeks. She had several falls in the past 2 months with pelvic fracture found in recent admission. Pelvic X-ray did not show any difference from her previous images. MRI of lower spine is shown here. What is likely the most significant new finding in this film? *(Figure Q132)*

    A. Osteoporosis

    B. Muscle strain

    C. Metastasis of cancer

    D. Fracture

    E. Bleeding

Figure Q132.

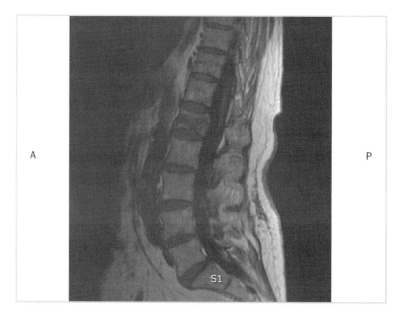

133. Which of the following congenital conditions is NOT caused by chromosomal abnormality

   A. Cri-du-Chat
   B. William's Syndrome
   C. Phenylketonuria
   D. Prader-Willi syndrome
   E. Dandy-Walker syndrome

134. A 25-year-old female social worker visited your office for depression. She reported chronic depression for over 2 years. She was treated by another physician who put her on fluoxetine at 60 mg/day for the past 6 months. Before she was treated with maprotiline intermittently. None of the medicines seemed to help her significantly. She also received psychotherapy for a while with no improvement. Her symptoms, besides chronic low mood, include overeating, over sleeping, feelings of heaviness on arms and legs, sensitivity to rejections, abdominal discomfort, joint and muscle ache. She also reported being happy for positive events in life, though the good mood usually lasted for no more than 1–2 days. She never had any suicidal or homicidal ideas or behaviors. Her extensive medical work-up had been generally negative besides moderate obesity. Though your examination there was no manic episode, nor psychotic symptoms were found. Which of the following regimen is most likely to induce clinical improvement in her depression?

   A. Stop fluoxetine and switch to another antidepressant
   B. Continue fluoxetine and add psychotherapy
   C. Tapering fluoxetine and switch to another antidepressant
   D. Continue fluoxetine and add alprazolam
   E. Continue fluoxetine and add olanzapine

135. Which of the following antiretroviral agents, when administered to patients already on benzodiazepine, may induce benzodiazepine withdrawal?

   A. Efavirenz
   B. Indinavir
   C. Nelfinavir
   D. Ritonavir
   E. Saquinavir

136. Codeine's analgesic effect is diminished when coadministered with the following agents EXCEPT

   A. Mirtazapine
   B. Amitriptyline
   C. Paroxetine
   D. Quinidine
   E. Ritonavir

137. Regarding valproic acid involved drug interaction, the following statements are correct EXCEPT

   A. Valproic acid increases serum level of warfarin through both metabolic inhibition and displacement of protein binding
   B. Valproic acid serum level is increased when coadministered with carbamazepine due to metabolic inhibition
   C. Valproic acid increases serum level of lamotrigine through metabolic inhibition

D. Valproic acid increases serum level of phenytoin through displacement of protein binding

E. Valproic acid serum level is decreased when coadministered with cimetidine due to metabolic induction

138. Which of the following antipsychotics bears lowest potential of weight gaining effect

   A. Risperidone
   B. Quetiapine
   C. Paliperidone
   D. Aripiprazole
   E. Olanzapine

139. Which of the following statements regarding electroconvulsive therapy is **INCORRECT**

   A. The highest static impedance in the electroconvulsive therapy (ECT) circuit is in the bony skull
   B. The combination of impedance in the skin and the brain tissue is only 1%–2% of the bony skull
   C. Approximately 60% of the electric stimulus enters the brain
   D. Brief-pulse stimuli drive neuronal firing more efficiently than either constant-step pulse or sine wave stimuli
   E. The preferred duration of a brief pulse is 0.5–2 milliseconds

140. Progressive multifocal leuko-encephalopathy is seen in approximately 5% of patients with acquired immune deficiency syndrome (AIDS). The following states regarding progressive multifocal leuko-encephalopathy are true **EXCEPT**

   A. It causes demyelination in CNS
   B. It presents with multifocal neurologic abnormalities
   C. It has white matter lesions without mass effect
   D. A CSF test using PCR technique may confirm the diagnosis
   E. It is associated with the secondary infection of a fungus

141. The following are etiological characteristics of nonfluent aphasia **EXCEPT**

   A. Usually associated with discrete structural lesion
   B. Location of lesion is in the frontal lobe, in or near Broca's area
   C. The lesion is in distribution area of left anterior cerebral artery
   D. Lesions often involve nearby motor and sensory cortex
   E. Lesions often extend to underlying white matters

142. The following are conditions appropriate for ECT **EXCEPT**

   A. Acute psychotic agitation
   B. Severe depression with suicidal ideas
   C. Bipolar mixed episode
   D. Intractable seizures
   E. Severe and frequent panic attacks

143. A 7-year-old boy was brought to the clinic for evaluation of recent onset recent "got lost" episodes. His episodes were described as abrupt loss of touch to reality, seemed in blank mind, staring to the space, blinking eyes at times. He would stop what he was doing for a few seconds. He could not recall what happened after recovery to normal status. He never fell or got any injury due to these spells. An EEG study found generalized 3 Hz spike-and-wave complexes. What is likely the first choice of treatment for this condition?

A. Lorazepam
B. Carbamazepine
C. Methylphenidate
D. Ethosuximide
E. Chlorpromazine

144. Which of the following condition is consistent with Brown-Sequard syndrome due to injury at right side?

A. Left side pain sense loss due to interruption of right spinothalamic tract
B. Right side hyperactive deep tendon responses and Babinski sign due to interruption of right spinothalamic tract
C. Right side position sense loss due to interruption of left dorsal column
D. Left side vibratory sense loss due to interruption of right dorsal column
E. Right side temperature sense loss due to interruption of right spinothalamic tract

145. The following statements regarding Huntington's chorea are correct **EXCEPT**

A. It is an autosomal dominant disease, carried on chromosome 4
B. Its mechanism is associated with abnormal expansion of CAG trinucleotide
C. Its usual onset age is between 18–25 years
D. Dementia appears within 1 year of onset of chorea
E. Brain image studies show atrophy of cerebral cortex and head of the caudate nuclei, and characteristic "bat-wing ventricles"

146. In 1957, A New York psychologist Leon Festinger proposed a theory. He found human being may sometimes have two cognitions that are incompatible, i.e., holding two conflicting thoughts at the same time. He proposed that the uncomfortable tension of having contradicting cognitions serve as a driving force that compels the mind to acquire or invent new thoughts or beliefs, or to modify existing beliefs. The contradicting cognitions in Festinger's theory were termed

A. Double binding
B. Learned helplessness
C. Strange situation
D. Cognitive dissonance
E. Anal fixation

147. The following are characteristic symptoms of amyotrophic lateral sclerosis **EXCEPT**

A. Asymmetric paresis
B. Pseudobulbar palsy
C. Dementia
D. Muscular atrophy with fasciculation
E. Bulbar palsy

148. According to John Bowlby, children of ages 6 weeks to 3 years start to develop emotional and behavioral dependence to caregiver or provider. This was termed "attachment," and believed to lasts through adult life. Attachment reactions present the children's feeling of being secure or insecure. Which is the following presents a secure attachment?

A. The child protests the mother's departure and quiets on the mother's return
B. Little to no signs of distress at the mother's departure and no visible response to the mother's return

C. Sad on the mother's departure but warmed up to a stranger, and ambivalent signs of anger on mother's return

D. The child becomes irritable, not eating well, and not making expected weight gains

E. Lack of coherent response, often stereotypes upon the mother's return after separation

149. When using emergency restraints, staffs should watch for the following rules **EXCEPT**

   A. At least four staffs should be used

   B. At least two restraints should be used

   C. When agitation improved, remove one restraint at a time at 5-minute intervals

   D. Proper documentation includes the reason for the restraints, the course of treatment, and the patient's response

   E. The restraining staff member should avoid being in the visual range of the patient

150. Psychiatrists have an ongoing obligation to treatment confidentiality. However, under the following situations the confidentiality can be legally breached **EXCEPT**

   A. When the case is heard in a military court

   B. When the patient asserts the testimonial privilege

   C. When it is a child abuse case

   D. When the physician is working on court-ordered exams

   E. When it is a malpractice case brought by the patient

Answers

1. Answer: **D.**

After a period of life-threatening experience in Iraq, the patient developed persistent reexperience, avoidance, and increased arousal symptoms, that did not present before the trauma. The symptoms caused significant distress. The duration of symptoms is more than 3 months. The onset of symptoms is more than 6 months after the stressor. The diagnosis is posttraumatic stress disorder (PTSD), chronic, with delayed onset.

The symptoms are prominently anxiety spectrum, and closely related to his traumatic experience. The depressive symptoms actually are not significant. Panic disorder with agoraphobia could not explain the flashback symptoms. Though there may be some degree of confusion, which is likely dissociative symptoms, there are no clear cut psychotic symptoms. Nightmare is only part of the PTSD, it dose not warrant a separate diagnosis.

2. Answer: **A.**

Nondeclarative memory is also known as implicit memory. It deals with skills, habits, and nonassociative learning. It does not require conscious awareness and concentration. Nondeclarative memory usually remains intact after brain injury. Brain structures involved in nondeclarative memory are – basal ganglia, limbic system, and perceptual cortex.

Declarative memory is also known as explicit memory. It deals with facts, events, and associative learning. It requires conscious awareness and concentration. Declarative memory is often impaired after brain injury. Brain structures involved in declarative memory are – hippocampus, orbitofrontal cortex, and parahippocampal gyrus.

Eidetic memory relies not on language codes as most people usually do, but on vivid visual memory.

Working memory is a temporal memory system where information is not necessarily prepared for long term storage, rather be ready for immediate use in managing cognitive tasks such as learning, reasoning, and comprehension. It is mostly associated with declarative memory.

3. Answer: **D.**

It is the hyponatremia, not hypernatremia, and the aggressive correction of hyponatremia, that are believed to be the essential etiology of central pontine myelinolysis (CPM).

CPM often presents with disturbances of consciousness, affect, and behavior. There are signs of damage in the corticobulbar and corticospinal tracts in the basis pontis. Paralysis of the lower cranial nerves often happens. Head computer tomography (CT) shows hypodense areas within the central pons, which can be confirmed by magnetic resonance imaging (MRI) on T1, while T2 shows hyperintense areas. Prevention and early diagnosis are crucial. Correcting electrolytes at proper rate is the key preventative strategy.

4. Answer: **E.**

Incestuous behavior has been associated with rural or isolative environment, not inner city. It is also associated with alcohol abuse, mental disorders, intellectual deficiencies, and overcrowded housing situations.

5. Answer: **C.**

The "4 Ds" in malpractice include – *Duty* to care, i.e., has established doctor–patient relationship; *D*eviation from the accepted standard of care; *D*amage happened to the patient; and the damage was *D*irectly caused by the deviation. Intentional deviation is not a required proof.

6. Answer: **C.**

Pupillary dilation is seen in intoxication of cocaine, amphetamine, and hallucinogen.

Opioid intoxication is associated with pupillary constriction, while lacrimation is seen in opioid withdrawal.

Hallucinogen intoxication is associated with pupillary dilation, not pupillary constriction.

Conjunctival injection is characteristic for cannabis intoxication.

Nystagmus is seen in the intoxication of alcohol, sedatives, phencyclidine (PCP), or inhalant.

Cannabis withdrawal has minimal physical signs and is not a DSM-IV-TR diagnosis.

7. Answer: **D.**

There is no evidence of epidural hemorrhage or subdural hemorrhage. The computer tomography (CT) picture shows a large right parietal scalp hematoma. The hematoma was likely due to his fall. But the scalp hematoma alone may not cause mental status change. There maybe accompanied brain contusion, which may well contribute to loss of conscious. However, the most prominent factor of cognitive impairment was alcohol intoxication. Alcohol withdrawal may present only when blood alcohol level is low or null.

8. Answer: **C.**

All patients must be assessed about suicidal thoughts. Assessment includes – intent, plans, means, perceived consequences, personal history of suicide, and family history of suicide. Studies have found that asking about suicide does NOT increase the risk of suicide. Personal history of suicide has shown to be the most relevant predictive factor for future suicidal behavior.

9. Answer: **D.**

Ganser syndrome is a unique behavior where the individual provides approximate answers to questions; e.g., 4 + 5 = 8. This is usually a manifestation of malingering, but may also be a sign of confusion or disinhibition status, such as dissociative status.

Abulia describes the mental status of indifference, lack of impulse and motivation to act or think spontaneously, and lack of ability to make decisions.

Circumstantiality is a thought process disorder. It presents with original difficulty in having goal-directed association in thoughts but eventually gets to the point.

Capgras syndrome is a delusion, where the patient believes that someone, usually a close relative or family member, has been replaced by an impostor.

Paramnesia is false memory usually due to distortion of recall. Commonly mentioned paramnesia includes jamais vu and déjà vu.

10. Answer: **E.**

La belle indifference is the inappropriately lack of concern about the deficit or disability. It typically appears in conversion disorders.

11. Answer: **D.**

Alexithymia is the inability to be aware of or express one's own mood and feeling.

Abulia is the mental status of indifference, lack of impulse and motivation to act or think spontaneously, and lack of ability to make decisions.

Blocking is the abrupt interruption in the train of thought. The individual is not able to recall of what was being said. Blocking is also known as thought deprivation.

Lethologica is a term coined by Carl Jung. It describes the inability of articulating the individual's thoughts by forgetting key words, phrases, or names in conversation.

Paramnesia is false memory, such as jamais vu and déjà vu.

12. Answer: **D.**

The scientific consensus in the United States is that reparative therapy is not effective at changing sexual orientation and is potentially harmful.

The rest of the statements are correct.

13. Answer: **C.**

Exact elements of executive function are not well defined. The generally accepted descriptions are the capacity of purposefully applying one's mental skills, or the capacity of accomplishing goal-directed behavior.

14. Answer: **B.**

Among elderly, the completed suicide is greater in the Caucasian, not the African-American, population.

The completed suicide rate in elderly is higher than in the general population. Suicide in elderly is usually precipitated by a loss. A completed suicide is usually accomplished by violent means.

15. Answer: **D.**

The question asks about construct validity, which refers to whether a test measures the unobservable that it purports to measure. Evaluation of construct validity include the test's theoretical grounds, its correlations from numerous studies using the test, whether it fits the expected pattern contribute, and its correlation of the measure with variables that are known to be related to the construct purpose.

Whether the test reproduces consistent result when used at different times and by different raters describes reliability, not construct validity.

16. Answer: **B.**

Déjà vu is an illusion in which a new situation is regarded as a previously experienced situation. It has no pathognomic meaning. Déjà vu may appear in seizure disorders, dissociative disorders, or people with no mental disorders.

With Jamais vu, a familiar situation is not recognized by the person as if he/she sees the situation the first time. Jamais vu may appear in amnesia, epilepsy, and migraine aura.

Folie à deux means "madness shared by two." The individual develops a delusion similar to another individual who already established a delusion. Usually the two individuals have a close relationship and a strong connection. In DSM-IV-TR, it is termed shared psychotic disorder.

Dissociative identity disorder was formerly known as "multiple personality disorder." The individual possesses two or more distinct personality states. At least two of these identities periodically take control of the person's behavior.

In Déjà pense, a completely new thought sounds familiar to the individual as if he/she had the same thought before.

17. Answer: **B.**

Y-BOCS, or Yale-Brown Obsessive-Compulsive Scale, is a test to measure the severity of obsessive-compulsive symptoms, and to monitor the response to treatment. It is not a projective test.

TAT, Draw-A-Person test, Rorschach test, and Sentence completion test are all projective test.

18. Answer: **A.**

The structured clinical interview for the DSM-IV (SCID) is a semistructured interview that is arguably the most reliable instrument for psychiatric diagnoses.

Abnormal involuntary movement scale (AIMS) measures late onset movement disorders, such as tardive dyskinesia. It is not a diagnostic tool.

Brief psychotic rating scale (BPRS) provides quantitative severity of psychotic symptoms. It is not a diagnostic tool.

Minnesota multiphasic personality inventory II (MMPI-2) is designed to help identify personal, social, and behavioral problems in psychiatric patients. It is not a diagnostic tool.

Positive and negative syndrome scale (PANNS) is a severity rating instrument designed for the assessment of schizophrenia. It is not a diagnostic tool.

19. Answer: **E.**

Amygdala has output to hypothalamus to activate the sympathetic nervous system; to nuclei of the CN-V and CN VII to regulate the facial expressions; to VTA to activate dopamine system; and to locus coeruleus to activate norepinephrine system.

Amygdala does not have output to the vagus nerve system.

20. Answer: **C.**

Beck depression inventory is a self-rating scale measuring severity of depression.

Brief psychotic rating scale, clinical global improvement scale, Hamilton rating scale for depression and Millon clinical multiaxial inventory are all administered by clinician.

21. Answer: **C.**

Lawrence Kohlberg described three major levels of morality

Preconventional – to avoid punishment, (A)

Conventional – to gain approval from others, (C)

Principle – to stand for ethical principles, (E)

Carol Gilligan proposed that girls concern more on relationships, and rely more on intuitive sense in decision making, rather than rules and reasoning as in boys, (B)

Attachment is associated with resources and security.

22. Answer: **D.**

"Bulb" is a term used to describe medulla and lower portion of pons. The nuclei of cranial nerves IX to XII locate in bulb, and are called bulbar cranial nerves. Lesions in bulb cause lower motor neuron injury of cranial nerves IX to XII. Symptoms of bulbar palsy are dysarthria and dysphagia, and hyporeflexia. Respiratory impairment appears in bulbar palsy.

Pseudobulbar palsy is a syndrome of dysarthria and dysphagia as though seen in bulbar palsy. However, the lesion is not in bulbar area, hence "pseudo." It is caused by lesions anywhere along the corticobulbar tract, usually in frontal lobe, and therefore is often associated with emotional and cognitive change. It is an upper motor neuron injury. Hyperactive jaw and gag reflexes are characteristic; usually no respiratory impairment.

In either bulbar or pseudobulbar palsy, dysarthria and dysphagia are not psychogenic.

23. Answer: **D.**

Double binding is a concept formulated by Gregory Bateson and Donald Jackson.

Basic trust vs. basic mistrust is Eric Erikson's first psychosocial developmental stage out of total of eight stages.

According to Kohut's self psychology, self-object function is the interaction between individuals (selves) and their mother and the other family members (objects). Selves need empathic interaction with objects.

Learned helplessness is a psychological condition in which an individual has learned to believe that any attempt to escape from the suffering will be useless. Seligman established the first animal model of depression based on the theory of learned helplessness.

Strange situation is a laboratory procedure designed to assess infant attachment style; developed by Mary Ainsworth and coauthors.

24. Answer: **E.**

Ethnicity is a preferred term by cross-cultural researchers. Ethnicity refers to individuals-shared characters that can be assessed clinically, such as – a sense of common identity, ancestry, belief, and shared history. Biological measurement does not define ethnicity.

25. Answer: **B.**

Projective identification is a psychological process that takes two steps – one person projects a thought, belief, or emotion to a second person; the second person is changed by the projection and begins to behave as though he or she is in fact actually characterized by those thoughts or beliefs that have been projected.

Splitting is a defense mechanism, in which the world is divided into simply good and bad. The individual rapidly shifts from one extreme to another.

Sublimation is a defense mechanism, as believed to be the healthiest and mature one. It is the refocusing of psychic energy away from negative outlets to healthy and creative behavior.

Suppression is a defense mechanisms to consciously held unwanted or unpleasant memory or thoughts out of conscious mind.

Passive aggression is a defense mechanism using passive resistance and uncooperativeness to avoid open confrontation.

26. Answer: **C.**

Eric Erikson proposed eight psychosocial developmental stages
Basic trust vs. basic mistrust (0–1 year)
Autonomy vs. shame and doubt (1–3 years)
Initiative vs. guilt (3–5 years), (E)
Industry vs. inferiority (6–11 years), (B)
Identity vs. role confusion (11–20 years)

Intimacy vs. self-absorption or isolation (21–40 years), (A)
Generativity vs. stagnation (40–65 years), (C)
Ego integrity vs. despair (65 years and beyond)
Repression vs. suppression is not one of Eric Erikson's stages.

27. Answer: **D.**

According to Pavlov's classical conditioning, a conditioned response can be established by the paired presentation of a neutral stimulus (conditioned stimulus) and a stimulus of significance (unconditioned stimulus). In this example, the dog usually salivates (unconditioned response) when served with food (unconditioned stimulus). After repeated exposure to bell sound (conditioned stimulus) paired with food, the dog may salivate (conditioned response) upon bell sound alone without food.

28. Answer: **C.**

Concrete operational stage is the third of Jean Piaget's developmental stages. It spans from 7–11 years old. Children in this stage possess rational and logical thought, and the ability to understand someone else's point of view. The concept of conservation is also development.

Phallic stage is the third of Sigmund Freud's five psychodynamic developmental stages; age 3–5 years. This stage has the most colorful psychodynamic description, including the famous Oedipal complex, castration anxiety, and penis envy.

Sensorimotor is the first of Jean Piaget's four stages for cognitive development. It spans from age 0–2 years. Children have stereotyped reaction to stimuli. They've development object permanency (8–9 months).

Rapprochement is the fifth developmental stage in Margaret Mahler's separation-individuation theory. Children constantly are concerned about the actual physical location of their mothers, and have great need for maternal love.

Formal operational stage is the last and most mature stage of Jean Piaget's developmental theory. It is beyond 11 years of age. Individuals in formal operational stage deal with concepts and ideas. Their thoughts are abstract, deductive, and conceptual. They are able to use synthesis, the integration of traits, attitudes, and impulses to create a total personality.

29. Answer: **B.**

Most common clinical capacity evaluation is regarding treatment decision making. A patient is capable of making treatment decision if he/she has – factual understanding of the information; appreciation of consequences of accepting or rejecting treatment; ability to manipulate the information rationally and come to a decision logically; and ability to communicate of a preference.

Competency is a legal status declared only by a judge, not a physician. A physician may perform clinical assessment on the capacity of decision making.

Loss of speaking ability can not preclude the ability of effective communication.

Psychotic patients may have residual ability of rationally manipulating treatment relevant information and therefore not necessarily incapable of decision making.

To be capable of decision making, a patient must appreciate the possible consequences of accepting treatment, and also the consequences of rejecting treatment.

30. Answer: **D.**

Dopamine neurons project to caudate originate mainly from the ventral tegmental area and the substantia nigra. Dopamine neurons in hypothalamus project to pituitary gland and form the tuberoinfundibular dopamine system, which regulates prolactin secretion.

The rest of the statements are correct.

31. The answer is **E.**

The choice of electroconvulsive therapy (ECT) should be made based upon the patient's need, not the physician's preference.

The rest of the choices are appropriate situations when ECT should be considered.

32. Answer: **C.**

Pseudocholinesterase is an enzyme hydrolyzes exogenous choline esters, such as succinylcholine. Individuals with pseudocholinesterase deficiency have slowed succinylcholine metabolism and prolonged apnea after electro convulsive therapy (ECT).

The rest of the choices are legitimate concerns during ECT, but not specific for pseudocholinesterase deficiency.

33. Answer: **D.**

Biological changes in posttraumatic stress disorder (PTSD) include – hyper-reactive in limbic/paralimbic structures, including amygdala, hippocampus, and anterior cingulated cortex. Physiological arousal after exposure to cues in individuals with PTSD, such as increase in heart rate, skin conduction, blood pressure, and electromyography (EMG) activity. Increase in norepinephrine turnover in the locus coeruleus, limbic regions, and cerebral cortex; and abnormalities of HPA axis.

34. Answer: **A.**

Apoptosis is programmed cell death. It involves expression of specific genes. It is associated with development, and neurodegenerative disease not acute trauma. In the process of apoptosis there is no inflammatory response. It may be prevented, not enhanced, by neurotrophins. Apoptosis is triggered by internal genetic programming, not external damage.

Choices B–E is characteristics of necrosis.

35. Answer: **B.**

Clinical effects of histamine blockade include – allergy relief; hypotension, not hypertension; sedation; weight gain; and decreased gastric acid production.

36. Answer: **C.**

This is a case of female orgasmic disorder. The proper next step is to rule out reversible factors, such as medication side effects and neurologic impairments.

Psychiatric evaluation on anxiety and relationship problems is also essential; however, the medical evaluation should take the first priority.

Pelvic diaphragm strengthening exercise, sensate focus exercise, tool-assisted sexual activity, and medication to improve sexual function are all viable options after a complete medical and psychiatric evaluation.

37. Answer: **B.**

Direct-coupled ion channels are one type of membrane-bound receptors, where ion channels are part of the receptors. These receptors respond fast to neurotransmitter activities. Binding of a ligand directly changes the ion channel; therefore no second messengers are needed.

Direct-coupled ion channels are constructed with multiple subunits, not single unit. Each subunit has 4–5 transmembrane domains. Examples of direct-coupled ion channel receptors include – nicotinic cholinergic receptor, 5-HT3, gamma-amino butyric acid (GABA)-A, and glutamate receptors.

G-protein coupled receptors are single unit receptors.

38. Answer: **C.**

The area of raphe nuclei is the central location of serotonin neurons. There is no significant dopamine secretion in this area.

The rest of the choices are correct.

39. Answer: **B.**

Na-K-ATPase pump moves Na$^+$ OUT and K$^+$ IN so to maintain the membrane potential.

Depolarization is to reduce the cytosol negative charge, makes the cell membrane ready to have action potential.

The action potential starts with depolarization by rapid influx of Na$^+$, not Cl$^-$.

Ca^{++} also has a higher concentration outside of cell, and enter cell during action potential with Na$^+$. Ca^{++} involves in many cytosol activities, also activates repolarization by outward K$^+$, not Na$^+$, current.

The outward K$^+$ current causes hyper polarization, not depolarization.

40. Answer: **E.**

Poor response to anxiolytic agents warrants further medical work-up to search for possible organic cause.

Factors imply organic etiology of anxiety include – onset of symptoms after the age of 35 years, lack of anticipatory anxiety, lack of avoidance behavior, and lack of personal or family history of anxiety disorders.

41. Answer: **A.**

Melatonin is secreted by the pineal gland.

The rest of the choices are correct statements.

42. Answer: **D.**

There are two subtypes of monoamine oxidase (MAO) – MAO-A and MAO-B. Both MAO-A and MAO-B appear in central nervous system.

MAO-A, not MAO-B, also appear in liver and intestine, where it breaks down tyramine from food.

No significant MAO activity is detected in blood vessel walls.

When MAO-A is inhibited, not induced, tyramine-rich food can cause surge of tyramine in blood and hypertensive crisis may occur.

43. Answer: **E.**

Atomoxetine is a norepinephrine reuptake inhibitor. It has not significant effect on *N*-methyl-*D*-aspartate (NMDA) receptor.

NMDA receptor is one of the five major types of glutamate receptors. When activated by two molecules of glutamate and one of glycine, it opens the integrated Ca^{++} channel to allow influx of calcium. It may be blocked by Mg^{++} and phencyclidine (PCP). NMDA receptor plays a key role in learning and memory. Down regulation of NMDA receptor may cause psychosis. Drugs bind to NMDA receptors include memantine, acamprosate, and the illicit substance PCP.

44. Answer: **A.**

Serotonin receptors in spinal cord, not brainstem, are associated with sexual side effects of serotonin selective receptor inhibitors (SSRIs).

Serotonin receptors at brainstem and in gastrointestinal system are associated with nausea and vomiting.

45. Answer: **E.**

Neurological conditions associated with trinucleotide repeat expansion include Huntington's disease, fragile X syndrome, myotonic dystrophy, spinobulbar muscular atrophy, spinocerebellar ataxia type 1, and Machado-Joseph disease.

Parkinson's disease is not related to Trinucleotide repeat expansion.

46. Answer: **D.**

Continuous treatment to enable chronic patients to attain best potential of functioning is an important part of tertiary, not secondary, prevention.

The rest of the choices are correct.

47. Answer: **D.**

Pseudotumor cerebri is also known as idiopathic intracranial hypertension.

It appears in young obese women, characterized by headache and papilledema due to increased intracranial pressure. Lumbar puncture is both diagnostic and therapeutic. Untreated, it may cause blindness and empty sella syndrome.

48. Answer: **D.**

Headache caused by space occupying lesion is usually progressive over days to weeks, may have focal signs, often unilateral, and often more severe in early morning, and awakening.

Migraine is also unilateral. It is a recurrent condition, but not progressive. It usually has pounding quality. It is exacerbated with activity. It should be accompanied by at least one of the following symptoms – photophobia, phonophobia, nausea and vomiting.

Cluster headache is recurrent, not progressive. It is also unilateral, but more often peri-orbital, and stabbing attacks in nature. Accompanying symptoms are ptosis, miosis, lacrimation, and congestion.

Headache due to meningitis is characterized by acute headache with fever and chills. Other possible symptoms include – nuchal rigidity, photophobia, vomiting, and seizure.

Headache due to subarachnoid hemorrhage is usually sudden onset, very severe headache, may have decreased level of consciousness.

49. Answer: **E.**

Triptans is an abortive treatment, not a prophylactic treatment for migraine headache.

The rest of the choices are correct.

50. Answer: **A.**

The 5-HT1b receptors are located on blood vessels. When activated, produces vasoconstriction, not vasodilation.

The 5-HT1d receptors are presynaptic nerve receptors. When activated, inhibits the release of vasoactive peptides, including substance P, histamine, bradykinins, etc.

The assumed inherited central migraine generator is activated by environmental migraine triggers, and sends impulses through trigeminal nerve.

Vasoactive and algogenic peptides are released through CN-V (trigeminal), and CN-V then sends the pain message back to the brain.

51. Answer: **D.**

Irritable heart is a term used during the civil war years. The condition is most close to the modern diagnosis of posttraumatic stress disorder.

Effort syndrome is another historical term to described similar conditions. It was used during the World War I.

52. Answer: **A.**

Shenjing shuairuo is a culture-bound syndromes found in China. Literally means "nerve weakness." Symptoms include – chronic fatigue, dizziness, headaches, sleep difficulties, nonspecific, and multiple somatic complaints. These conditions are likely related to depression, anxiety, fibromyalgia, chronic fatigue, and irritable bowel syndromes.

Mal de mojo is a culture-bound syndrome in Mediterranean cultures. Symptoms are crying without a reason, vomiting, diarrhea. Often occurs in children.

Koro is found in males of China and Malaysia. Symptoms – intense anxiety, senses as if genital retracted back into the body. Some patients use devices to attach the genital to the wall to prevent such retraction.

Amafufanyane occurs in Zulu population of southern Africa. Clinical features – sleep paralysis, abdominal pain, blindness, shouting and sobbing, amnesia, and pseudoseizure. Often occurs in young females, influenced by witchcraft, contains sexual content.

Ataque de nervios occurs among Latinos from the Caribbean. Clinical features – uncontrollable shouting, crying episodes, trembling, sense of heat rising from chest moving toward head. Usually has Amnesia of the episode.

53. Answer: **E.**

Poverty is not a risk factor of child abuse.

54. Answer: **C.**

In contrast to primary anxiety, organic anxiety usually has little or no anticipatory anxiety, no avoidance behavior, and no personal or family history of anxiety disorders. Onset of symptoms after the age of 35 years warrants further investigation for organic etiology. Organic anxiety often has poor response to anxiolytic medications.

55. Answer: **E.**

The location of injury is at temporal and/or parietal lobe, therefore the motor cortex is not affected. Hemiparesis is often associated with nonfluent aphasia, but rarely with fluent aphasia.

The rest of the choices are correct statements.

56. Answer: **C.**

Electroconvulsive therapy (ECT) was introduced in 1938 as the first biological treatment.
  The introduction of landmark psychopharmacological agents are as following
  1949 – lithium, the first psychotropic agent
  1953 – chlorpromazine, the first antipsychotic
  1957 – imipramine, the first antidepressant
  1985 – fluoxetine, the first serotonin selective reuptake inhibitor (SSRI)

57. Answer: **D.**

Boufee delirante is a culture-bound syndrome found in West Africa and Haiti. Clinical symptoms include – sudden outburst of agitation, aggressive behavior, and confusion.

Shenjing shuairuo is a culture-bound syndrome found in China. Clinical symptoms include – chronic fatigue, dizziness and headaches, sleep difficulties and nonspecific somatic complaints.

Koro is a culture-bound syndrome found in males of China and Malaysia. Characteristic symptoms are intense anxiety accompanied with senses as if genital retracted back into the body.

Latah is a culture-bound syndrome occurring in Malaysia and Indonesia. Symptoms include – startle response, intense light reactions, echolalia and echopraxis.

Amok is a culture-bound syndrome occurring in the population of Malaysia, Indonesia, Laos, and Philippines. Clinical features – sudden outburst of rage, running out, aggressive and violent behavior toward people and self.

58. Answer: **D.**

Nonfluent aphasia is associated with lesions in or near Broca's area in motor cortex. Temporal and parietal lobes are usually not impaired. Therefore receptive language and comprehension are not usually impaired in nonfluent aphasia.

The rest of the choices are correct statements.

59. Answer: **B.**

Schneider's first rank symptoms include – audible thoughts, voices arguing or discussing, voices commenting, somatic passivity experiences, thought withdrawal, thought broadcasting, delusional perceptions, volition, made affects, and made impulses.

Emotional impoverishment is not a first rank symptom.

60. Answer: **D.**

Volume reduction has been found in prefrontal cortex, thalamus, hippocampus, and superior temporal cortex. There is no consistent finding of occipital atrophy in individuals with schizophrenia.

61. Answer: **C.**

Delusional disorder presents prominently nonbizarre delusions with relatively less extent of other thought and behavior disturbances. The clinical presentation should never meet symptomatic criteria for schizophrenia.

The diagnosis of delusional disorder requires nonbizarre delusions for at least 1 month, not 6 months. Comparing with other psychotic disorders, delusional disorder preserves functioning level relatively well; may have olfactory and tactile hallucinations congruent with delusional theme.

Identified subtypes are – erotomanic, grandiose, jealous, persecutory, somatic, mixed, and unspecified.

Nihilistic is not an identified subtype of delusional disorder.

62. Answer: **C.**

Klinefelter's syndrome has the chromosomal pattern of 47, XXY. Patients usually have a normal intelligence quotient (IQ), with weakened male habitus. Behavior and mood symptoms are impulsivity, anxiety, aggression, and difficulty in socialization.

Sturge-Weber syndrome is remarkable for its cutaneous angioma looks like port wine stain in trigeminal distribution. Physical features are limited to central nervous system – seizure, glaucoma, and buphthalmos (the eyeball enlarges and bulges out of its socket) due to higher intraocular pressure. Characterized by possible developmental delay and mental retardation. It has characteristic pattern of railroad track clacifications on skull X-ray.

Seckel syndrome is also known as "bird-headed dwarfism." It is a congenital condition with mental retardation, inherited in autosomal recessive manner. It has probable genes on chromosomes 3 and 18. Clinical features include low birth weight, short stature, microcephaly, receding forehead, large eyes, low ears, prominent beaklike protrusion of the nose, and smallish chin. Behavior is usually friendly and pleasant.

Turner's syndrome's chromosomal pattern is monosomy X. Physical features – short stature, obesity, low hairline, low-set ears, simian crease, drooping eyelids, and webbed neck. Patients also have lymphoedema and amenorrhea.

William's Syndrome has chromosome 7 deletion. Patients have distinctive facial appearance and Broad range of vascular stenosis, including supravalvular aortic stenos and pulmonary artery stenosis. Mental features include mild to moderate mental retardation, learning difficulties and unique personality that combines overfriendliness and high levels of empathy with anxiety.

63. Answer: **E.**

Presence of obvious precipitating factors is a good prognostic factor.

Other good prognostic factors are – female, later age of onset, married status, negative family history of schizophrenia, absence of perinatal complications, acute onset, predominance of positive symptoms, affective symptoms, confusion or other organic symptoms, paranoid subtype, family history of affective disorder, good premorbid functioning, and high intelligence quotient (IQ).

64. Answer: **A.**

Hieroglyphics, i.e., using pictorial symbols to represent meaning or sounds, is a function of dominant hemisphere. Other dominant language forms are – speaking, writing, listening, reading, and sign language.

Language forms of nondominant hemisphere are – singing, prosody (tone of speaking), gestures (body language), cursing, and music.

65. Answer: **D.**

Verbal input pathway – CN VIII → lateral lemniscus → medial geniculate body → Heschl's gyri → Wernicke's area.

Occipital cortex is a component of visual input, not verbal input.

66. Answer: **A.**

Lesions associated with pseudobulbar palsy are located in frontal lobes or any location along the corticobulbar tract. Lesions at medulla and lower portion of pons may cause impairment to nucleus of cranial nerves IX (Glossopharyngeal), X (vagus), XI (accessory), and XII (hypoglossal), which are associated with bulbar, not pseudobulbar, palsy. Bulbar palsy, in contrast to pseudobulbar palsy, is a lower motor neuron injury.

The rest of the choices are correct statements.

67. Answer: **E.**

Medications that may cause sexual dysfunction include – tricyclic antidepressants, serotonin selective reuptake inhibitors (SSRIs), β-blockers, antipsychotics, corticosteroids, and estrogens.

Among the new antidepressants, mirtazapine (Remeron), venlafaxine (Effexor) and bupropion (Wellbutrin) have minimum negative influence on sexual function.

68. Answer: **C.**

Transcortical aphasia is also known as isolation aphasia. It is a fluent aphasia with echolalia, while global aphasia is a nonfluent aphasia.

The lesion isolates language arc from the remaining cortex, and preserves areas surrounding perisylvian arc.

Common causes of transcortical aphasia include – anoxia, CO poisoning, and Alzheimer's disease.

69. Answer: **A.**

The question describes alpha wave, which appears when the subject is awake, relaxed, with eyes closed.

When drowsy, in stage 1 sleep, or in meditation, the electroencephalogram (EEG) shows theta wave, with frequency of 3–7 Hz.

In stage 2 sleep, the EEG shows sleep spindles with frequency of 12–16 Hz, and the characteristic K-complexes.

Stages 3 and 4 are the deepest sleep stage. The EEG is the highest in amplitude and lowest in frequency. It is also called slow-wave sleep. The EEG frequency is up to 3 Hz.

In rapid eye movement (REM) sleep, the EEG has low voltage, random, fast, with sawtooth waves.

70. Answer: **B.**

When the wrist is hyperflexed, the patient experiences painful paresthesias. This is characteristic for carpel tunnel syndrome. This test is named after George Phalen (1911–1998), an American orthopaedist.

None of the rest conditions mentioned is associated with Phalen's test.

Eaton-Lambert syndrome is a paraneoplastic disorder associated with small-cell lung cancer. It presents with progressive weakness due to the antibodies to presynaptic voltage-gated calcium channels, which impairs the release of acetylcholine.

Guillain-Barré syndrome is an acute inflammatory demyelinating polyneuropathy with often severe weakness including quadriplegia and respiratory paralysis,

Locked-in syndrome is a syndrome of quadriplegia and bulbar palsy with preserved eye movement and general cognition. It is due to the impairment of corticospinal tracts and cranial nerves IX to XII, usually associated with infarction at the ventral portion of pons and medulla.

Cauda equine syndrome present the combination of pain in legs and lower back, flaccid areflexic paraparesis, and incontinence. It is caused by L2–S5 injury.

71. Answer: **D.**

Monoamine oxidases inhibitors (MAOIs), including phenelzine, may cause hypertensive crisis when interacted with a variety of medicines. However, hypertension is not a common side effect when MAOIs are used alone. The most common side effect of MAOIs is orthostatic hypotension.

Other side effects include – most common – insomnia, sedation, weight gain, sexual dysfunction (anorgasmia or impotence), headache, and dry mouth.

72. Answer: **E.**

Memantine's binds to a different binding site than that of glutamate, and therefore does not compete with glutamate. It is a noncompetitive N-methyl D-aspatate (NMDA) receptor antagonist.

The rest of the statements are correct.

73. Answer: **C.**

Lewy bodies are eosinophilic neuronal inclusions appear in Lewy body dementia, Parkinson's disease, and Lewy body variant of Alzheimer's disease. These structures are composed of α-synuclein, ubiquitin, neurofilament protein, and α B crystallin.

β amyloid is a component of senile plaque in Alzheimer's disease.

74. Answer: **C.**

In patients with chronic alcohol consumption, rapid eye movement (REM) sleep is increased in the early morning, but overall decreased.

Other sleep changes in individuals with chronic alcohol consumptions include

- ▶ Increased sleep latency
- ▶ Decreased slow-wave sleep; however, increased early in night
- ▶ Decreased total sleep time
- ▶ Sleep fragmentation
- ▶ Reduction of restful sleep and day time fatigue

Note that sleep disturbances may continue even with prolonged abstinence, and relapse may temporally reduce the sleep disturbances.

75. Answer: **B.**

Risk factors for cerebrovascular accidents include – age, hypertension, cardiac condition, diabetes, cholesterol elevation, cigarette smoking, heavy alcohol use, physical inactivity, drug abuse, C-reactive protein elevation, and homocysteine elevation.

Malnutrition is not directly associated with cerebrovascular accident.

76. Answer: **E.**

In chronic schizophrenic patients, brain volume reduction is found in prefrontal cortex, thalamus, hippocampus, and superior temporal cortex. Lateral and third ventricles are found to be enlarged.

77. Answer: **C.**

St. John's word should not be used with serotonin selective reuptake inhibitors (SSRIs) and monoamine oxidase inhibitors (MAOIs). The combination may cause serotonin syndrome, and there were reports of manic reaction when St. John's wort was used with sertraline.

St. John's wort is an inducer of P450 3A4. Other complicated drug interaction may also occur. It may decrease blood levels of protease inhibitors. Owing to its interaction with alcohol and opioids, the combination should be avoided. St. John's wort should be discontinued 5 days before surgery.

78. Answer: **D.**

Safe over-the-counter (OTC) medications – guaifenesin (Robitussin), chlorpheniramine (Chlor-Trimeton), brompheniramine (Dimetane).

Dextromethorphan (Robitussin DM) is contraindicated in combination with monoamine oxidase inhibitors (MAOIs) due to the risk of serotonin syndrome.

Oxymetazoline (Afrin) is contraindicated in combination with MAOIs due to potential hypertensive crisis.

Pseudoephedrine (Sudafed) is contraindicated in combination with MAOIs due to the risk of causing hypertensive crisis.

Phenylephrine (Sudafed PE, Neo-Synephrine) is not contraindicated in combination with MAOIs but cautions required due to synergistic effect on blood pressure.

79. Answer: **A.**

In Wada test, the tester observes the step-wise transient aphasia in seconds to minutes following infusion of a barbiturate into the carotid artery. The test is designed to confirm cerebral dominance to help decision on destructive brain surgery.

80. Answer: **B.**

Locked-in syndrome is associated with occlusion of a branch of the basilar artery, not the internal carotid artery.

Location of lesion is at the ventral portion of pons and medulla.

Impairment of cranial nerves IX (glossopharyngeal), X (vagus), XI (accessory) and XII (hypoglossal) is associated with bulbar palsy.

Impairment of corticospinal tracts causes quadriplegia.

81. Answer: **C.**

Propranolol is a nonselective β 1 and β 2 adrenergic antagonist.

It is indicated for hypertension, angina, myocardial infarction, cardiac arrhythmia, migraine headache, essential tremor, and pheochromocytoma.

It is also found to be effective for

▶ Akathisia and tremor induced by antipsychotics and lithium
▶ Posttraumatic stress disorder (PTSD), especially nightmares and exaggerated startle response
▶ Restless leg syndrome

82. Answer: **B**

Most psychotropic drugs are moderate to high protein-bound. For most drugs, only the unbound state is available for pharmacological activity. Protein-binding drugs may displace other protein-bound drugs, and potentially vital to the dosing and monitoring. Among psychotropic medicines, lithium is known to have no protein-binding ability. Gabapentin, oxcarbazepine, topiramate, and venlafaxine have minimum protein-binding potential. Valproate is medium to high protein-binding.

83. Answer: **B.**

This is a case of Arnold-Chiari malformation. The recommended treatment for symptomatic cases is surgical decompression. Given the significant and debilitating symptoms, conservative observation is inappropriate.

Lumber puncture may be helpful for normal pressure hydrocephalus, but should be avoided in this case. The elongated cerebellar tonsils may block cerebrospinal fluid (CSF) and lumber puncture may induce hernia.

Ventriculoperitoneal shunt is a definite treatment for normal pressure hydrocephalus, but not a choice for Arnold-Chiari malformation.

There is no sign of infection, therefore intravenous (IV) antibiotics is not indicated.

84. Answer: **D.**

In combined system disease, serum homocysteine is elevated. The rest of the choices are correct.

85. Answer: **A.**

This case describes Guillain-Barré syndrome, and inflammatory condition. The cerebrospinal fluid (CSF) is clear in color, minimally increased white blood cells (WBC) (5–20), mildly to moderately increased protein (80–200), and normal glucose (60–100).

Choice B shows normal CSF, where the color is clear, WBC is 0–4, protein is 30–45, glucose is 60–100.

Choice C shows CSF of bacterial meningitis, where the color is turbid, WBC significantly elevated WBC (100–500), protein also elevated (75–200).

Choice D shows viral meningitis, where the color is turbid, WBC moderately elevated (50–100), protein mild increased; glucose is normal or slightly decreased (40–60).

Choice E is subarachnoid hemorrhage.

86. Answer: **B.**

High prolactin, not low prolactin, is associated with sexual dysfunction.

The rest of the choices are possible causes of sexual dysfunction.

87. Answer: **A.**

The case describes characteristic features of fragile X syndrome.

Abnormality on short arm of chromosome 5 is the deficit of Cri-du-Chat. Patients have moderate to severe mental retardation, and cat-like cry.

Klinefelter's syndrome has XXY chromosomal pattern. Patients usually have a normal intelligence quotient (IQ), and weakened male habitus. Behavior and mood symptoms include impulsivity, anxiety, aggressiveness, and difficulty in socialization.

Prader-Willi syndrome has deletions in chromosome 15. Patients are usually obese and short, with small hands and feet. Other features include inability of conjugation, hypotonia, and hypogonadism.

Monosomy X is the chromosomal deficit of Turner's syndrome. Physical features – short stature, obesity, low hairline, low-set ears, simian crease, drooping eyelids, webbed neck. Patients also have lymphoedema and amenorrhea.

88. Answer: **E.**

Medial frontal lesions are associated with apathy. Emotional lability is associated with orbitofrontal lobe lesions.

The rest of the choices are correct statements.

89. Answer: **D.**

Introjection is an immature defense mechanism. To internalize the qualities of an object, the subject replicates behaviors, attributes or other fragments of the external world. According to Freud, the ego and the superego are constructed by introjecting external behavior into the personality. Introjection of a feared object serves to avoid anxiety when the aggressive characteristics of the object are internalized, thus placing the aggression under one's own control. Identification is believed by some to be a presentation of introjection. Introjection is the most common defense mechanism in depression.

Projection is to attribute the undesirable impulses and feelings to another person.

Suppression is a defense mechanism that, through a conscious effort, holds unwanted or unpleasant memory or thoughts out of the conscious mind.

Sublimation is believed to be the healthiest and the most mature one. It is to refocus the psychic energy away from negative outlets to healthy and creative behavior.

Repression is a defense mechanism that, through an unconscious act, holds unwanted or unpleasant memory or thoughts out of conscious mind.

90. Answer: **D.**

The ventral tegmental area plays an important role in the dopamine reward system, in emotion regulation, and in avoidance reactions. It is not part of basal ganglia.

Anatomical components of basal ganglia are – putamen, caudate nucleus, nucleus accumbens, globus pallidus, subthalamic nucleus, and substantia nigra.

91. Answer: **D.**

Dopa-responsive dystonia is an autosomal dominant disorder. Its genetic defect is on chromosome 14q.

The onset of dystonia is usually in childhood. It is more frequent in females. It is characteristic in diurnal fluctuation – asymptomatic in morning and dystonia or Parkinsonism in evening. The mechanism of the condition is deficiency of guanosine triphosphate (GTP).

The symptoms respond dramatically to L-dopa, hence the name of the condition.

92. Answer: **B.**

This is a typical case of Huntington's disease. The average onset is between ages 30–50 years. It is an autosomal dominant disease, carried on chromosome 4. Expansion of CAG trinucleotide is proved to be the pathophysiology of Huntington's disease. The typical clinical features are chorea – rapid, jerky motions of trunk and limbs. The movement appears as if the patient is dancing in a bizarre manner with loss of control. Dementia appears within 1 year of onset of chorea. Brain images show atrophy of cerebral cortex and head of the caudate nuclei. Compensatory enlargement of lateral ventricles results in the characteristic bat-wing ventricles.

Accumulation of copper in tissues is the mechanism of Wilson's disease. The onset of Wilson's disease is in average at the age of 16 years, though later onset is possible. Clinical features of Wilson's disease include hepatic cirrhosis, Kayser-Fleischer ring and movement symptoms. Among a variety of involuntary movements, the "wing-beating tremor" is characteristic in Wilson's disease. Parkinsonian movements may also appear. However, the dance-like chorea is not a feature of Wilson's disease. Dementia may start early, even before the movement symptoms appeared.

The eosinophilic neuronal inclusions composed of α-synuclein is Lewy body. Though Lewy body may appear in Parkinson's disease and Alzheimer's disease (Lewy body variant of Alzheimer's disease), it appears prominently in Lewy body dementia. The clinical presentation is prominently visual hallucinations and delusions appeared with dementia. The patients are sensitive to extrapyramidal symptoms (EPS) from antipsychotics, making the treatment for psychotic symptoms difficult. Abnormal movement is characterized by Parkinsonism, not chorea.

High normal level of intracranial pressure is a description for normal pressure hydrocephalus. The clinical features are gait disturbance, dementia, and urinary incontinence. Computer tomography (CT) or magnetic resonance imaging (MRI) scan shows enlarged ventricles without convolutional atrophy.

Senile plaques with β amyloid in center and neurofibrillary tangles with tau protein are pathological changes in Alzheimer's disease. The onset age is much older. The progress is slow, usually in a few years. Cortical atrophy involves all cerebral lobes. Movement abnormality is usually nonspecific, and often Parkinsonian-like.

93. Answer: **C.**

Among all the specialists, psychiatrists are at greatest risk of suicide, followed by ophthalmologists and anesthesiologists.

Physician has higher suicide rate than general population. Female physicians are at higher risk. Physicians who commit suicide often have a mental disorder, most often depressive disorder, substance dependence, or both. Physicians commit suicide more often by substance overdoses and less often by firearms than general population.

94. Answer: **B.**

The minimum required duration of seizure is controversial. There is no objective criteria are established. Many agreed on the range 25–30 seconds.

Though lack of data, consensus of expert opinion agreed that a good quality of seizure is – symmetrical, synchronous, with high-amplitude, with high interhemispheric coherence, with marked postictal suppression, accompanied by a prominent tachycardia response.

95. Answer: **A.**

The tasks of bereavement in children with deceased parents are – accepting the reality of loss, experiencing the pain or emotional aspects of loss, adjusting to an environment in which the deceased is missing, relocating the deceased within the child's life, finding ways to memorialize the deceased. The apparent difficult task is to deal with a prior conflictual relationship between the child and the deceased parent.

96. Answer: **D.**

Down's syndrome is associated with increased risk of congenital heart defects, gastroesophageal reflux disease, recurrent ear infections, obstructive sleep apnea, and thyroid dysfunctions.

The rest of the choices are correct.

97. Answer: **E.**

DSM-IV workforce established a work model hopefully will guide the future revision, which includes – designated work groups on each category to conduct extensive review of published literature, reanalysis of the research data, and issue-focused field trials.

Treatment trial was not one of the tasks demanded by DSM-IV workforce.

98. Answer: **A.**

Alcohol may temporally decrease the sleep latency for people with no chronic consumption. People cosuming alcohol chronically have the following change in their sleep pattern – increased sleep latency; increased early night slow-wave sleep, but decreased overall slow-wave sleep; decreased total sleep time; increased early morning rapid eye movement (REM) sleep, but decreased overall REM sleep; sleep fragmentation; reduction of restful sleep; sleep disturbances may continue even with prolonged abstinence; relapse may temporally reduce the sleep disturbances.

99. Answer: **D.**

Depression is associated with increased rapid eye movement (REM) density, shortened REM latency, low sleep efficiency, and early morning awakening. REM density is sometimes termed REM frequency.

100. Answer: **C.**

Antipsychotics, as well as serotonin selective reuptake inhibitors (SSRIs) and norepinephrine reuptake inhibitors, promote melatonin synthesis.

Melatonin synthesis receives negative feedback from the retinohypothalamic tract. The darkness stimulates the synthesis, while the daylight suppresses it.

The location of melatonin synthesis is the pineal gland.

Tryptophan is an essential amino acid and a precursor of serotonin synthesis. Melatonin is synthesized from 5-HIAA, a major metabolite of serotonin.

101. Answer: D.

Orexin receptors are G-protein coupled receptors, not direct-coupled ion channels. Orexins are highly excitatory neuropeptides produced by a small group of neurons in hypothalamus. Orexins are also known as hypocretins. Medical use is under investigation.

102. Answer: A.

Schizophrenia is associated with brain volume reduction in prefrontal cortex, thalamus, hippocampus, superior (not inferior) temporal cortex. The loss of parenchymal volume can cause enlarged ventricular space.

103. Answer: B.

According to Adolf Meyer's view of psychobiology, schizophrenia was a maladaptive reaction to stresses. The condition results from personality dysfunction rather than brain pathology.

Dementia precox and manic-depressive psychoses are Emil Kraepelin's terms.

Ego disintegration represents a regression to the time when the ego was not yet established. According to Sigmund Freud, ego disintegration appears in the development of schizophrenia.

Paraphrenia is a historical term refers to paranoid schizophrenia or schizophrenia with progressively deteriorating course. It is no longer a preferred term.

104. Answer: C.

Symptoms of amphetamine intoxication include – tachy- or bradycardia, pupillary dilation, weight loss, hyper- or hypotension, perspiration and chills, nausea and vomiting, confusion, and respiratory failure.

Amphetamine tends to increase energy and wakefulness. Fatigue is a symptom of amphetamine withdrawal.

105. Answer: C.

Cannabinoid receptors are G-protein associated receptors, not direct-coupled ion channels. Activation of CB1 blocks voltage-dependent calcium channels and reduces, not increases, the calcium influx. CB1 may also modulate potassium channels. THC is the major element from natural cannabis. It is not an endocannabinoid. Endocannabinoids are arachidonate-based lipids, not peptides.

106. Answer: E.

Cocaine in the milk may cause elevated blood pressure, tachycardia, and mydriasis (not miosis) in the newborn.

Cocaine can cause brain developmental disturbance due to hypoperfusion of the brain, fetal growth retardation, decreased birth weight, and malformations of the urogenital system of the newborn.

107. Answer: B.

Structures in the limbic system, particularly amygdale, mediate anxiety response. Gamma-aminobutyric acid (GABA) receptors are concentrated in limbic system.

Stimulation of locus coeruleus, not blockade of locus coeruleus, may generate panic attacks. Serotonin and norepinephrine are regulatory transmitters that may influence the GABAergic system. GABAergic system is widely distributed with highest density at the limbic system, not the frontal cortex. Binding with benzodiazepines reduces, not induces, anxiety.

108. Answer: **E.**

In Alzheimer's disease, the decreased, not increased, neuronal projections from the nucleus basalis of Meynert are associated decreased cholinergic transmission.

Senile plaques are quantitatively correlated with the severity of the dementia. Senile plaques are composed of Aβ, astrocytes, dystrophic neuronal processes, and microglia. Neurofibrillary tangles are cytoskeletal elements including phosphorylated tau protein. Other changes include neuronal loss in the cortex and the hippocampus, synaptic loss, and granulovascular degeneration of the neurons.

109. Answer: **B.**

For conversion disorder, interview with assistance of amobarbital or lorazepam may be helpful in obtaining information, but not always reliable for diagnosis.

The most important issue of the therapy is the therapeutic relationship between the patient and the therapist. Psychotherapies that may be applied to conversion disorder include insight-oriented supportive therapy, behavior therapy, and brief psychotherapy. Therapy should focus on stress and coping. Hypnosis and anxiolytics may be effective in some cases.

110. Answer: **E.**

Characteristics of uncompleted suicide – female, under age of 35 years, using low lethality of method such as overdose or wrist cut, and approximately 10% will finally be successful.

Characteristics of completed suicide – male, greater rate in Caucasian population, over 60 years of age, usually precipitated by a loss, and using lethal method such as firearms or hanging.

111. Answer: **B.**

Central nervous system (CNS) lymphoma is the most common neoplasm in acquired immunodeficiency syndrome (AIDS). It is a highly malignant B-cell tumor, associated with Epstein-Barré (EB) virus infection. Clinically, it produces slowly progressing multifocal deficits. In head computer tomography (CT), lymphoma has multiple enhancing lesions with diffuse or ring pattern, appears similar to toxoplasmosis. Unlike toxoplasmosis, lymphoma usually is not associated with fever, headache, and seizures. Focal signs are minimal to moderate. In single photon emission computer tomography (SPECT), lymphoma is hot, while toxoplasmosis is cold.

Human immuno virus (HIV) meningitis occurs in 5% of HIV patients. It usually occurs at the seroconversion, but may appear in later the stage of the illness. The process is brief and benign. There is no change in brain image.

Cryptococcus is the most common CNS fungal infection in AIDS. Its clinical characteristics are – headache, fever, meningeal signs, and mental status changes. Diagnosis is through CSF culture and cryptococcal antigen detection.

Neurosyphilis is rare in the post-penicillin era. It may rise among individuals with AIDS. Classic neurological signs include – tremor, dysarthria, hyperreflexia, hypotonia, and ataxia.

112. Answer: **D.**

Child in the home is a protective factor for suicide.

Risk factors for suicide include – unemployment, living alone, lack of social support, domestic violence, recent deterioration in socioeconomic status, and recent life stressors.

113. Answer: **B.**

Suicidal risk in ethnic groups in descending order
    Caucasians, with highest risk in elderly white males
    Native Americans
    African-Americans
    Hispanic Americans
    Asian-Americans

114. Answer: **E.**

The question gives the description of Food and Drug Administration (FDA) pregnancy category C. Among the five antidepressants listed, only bupropion belongs to category C. (Bupropion used to be category B.)
    Paroxetine, imipramine, and desipramine are category D.
    Maprotiline is the only antidepressant that belongs to category B.
    Antidepressants that are not mentioned in this question all belong to pregnancy category C.

115. Answer: **A.**

Nondeclarative memory deals with skills, habits, and nonassociative learning. It is also known as implicit memory. It does not require conscious awareness and concentration. It usually remains intact after brain injury. Structures involved in nondeclarative memory are basal ganglia, limbic system, and perceptual cortex.
    Declarative memory is also known as explicit memory. It deals with facts, events, and associative learning. Declarative memory requires conscious awareness and concentration, and is impaired after brain injury. Structures involved in declarative memory are hippocampus, orbitofrontal cortex, and parahippocampal gyrus.

116. Answer: **B.**

Pregnancy should be avoided until symptoms of anorexia nervosa are stabilized.
    The rest of choices are appropriate medical treatments for anorexia nervosa.

117. Answer: **C.**

Ecstasy is a serotonin reuptake blocker.
    LSD has effect of serotonergic and dopaminergic stimulation.
    Cannabis acts on cannabinoid receptors.
    Opioids act on opioid receptors.
    PCP binds to N-methyl D-aspartate (NMDA) receptor and blocks the calcium channel.
    Another possible answer is cocaine, which blocks reuptake of dopamine, serotonin, and norepinephrine.

118. Answer: **B.**

The making of DSM-III was a historical major revision known as "neo-Kraepelinian," focused on improving the scientific reliability of psychiatric diagnosis. Psychodynamic view was abandoned in favor of a biomedical model. Categorization was based on description rather than assumptions of etiology. Field trials supported by National Institute of Mental Health (NIMH) were conducted to test the reliability of the new diagnoses.

119. Answer: **C.**

Word comprehension happens approximately 3 months before word production.

Language development milestones
▶ 0–2 month – vegetative sounds
▶ 2–6 month – vowel sounds
▶ 6–8 month – babbling
▶ 8–10 month – word comprehension
▶ 11–13 month – word production
▶ 20–24 month – word combination
▶ 30 month – grammar

120. Answer: **D.**

CYP 2D6 is involved in the metabolisms of tricyclic antidepressants. Codeine is a prodrug which requires CYP 2D6 to convert to morphine. Without this conversion, codeine is not an effective pain reliever by itself.

121. Answer: **A.**

Drugs that increase lithium level – angiotensin converting enzyme inhibitors including captopril, enalapril, and lisinopril; fluoxetine; ibuprofen; indomethacin; Spironolactone; and thiazide diuretics.

Drugs that decrease lithium level include theophylline, caffeine, and laxatives.

122. Answer: **D**

Ego spans over unconscious, preconscious, and conscious. The conscious and preconscious part of ego deals with abstract thinking and verbal expression, while the unconscious part deals with defense mechanisms.

Id is dominated by primary process. It is unorganized, and lacks the capacity to delay or modify the instinctual drives.

Superego dictates moral conscience and value.

Both id and superego function largely unconsciously.

123. Answer: **C.**

Abraham Kardiner, a U.S. psychoanalyst, believed that each culture is associated with a common personality structure, or national character. His theory was, however, used to foster political and discriminatory attitude.

Bronislaw Malinowski, a polish anthropologist, challenged the universality of the Oedipus complex. Margaret Mead, a U.S. anthropologist, believed that a society can create deviance by encouraging or condemning certain behavior patterns. Mead argued that the general casualness of the whole society may make personality maturation easier and healthier. By this she referred mainly to the societal acceptance of open, nonpossessive sexual relationship. Sigmund Freud and Carl Jung believed that adult personality is determined mainly by childhood experience.

124. Answer: **A.**

Choice A describes shen-k'uei or shenkui.
Choice B describes koro.
Choice C describes dhat.
Choice D describes shenjing shuairuo or neurasthenia.
Choice E describes susto.

125. Answer: **D.**

Insidious onset implies poor prognosis.

Good prognostic factors for schizophrenia include – paranoid subtype, high intelligence quotient (IQ), affective symptoms, acute onset, confusion or other organic symptoms, female, later age of onset, married status, negative family history of schizophrenia, absence of perinatal complications, predominance of positive symptoms, obvious precipitating factors, family history of affective disorder, and good premorbid functioning.

126. Answer: **B.**

Three benzodiazepines require no oxidation in hepatic metabolism. These are – temazepam (Restoril), oxazepam (Serax), and Lorazepam (Ativan). These benzodiazepines are relatively safe for liver-impaired patients.

127. Answer: **E.**

The case describes Lennox-Gastaut syndrome, a form of childhood-onset epilepsy. The onset is usually between ages 2–4 years. Symptoms are frequent, sometimes daily frequent seizures with different seizure types. Psychomotor development is often slowed down. Interictal electroencephalogram (EEG) has characteristic slow spike-wave complexes. The common causes are encephalopathy, tuberous sclerosis, encephalitis, meningitis, hypoxia, and ischemia. The condition is often treatment resistant. Valproic acid and benzodiazepines are first line options. Alternative treatments include ketogenic diet, other anticonvulsants, and vagus nerve stimulation. Surgical intervene such as corpus callosotomy may be helpful.

128. Answer: **C.**

Interictal psychosis appears more common in patients with female gender, left-handedness, puberty onset of seizures, and with left-sided lesion. The symptoms are usually preceded by personality change. Patients usually remain appropriate affect. Common thought disorders are conceptualization and circumstantiality, while blocking and looseness are relatively uncommon.

129. Answer: **D.**

Topiramate (Topamax) and zonisamide (Zonegran) may cause renal stones. Proper hydration may prevent renal stones.

130. Answer: **E.**

High-dose folate, not vitamin D, may reduce the risk of neural tube defects induced by antiepileptic drugs.

The rest of the choices are correct statements.

131. Answer: **B.**

Except in severe cases, protein and albumin levels are usually normal in anorexic patients.

Hypokalemic alkalosis, leukopenia with relative lymphocytosis, hypersecretion of CRH, and elevated β-carotene are usual findings. Other laboratory findings include hypoglycemia and hypothyroidism. Serum salivary amylase is found to be elevated in patients who purge, with either anorexia or bulimia.

132. Answer: **D.**

The magnetic resonance imaging (MRI) image shows L1 compressed fracture. The vertebral body has lost approximately 20% of its height. There is a retropulsion from the posterior superior wall of L1 into the spinal canal.

Some degree of osteoporosis is seen, but this is likely chronic and not a new significant
finding. There is no evidence of muscle strain, bleeding, or metastasis.

133. Answer: **E.**

Dandy-Walker syndrome does not have known connection to chromosomal abnormality.
Cri-du-Chat is associated with chromosome 5 abnormality.
William's Syndrome is associated with chromosome 7 deletion.
Phenylketonuria is found to have genetic location on chromosome 12.
Prader-Willi syndrome is associated with chromosome 15 abnormality.

134. Answer: **C.**

The case described typical features of atypical depression. The traditional treatment of
choice is monoamine oxidase inhibitor (MAOI), which requires discontinuation of fluoxetine for 5 weeks before initiation of treatment. The patient had a job at the time and
never had any suicidal or homicidal ideas or behaviors. She should be able to tolerate a
few weeks without any antidepressant. If there is any concern of starting an MAOI, some
change of the regimen should still be considered. Fluoxetine was in high dosage with no
response. Therefore tapering fluoxetine is a reasonable choice.

Abrupt discontinuation of an serotonin selective reuptake inhibitor (SSRI) is not as
well tolerated as tapering, due to discontinuation symptoms.

Adding psychotherapy is another reasonable choice. However, due to the previous
failed experience, this is not as good a choice as changing medication.

Though panic disorder is a common comorbid condition to atypical depression, anxiety is not a prominent complaint in the described case. In addition to that, alprazolam is
no longer a top choice for panic disorder.

Atypical depression may present in major depressive disorders or bipolar disorders.
However, olanzapine is not a good choice not only because this patient did not have
manic or psychotic symptoms, but also because she was moderately obese.

135. Answer: **A.**

Among antiretroviral agents, efavirenz and nevirapine induce, not inhibit, CYP 3A4. This
may cause abrupt increase of benzodiazepine metabolism and induce withdrawal.

Many protease inhibitors can inhibit CYP 3A4. Most of these agents have a name end
with "-navir," including – indinavir, nelfinavir, ritonavir, saquinavir, and amprenavir.

136. Answer: **A.**

Codeine is a prodrug with minimal analgesic effect by itself. CYP 2D6 converts codeine to
morphine. When CYP 2D6 is inhibited, the conversion is slowed, and the analgesic effect
of codeine is diminished. Most tricyclic antidepressants and several serotonin selective
reuptake inhibitors (SSRIs) (paroxetine, fluoxetine, and sertraline) are CYP 2D6 inhibitors.
Antiretroviral agent ritonavir is a 2D6 and 3A4 inhibitor. Quinidine is also a 2D6 inhibitor.

137. Answer: **B.**

Carbamazepine decreases valproic acid level through metabolic induction, while valproic acid increases carbamazepine level through both metabolic inhibition and protein-
binding competition.

The rest of the choices are correct statements.

138. Answer: **D.**

Antipsychotics with high probability of weight gaining – clozapine and olanzapine.

Antipsychotics with moderate probability of weight gaining – risperidone, quetiapine, and paliperidone.

Antipsychotics with low probability of weight gaining – ziprasidone and aripiprazole.

139. Answer: **C.**

Only less than 20% of the stimulus enters the brain.

The rest of the choices are correct statements.

140. Answer: **E.**

Progressive multifocal leuko-encephalopathy is a central nervous system (CNS) infection caused by John Cunningham (JC) virus, a papovarirus, not a fungus.

It is a demyelinating disorder of the CNS. It is manifested with multifocal neurologic abnormalities. It causes white matter lesions without mass effect. The diagnostic test is polymerase chain reation (PCR) in cerebrospinal fluid (CSF), which shows positive for JC virus.

141. Answer: **C.**

Broca's area is supplied by middle cerebral artery, not the anterior cerebral artery.

The rest of the choices are correct statements.

142. Answer: **E.**

The conditions appropriate for electroconvulsive therapy (ECT) are – depression, unipolar or bipolar, particularly psychotic and catatonic depression; mania; psychotic agitation; treatment resistant positive symptoms; Parkinson's disease; organic affective disorders; intractable seizures; and chronic pain.

ECT is not effective for anxiety disorders.

143. Answer: **D.**

The case described absence seizure, also known as petit mal. It usually begins at ages of 2–10 years and disappears in early adulthood. It presents with abrupt loss and resolution of consciousness, blinking, facial and finger automatisms. It usually lasts for 1–10 seconds. Characteristic electroencephalogram (EEG) finding is generalized 3 Hz spike-and-wave complexes. The patient is unaware of episode. Usually no postictal abnormal behavior is noted. The first choice of treatment is ethosuximide. Valproic acid is an alternative option.

Lorazepam and carbamazepine are not as effective for absence seizure.

Methylphenidate and chlorpromazine should be avoided due to potential of decreasing seizure threshold.

144. Answer: **A.**

Brown-Sequard syndrome is lateral hemitransection of spinal cord. The right side injury causes interruption of all major tracts at the right side (therefore C is wrong).

Interruption of corticospinal tract causes upper motor neuron paresis. Since the corticospinal tracts are already crossed at the pyramid level, the motor symptoms are ipsilateral.

Fibers in the dorsal columns will cross at in the brain stem, so the position and vibratory sense loss are ipsilateral (therefore D is wrong).

The pain and temperature sense loss are the only two symptoms that are contralateral, because spinothalamic tract crosses at 1–2 sections ascending (Figure 43-5, and therefore A is right and E is wrong.)

Spinothalamic tracts do not have motor components therefore B is wrong.

115. Answer: **C.**

The onset age of Huntington's disease is between 30–50 years.

It is an autosomal dominant disease, carried on chromosome 4. The mechanism is the expansion of CAG trinucleotide – N ≥36 → Huntington's disease; N ≥60 → juvenile Huntington's disease.

Dementia appears within 1 year of onset of chorea. Brain images show trophy of cerebral cortex and head of the caudate nuclei, and bat-wing ventricles caused by compensatory enlargement of lateral ventricles.

146. Answer: **D.**

The passage describes Festinger's theory of cognitive dissonance.

Double binding is a concept formulated by Gregory Bateson and Donald Jackson, referring to children's dilemma when receiving contradictory parental demands about their behavior, where they are not possibly able to fulfill both.

Learned helplessness is a psychological condition in which a human being or an animal has learned to believe that any attempt to escape from the suffering will be useless. Seligman established the first animal model of depression based on this concept.

Strange situation is a laboratory procedure designed to assess infant attachment style. It was developed by Mary Ainsworth and her coauthors.

Anal fixation is a behavioral regression, according to Freud, to anal stage. It is characterized by obsession to details and orderliness, often becomes annoyance to others.

147. Answer: **C.**

Amyotrophic lateral sclerosis is a motor neuron disease that causes both upper and lower neuron degeneration. Characteristic features are asymmetric paresis, atrophy with fasciculation, and both bulbar and pseudobulbar palsy. There is no direct mental impairment, though secondary depression and anxiety are common.

148. Answer: **A.**

Four types of attachment style are identified (types A–D). Types B–D is also called "insecure attachments," and are associated with development of personality disorders.

Choice A decribes type A – secure attachment.

Choice B decribes type B – avoidant attachment.

Choice C decribes type C – ambivalent attachment.

Choice D decribes childhood depression, not a type of attachment.

Choice E decribes type D – disorganized attachment.

149. Answer: **E.**

In emergency restraining, at least one staff should always be visible to the patient so to reduce the paranoia and traumatic feeling. At least four staffs should be used. At least two restraints should be used. When agitation improved, remove one restraint at a time at 5-minute intervals. Proper documentation includes the reason for the restraints, the course of treatment, and the patient's response.

150. Answer: **B.**

"Testimonial privilege" refers to a patient's right to exclude certain material from judicial settings testimony. This is exactly the time the physician is obligated to protect the patient's confidentiality.

Exceptions to testimonial privilege include – military court, child abuse case, court-ordered examinations, malpractice case brought by the patient, civil commitment, competency proceedings, and situation in which patient enters mental condition into proceedings, e.g., not guilty due to insanity.

Bibliography

Abrams, R. (2002). *Electroconvulsive therapy* (4th ed.). New York: Oxford University Press.

American College of Psychiatrists: Psychiatry Resident In-Training Examination, 2003–2008. Chicago: American College of Psychiatrists.

American Psychiatric Association. (2000). *Diagnostic and statistical manual of mental disorders* (4th ed.). *Text revision*. Washington, DC: American Psychiatric Association.

American Psychiatric Association. (2007). *Practice guideline for the treatment of patients with Alzheimer's disease and other dementias.*Washington, DC: American Psychiatric Association.

Appelbaum, P. S., & Gutheil, T. G. (2006). *Clinical handbook of psychiatry and the law* (4th ed.). Philadelphia, PA: Lippincott Williams & Wilkins.

Galanter, M., & Kleber, H. D. (2008) *The American psychiatric publishing textbook of substance abuse treatment*. Washington, DC: American Psychiatric Publishing.

Green, G. B., Harris, I. S., Lin, G. A., & Moylan, K. C. (Ed.). (2004). *The Washington manual of medical therapeutics* (31st ed.). Philadelphia: Lippincott Williams & Wilkins.

Kaufman, D. M. (2007). *Clinical neurology for psychiatrists* (6th ed.). Philadelphia, PA: W.B. Saunders.

Leo, R. J. (2008). *Clinical manual of pain management in psychiatry*, Washington, DC: American Psychiatric Publishing.

Martin, J. H. (2003). *Neuroanatomy* (3rd ed.). New York: McGraw-Hill.

Othmer, E., & Othmer, S. C. (2002). *The clinical interview using DSM-IV-TR*, Washington, DC: American Psychiatric Publishing.

Purves, D., Augustine, G. J., Fitzpatrick, D., Katz, L., LaMantia, A. S., McNamara, J., et al. (Ed.). (2007). *Neuroscience* (4th ed.). Sunderland, MA: Sinauer Associates.

Sadock, B. J., & Sadock, V. A. (Ed.) (2006). *Kaplan & Sadock's comprehensive textbook of psychiatry* (8th ed.). Philadelphia, PA: Lippincott Williams & Wilkins.

Sadock, B. J., & Sadock, V. A. (2007). *Kaplan & Sadock's synopsis of psychiatry* (10th ed.). Philadelphia, PA: Lippincott Williams & Wilkins.

Stahl, S. M. (2008). *Stahl's essential psychopharmacology: neuroscientific basis and practical applications* (3rd ed.). New York, Cambridge University Press.

Index